T0259359

Best Practices in High-Risk Pregnancy

Editor

LYNN L. SIMPSON

OBSTETRICS AND GYNECOLOGY CLINICS OF NORTH AMERICA

www.obgyn.theclinics.com

Consulting Editor
WILLIAM F. RAYBURN

June 2015 • Volume 42 • Number 2

ELSEVIER

1600 John F. Kennedy Boulevard • Suite 1800 • Philadelphia, Pennsylvania, 19103-2899

http://www.theclinics.com

OBSTETRICS AND GYNECOLOGY CLINICS OF NORTH AMERICA Volume 42, Number 2
June 2015 ISSN 0889-8545, ISBN-13: 978-0-323-38898-6

Editor: Kerry Holland
Developmental Editor: Stephanie Wissler

Obstetrics and Gynecology Clinics (ISSN 0889-8545) is published quarterly by Elsevier Inc., 360 Park Avenue South, New York, NY 10010-1710. Months of issue are March, June, September, and December. Periodicals postage paid at New York, NY, and additional mailing offices. Subscription price per year is $310.00 (US individuals), $545.00 (US institutions), $155.00 (US students), $370.00 (Canadian individuals), $688.00 (Canadian institutions), $225.00 (Canadian students), $450.00 (international individuals), $688.00 (international institutions), and $225.00 (international students). To receive student/resident rate, orders must be accompanied by name of affiliated institution, date of term, and the signature of program/residency coordinator on institution letterhead. Orders will be billed at individual rate until proof of status is received. Foreign air speed delivery is included in all *Clinics* subscription prices. All prices are subject to change without notice. POSTMASTER: Send address changes to *Obstetrics and Gynecology Clinics*, Elsevier Health Sciences Division, Subscription Customer Service, 3251 Riverport Lane, Maryland Heights, MO 63043. **Customer Service: Telephone: 1-800-654-2452 (U.S. and Canada); 314-447-8871 (outside U.S. and Canada). Fax: 314-447-8029. E-mail: journalscustomerservice-usa@elsevier.com (for print support); journalsonlinesupport-usa@elsevier. com (for online support).**

Reprints. For copies of 100 or more of articles in this publication, please contact the Commercial Reprints Department, Elsevier Inc., 360 Park Avenue South, New York, New York 10010-1710. Tel.: 212-633-3874; Fax: 212-633-3820; E-mail: reprints@elsevier.com.

Obstetrics and Gynecology Clinics of North America is also published in Spanish by McGraw-Hill Interamericana Editores S.A., P.O. Box 5-237, 06500, Mexico; in Portuguese by Reichmann and Affonso Editores, Rio de Janeiro, Brazil; and in Greek by Paschalidis Medical Publications, Athens, Greece.

Obstetrics and Gynecology Clinics of North America is covered in MEDLINE/PubMed (Index Medicus), Excerpta Medica, Current Concepts/Clinical Medicine, Science Citation Index, BIOSIS, CINAHL, and ISI/BIOMED.

Contributors

CONSULTING EDITOR

WILLIAM F. RAYBURN, MD, MBA
Associate Dean, Continuing Medical Education and Professional Development; Distinguished Professor and Emeritus Chair, Obstetrics and Gynecology, University of New Mexico School of Medicine, Albuquerque, New Mexico

EDITOR

LYNN L. SIMPSON, MSc, MD
Hillary Rodham Clinton Professor of Women's Health, Professor of Obstetrics and Gynecology, Department of Obstetrics and Gynecology, Columbia University Medical Center, New York, New York

AUTHORS

STEPHANIE ANDRIOLE, MS, CGC
Comprehensive Genetics, PLLC and Fetal Medicine Foundation of America, New York, New York

MERT OZAN BAHTIYAR, MD
Associate Professor, Maternal-Fetal Medicine, Department of Obstetrics, Gynecology and Reproductive Sciences; Yale Fetal Cardiovascular Center; Director, Yale Fetal Care Center, Yale School of Medicine, New Haven, Connecticut

KELLI D. BARBOUR, MD, MSc
Maternal-Fetal Medicine Fellow, Division of Maternal-Fetal Medicine, Department of Obstetrics and Gynecology, University of Utah Health Sciences Center, Salt Lake City, Utah

AHMET A. BASCHAT, MD
Director of The Johns Hopkins Center for Fetal Therapy, Department of Gynecology and Obstetrics, The Johns Hopkins Hospital, Baltimore, Maryland

VINCENZO BERGHELLA, MD
Division of Maternal-Fetal Medicine, Department of Obstetrics and Gynecology, Sidney Kimmel Medical College, Thomas Jefferson University, Philadelphia, Pennsylvania

AARON B. CAUGHEY, MD, PhD
Department of Obstetrics and Gynecology, Oregon Health & Science University, Portland, Oregon

STEVEN L. CLARK, MD
Texas Children's Hospital, Baylor College of Medicine, Houston, Texas

SARA CONSONNI, MD
Department of Obstetrics and Gynecology, University of Milano-Bicocca, Milano-Bicocca, Italy

JOSHUA A. COPEL, MD
Maternal-Fetal Medicine, Department of Obstetrics, Gynecology and Reproductive Sciences; Yale Fetal Cardiovascular Center; Yale Fetal Care Center; Department of Pediatrics, Yale School of Medicine, New Haven, Connecticut

ELAINE L. DURYEA, MD
Department of Obstetrics and Gynecology, University of Texas Southwestern Medical Center, Dallas, Texas

MARK I. EVANS, MD
Comprehensive Genetics, PLLC and Fetal Medicine Foundation of America; Department of Obstetrics and Gynecology, Mt. Sinai School of Medicine, New York, New York

SHARA M. EVANS, MSc, MPH
Comprehensive Genetics, PLLC and Fetal Medicine Foundation of America, New York, New York

ALEXANDER M. FRIEDMAN, MD
Division of Maternal-Fetal Medicine, Department of Obstetrics and Gynecology, College of Physicians and Surgeons, Columbia University, New York, New York

MANISHA GANDHI, MD
Assistant Professor, Division of Maternal-Fetal Medicine, Department of Obstetrics and Gynecology, Baylor College of Medicine, Texas Children's Pavilion for Women, Houston, Texas

ALESSANDRO GHIDINI, MD
Inova Alexandria Hospital, Alexandria, Virginia

ANNA LOCATELLI, MD
Department Obstetrics and Gynecology, University of Milano-Bicocca, Milano-Bicocca, Italy

NICOLE E. MARSHALL, MD, MCR
Department of Obstetrics and Gynecology, Oregon Health & Science University, Portland, Oregon

STEPHANIE R. MARTIN, DO
Director, Southern Colorado Maternal Fetal Medicine; Director, Maternal Fetal Medicine Services St Francis Medical Center/Centura Southstate; Visiting Associate Clinical Professor, Department of Obstetrics and Gynecology, University of Colorado, Colorado Springs, Colorado

JOHN F. MISSION, MD
Maternal-Fetal Medicine, Department of Obstetrics, Gynecology and Reproductive Sciences, Magee-Womens Hospital of University of Pittsburgh Medical Center, Pittsburgh, Pennsylvania

JAIMEY M. PAULI, MD, FACOG
Assistant Professor, Division of Maternal-Fetal Medicine, Department of Obstetrics and Gynecology, Penn State University, College of Medicine; Attending Perinatologist, The Milton S. Hershey Medical Center, Hershey, Pennsylvania

JOHN T. REPKE, MD, FACOG
University Professor and Chairman, Department of Obstetrics and Gynecology,
Penn State University, College of Medicine; Obstetrician-Gynecologist-In-Chief, The
Milton S. Hershey Medical Center, Hershey, Pennsylvania

VIOLA SERAVALLI, MD
Department of Gynecology and Obstetrics, The Johns Hopkins Center for Fetal Therapy,
The Johns Hopkins Hospital, Baltimore, Maryland

JEANNE S. SHEFFIELD, MD
Department of Obstetrics and Gynecology, University of Texas Southwestern Medical
Center, Dallas, Texas

ROBERT M. SILVER, MD
Division Chair, Division of Maternal-Fetal Medicine, Department of Obstetrics and
Gynecology, University of Utah Health Sciences Center, Salt Lake City, Utah

LYNN L. SIMPSON, MSc, MD
Hillary Rodham Clinton Professor of Women's Health, Professor of Obstetrics and
Gynecology, Department of Obstetrics and Gynecology, Columbia University Medical
Center, New York, New York

CATHERINE Y. SPONG, MD
Deputy Director, National Institute of Child Health and Human Development, National
Institutes of Health, Bethesda, Maryland

ANJU SUHAG, MD
Division of Maternal-Fetal Medicine, Department of Obstetrics and Gynecology, Sidney
Kimmel Medical College, Thomas Jefferson University, Philadelphia, Pennsylvania

AUDRA E. TIMMINS, MD, MBA
Texas Children's Hospital, Baylor College of Medicine, Houston, Texas

Contents

> Preeclampsia is a hypertensive disorder that affects 4% of pregnancies and has a high risk of maternal, fetal, and neonatal morbidity and mortality, as well as long-term cardiovascular risk. Recent updates in the definition, diagnosis, and management guidelines for preeclampsia warrant review by general obstetrician-gynecologists. Screening and prevention algorithms for preeclampsia are available, but ultimately the cure remains delivery of the fetus and placenta. Close monitoring for the development and worsening of preeclampsia during pregnancy is essential to optimize both maternal and fetal/neonatal outcomes.

> Physiologic changes in pregnancy can place extra demands on cardiac function. Preconception counseling is key to improving pregnancy outcomes. The most commonly encountered cardiac events are pulmonary edema and dysrhythmias. A team approach to antepartum care is recommended and should include maternal-fetal medicine, cardiology, and anesthesia as indicated, particularly for patients with congenital cardiac disease.

> Obesity has increased dramatically in the United States over the last several decades, with approximately 40% of pregnant women now considered overweight or obese. Obesity has been shown to be associated with numerous poor pregnancy outcomes, including increased rates of preeclampsia, gestational diabetes, fetal macrosomia, stillbirth, postterm pregnancy, and increased rates of cesarean delivery. Many of these complications have been found to increase even further with increasing body mass index in a dose-response fashion. In this review, the association of obesity with maternal, fetal, and pregnancy outcomes is discussed as are the recommendations for caring for the obese gravida.

> A maternal mortality rate of 1% was reported during the 2009–2010 influenza pandemic, with influenza in pregnancy posing a serious risk to maternal health. A high level of suspicion coupled with prompt diagnosis and treatment is paramount to minimizing morbidity and mortality. Vaccination during pregnancy should be of high priority to improve both maternal and neonatal outcomes.

> Since its inception, many have questioned the utility of electronic fetal heart rate (FHR) monitoring. However, it arrived without the benefit of clear,

standard nomenclature, leading to difficulty interpreting studies regarding its benefit. In 2008, the National Institute of Child Health and Human Development (NICHD) developed standard nomenclature for interpreting eFHR tracings. Understanding what drives the tracings is key to managing them. Category II FHR patterns are by far the most common and most diverse patterns, leading to broad variation in care. Presented here is an algorithm for standardization of management of category II FHR tracings, based on the pathophysiology of decelerations, that can be followed in any labor unit.

Education of providers and patients on the importance of vaginal delivery, for the current pregnancy as well as future pregnancies, is essential to reverse the current trend of primary cesareans. When discussing cesarean with patients, counseling should include the effect on subsequent pregnancy risks including the possibility of uterine rupture and placentation abnormalities. In addition, counseling must include the concept that normal labor takes time. Re-education on the natural process of labor, the importance of allowing the time needed, and patience with the duration of pregnancy and process of labor is essential.

Placenta accreta can lead to hemorrhage, resulting in hysterectomy, blood transfusion, multiple organ failure, and death. Accreta has been increasing steadily in incidence owing to an increase in the cesarean delivery rate. Major risk factors are placenta previa in women with prior cesarean deliveries. Obstetric ultrasonography can be used to diagnose placenta accreta antenatally, which allows for scheduled delivery in a multidisciplinary center of excellence for accreta. Controversies exist regarding optimal management, including optimal timing of delivery, surgical approach, use of adjunctive measures, and conservative (uterine-sparing) therapy. We review the definition, risk factors, diagnosis, management, and controversies regarding placenta accreta.

OBSTETRICS AND GYNECOLOGY CLINICS

ISSUE OF RELATED INTEREST

THE CLINICS ARE AVAILABLE ONLINE!
Access your subscription at:
www.theclinics.com

Foreword
At-Risk Pregnancies

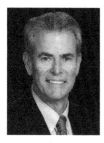

William F. Rayburn, MD, MBA
Consulting Editor

This issue of *Obstetrics and Gynecology Clinics of North America* provides a management update for pregnancies at-risk. The editor, Dr Lynn Simpson, has compiled a list of topics that have much relevance to contemporary obstetrics. Care of the at-risk pregnancy is often complex and demanding. Providers must be aware of those women's unique medical and emotional needs and their desire for open communication about events surrounding a successful pregnancy.

This issue consists of a well-qualified team of maternal-fetal medicine specialists who focus on various subjects related directly to management dilemmas of at-risk pregnancies. Topics of interest begin with updates on prenatal screening and diagnosis and end with the prevention of the first cesarean delivery and the placenta accreta spectrum. Fresh focuses are provided on subjects relating to maternal warning systems (hypertensive disorders, cardiac disease, obesity, influenza) and on fetal evaluation and surveillance (congenital heart disease, growth restriction and Doppler velocimetry, category II fetal monitoring). Emphasized are scientific underpinnings of clinical obstetrics decision-making, which includes the latest biochemical and physiological principles.

Articles in this issue incorporate guidelines from leading professional and academic organizations, such as the American College of Obstetricians and Gynecologists, Society for Maternal-Fetal Medicine, National Institutes of Health, and Centers for Disease Control and Prevention. Summaries of current management strategies reflect and bear witness to the ever-expanding knowledge from proper evaluations of appropriate clinical studies.

Dr Simpson and her talented group of authors have provided valuable knowledge from both evidence-based publications and the bedside. It is hoped that the practical information provided herein will offer management guidelines to optimize team-based care for this at-risk population and their unborn infants. I am grateful to those who

Obstet Gynecol Clin N Am 42 (2015) xiii–xiv
http://dx.doi.org/10.1016/j.ogc.2015.02.002
0889-8545/15/$ – see front matter © 2015 Published by Elsevier Inc.

obgyn.theclinics.com

contributed their time and expertise for the completion of this issue. Their commitment to quality care and performance measures is exemplary.

William F. Rayburn, MD, MBA
Department of Obstetrics and Gynecology
Office of Continuing Medical Education and Professional Development
University of New Mexico School of Medicine
MSC10 5580, 1 University of New Mexico
Albuquerque, NM 87131-0001, USA

E-mail address:
wrayburn@salud.unm.edu

Preface

At-Risk Pregnancies: Update on Management

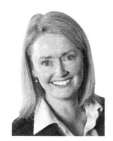

Lynn L. Simpson, MSc, MD
Editor

Obstetric care continues to evolve with the incorporation of evidence-based recommendations to optimize maternal and perinatal outcomes. Today, all women should be offered prenatal diagnosis, moving away from a time when chorionic villus sampling and amniocentesis were only offered to patients identified to be at risk of fetal aneuploidy. Noninvasive prenatal testing is now a reality, increasing screening options with improved detection rates for Down syndrome. Screening for congenital heart disease these days warrants an evaluation of multiple views of the fetal heart, and the indications for fetal echocardiography have expanded, all in an effort to increase the prenatal detection of major heart anomalies. The use of reproductive technologies continues to bolster multiple births and their related complications, particularly those associated with monochorionic placentation. The role of cervical length assessment in both multiple and single gestations has gained acceptance in patients at risk of preterm birth. A major emphasis of contemporary obstetrics has been to decrease prematurity, and the approach to preterm labor has changed significantly based on recent clinical studies. The management of suspected intrauterine fetal growth restriction has also been modified, incorporating Doppler velocimetry into serial surveillance of fetal well-being.

A fresh focus on women's health has come about with the recognition of our nation's unabating maternal mortality rate. Maternal early warning systems have been introduced into clinical practice to promote the early recognition of women at risk with prompt interventions to improve outcomes. Hypertensive disorders of pregnancy, maternal cardiac disease, obesity, and complications related to influenza all contribute to maternal morbidity and mortality and, unfortunately, these conditions are on the upswing. Preeclampsia can impact immediate and long-term health of women. Patients with congenital heart disease are now surviving into their reproductive years and, despite the risks, are interested in having families of their own. Obesity rates continue to climb, impacting all aspects of obstetric care, and influenza remains an

Obstet Gynecol Clin N Am 42 (2015) xv–xvi
http://dx.doi.org/10.1016/j.ogc.2015.02.001
0889-8545/15/$ – see front matter © 2015 Published by Elsevier Inc.

obgyn.theclinics.com

incessant risk to pregnant women during the flu season. Obstetric providers need to recognize these conditions and their risks to maternal health and adjust their approach accordingly.

The potential for maternal or perinatal injury continues into the intrapartum period. Electronic fetal monitoring is commonly utilized during labor to evaluate fetal well-being, and new guidelines are now available for the interpretation, categorization, and management of various patterns that may be predictive of perinatal asphyxia. Correct interpretation of fetal tracings is key to avoid unnecessary cesarean deliveries, particularly a patient's first. A prior cesarean delivery is the most common reason for a repeat cesarean, which places the patient at risk for intraoperative and postoperative complications as well as an increased risk of abnormal placentation in a future pregnancy. The recognition of risk factors and placental evaluation is critical to the diagnosis and management of placenta accreta, which can be life-threatening even when detected prior to delivery.

This issue of *Obstetrics and Gynecology Clinics of North America* is an update for clinicians on current best practices in high-risk pregnancies. Articles were written by experts in the field, incorporating evidence-based substantiation to support present-day recommendations. While there are many conditions that threaten maternal and perinatal outcomes, sometimes seemingly low-risk patients become high-risk due to antepartum, intrapartum, or postpartum events. We all need to be prepared!

Lynn L. Simpson, MSc, MD
Department of Obstetrics & Gynecology
Columbia University Medical Center
622 West 168th Street, PH-16
New York, NY 10032, USA

E-mail address:
ls731@cumc.columbia.edu

Genetics

Update on Prenatal Screening and Diagnosis

Mark I. Evans, MD[a,b,*], Stephanie Andriole, MS, CGC[a],
Shara M. Evans, MSc, MPH[a]

KEYWORDS

- Genetic disorder • Mendelian • Chromosomal • Chorionic villus sampling
- Multiple pregnancies • Fetal reduction • Pre-implantation diagnosis • Amniocentesis

KEY POINTS

- There have been tremendous advances in the ability to screen for the "odds" of having a genetic disorder (both Mendelian and chromosomal). At the same time, diagnostic capabilities have in parallel logarithmically increased as genetics advances moves from cytogenetic to molecular techniques for both chromosomes and Mendelian disorders.
- With microarray analyses on fetal tissue now showing a minimum risk for any pregnancy being at least 1 in 150 and ultimately greater than 1%, it is thought that all patients, regardless of age, should be offered chorionic villus sampling/amniocentesis and microarray analysis.
- As sequencing techniques replace other laboratory methods, the only question will be whether these tests are performed on villi, amniotic fluid cells, or maternal blood.

INTRODUCTION

Over the last past 4 decades, there have been revolutionary changes in the approach to prenatal diagnosis and screening.[1] In the 1960s and 1970s, prenatal diagnosis and screening evolved from merely wishing patients "good luck" to then asking "how old are you?" Maternal age was, and still is, a cheap screening test for aneuploidy. However, an explosion of techniques has dramatically enhanced the statistical performance of screening tests to identify high-risk patients. Biochemical and ultrasound (US) screens have gone through multiple generations with increasing sensitivities

---

The authors have nothing to disclose.
[a] Comprehensive Genetics, PLLC and Fetal Medicine Foundation of America, 131 E65th Street, New York, NY 10065, USA; [b] Department of Obstetrics & Gynecology, Mt. Sinai School of Medicine, 131 E65th Street, New York, NY 10065, USA
* Corresponding author. Comprehensive Genetics, PLLC and Fetal Medicine Foundation of America, 131 E65th Street, New York, NY 10065.
E-mail address: Evans@compregen.com

and specificities to the point where there has been considerable (and sometimes deliberate) confusion as to the distinction between screening and diagnosis.

A pendulum has swung back and forth between screening and testing primacy as new technologies have been developed. Overall, prenatal diagnosis has moved along 2 parallel paths (ie, imaging and tissue diagnoses) that sometimes converge. Often, clinicians are experts in one diagnostic modality or the other; there are a very limited number who are experts in both. As a result, there is often huge variability in approach to screening and diagnosis depending on by whom and where a patient is seen.

Thousands of articles and hundreds of textbooks have been written over the past decades about the subjects addressed here, but only a miniscule percentage of the available literature can be cited here. Here, the focus is on the leading edge changes in approach because a comprehensive review would go far beyond space limitations.

GENETIC COUNSELING

There has never been more need for genetic counseling for all pregnancies both to educate patients and to document that the patient was provided adequate information with which to make decisions. As the complexity of genetic information has increased massively in scope and amount, front-line obstetrician gynecologists generally have neither the time nor often the expertise to explain the nuances of new technologies. Genetic counselors are master's-trained individuals who have both an in-depth knowledge of genetic fundamentals and an understanding of screening principles and testing options. Genetic counseling as a profession emerged over the past few decades. In many settings, the counselors have far more understanding of genetic issues than do the attending physicians. It is optimum to have a coordinated team approach to patient care.

What too frequently occurs in obstetric practice is that, without adequate guidance, a "vending machine" selection of possible screening and testing options is offered to the patient. Only when there is an abnormal result does the primary medical provider first call for help to explain to an often panicked patient what the results actually mean. Thus, when possible, dedicated centers providing the continuum of genetic counseling, diagnosis, and treatment are optimal.

PRENATAL SCREENING
Mendelian Disorders

In the 1970s, prenatal screening for Mendelian disorders was simple: sickle cell for Africans, Tay-Sachs for Ashkenazi Jews, β-thalassemia for Mediterraneans, and α-thalassemia for Asians.[2] Since then, there has been an explosion of testing possibilities but also a serious disconnect between actual risks for a specific disorder and whether such risks constitute "high risk." For example, the Ashkenazi panel has increased from 1 to 3 available tests in the 1970s to 18 current "routine" test offerings,[3] and more tests are being developed. For many of the diseases tested for, the incidence in the Jewish population is actually no higher than in other ethnic groups, and the incidence of some is less than 1/100,000. Patients have been called "high risk" when a couple's risk has gone from 1 in one million to 1 in 10,000.

Several companies are now offering pan-ethnic screening for dozens of disorders.[4] Although there have been some serious problems in the implementation of these screens, including confusion regarding the actual risks of a disease for individual couples, it may ultimately prove more cost-effective to offer screening for "everything" to "everyone." However, such expansion of screening will require an increase in the understanding of genetic testing and the ability to appropriately communicate the information far beyond the level currently available. Frequently, new patients are seen who state that they have already been screened for "everything" and who are upset to learn that there is no such thing.

Public policy will also have to catch up with technologic reality.[5] At the same time that there has been at least partial acceptance of screening for rare disorders such as Usher syndrome, national organizations such as the American Congress of Obstetrics and Gynecology have declined to endorse offering universal screening for disorders such as Fragile X and spinal muscular atrophy, of which incidences are far higher. With rapid advances in testing technologies, the cost/benefit analyses of how much it is "worth doing" can be expected to change many times over the next several years.

Chromosomal Disorders

In 1970, only about 5% of births were to women 35 years of age or older, but the percentage increased to 10% by 1990. In the United States today, the number of births to women 35 years of age and older has reached almost 15%, and in selected areas such as Manhattan, it is approximately 20%.[6] In 1970, the typical 40-year-old pregnant woman had been married for 20 years and was having her fourth child. Today, the 40-year-old is more likely to be a professional woman having her first child. Not surprisingly, there are dramatic differences in approach, including acceptance and tolerance of genetic risk, between the 40-year-old grand-multipara and the 40-year-old primipara.

Much of the change in attitude has come from improvements in the ability to accurately detect genetic health status of the fetus. Although Down syndrome (DS) represents only a small proportion of the serious genetic disorders observed worldwide, it continues to be at the forefront of patient concern because that is the name "they know" (**Box 1**).

Efficacy of DS screening has evolved over a period 50 years, using many steps with evolving protocols. The unifying theme of all these advances has been the attempt to obtain a higher sensitivity with lower false positive rates by using one or more of 3 different categories of technique (biochemical, US, and now molecular markers) (**Table 1**).

Available second-trimester biochemical testing increased from single screening using maternal serum α-fetoprotein (MSAFP) in the early 1990s to double screening for MSAFP and human chorionic gonadotropin (hCG), triple screening by adding testing for unconjugated estriol, and currently to quadruple testing by adding Inhibin A. In the mid to late 1990s came the beginning of the shift of focus to the first trimester, and the best markers have proven to be pregnancy-associated plasma protein-A

Box 1
Worldwide birth defects

Congenital heart defects: 1,040,835

Neural tube defects: 323,904

Hemoglobin disorders: 307,897

Down syndrome: 217,293

Glucose-6-phosphate dehydrogenase deficiency: 177,032

Data from Global report on birth defects: the hidden toll of dying and disabled children. White Plains (NY): March of Dimes Birth Defects Foundation; 2006.

Table 1
Down syndrome screening protocols over the past 50 years

Method	Components	Time Frame	Sensitivity (%)	FPR* (%)
Maternal age	Birthday	1960s to present	35	15
Low MSAFP + age	AFP	1980s	50	~5
Double	AFP/HCG	1990s	55	~5
Triple	AFP/HCG/estriol	1990s	60	~5
Quad	AFP/HCG/estriol/inhibin	1990s/2000s	65	~5
NT	US measurements	1990s to present	60	~5
Combined	Free B HCG/PAPP-A/NT	2000s to present	85	~5
Sequential	Combined + quad	2000s to present	85–90	~5
Free fetal DNA	Sequencing/targeted	Since 2011	98	0.2–1

Abbreviation: FPR, false positive rate.

(PAPP-A) and the free β component of hCG.[7] Emerging protocols for the next few years will include α-fetal protein (AFP), placental growth factor, and possibly others as attempts are made to simultaneously screen for various aneuploidies, preeclampsia, and potentially preterm labor.[8]

Over the years, a change in the pattern of indications for chromosomal prenatal diagnosis has been observed. Overall, the most common indication for genetic counseling and prenatal diagnosis is still the risk for non-disjunctional aneuploidy stemming from "advanced maternal age," which is still defined as being 35 years of age or older at delivery or having a risk equivalent to that. Other "classic" indications to evaluate fetal karyotype include a previous affected offspring, patients with a balanced structural rearrangement of parental chromosomes, or diagnosed US abnormality.[1]

In the second trimester, US markers for fetal chromosome anomalies are observed in 3% to 5% of pregnancies.[9] There are also many "soft" US markers that have sometimes been associated with increased risk, but whose statistics are not adequate to become incorporated into routine use.[10] Merely because a given finding has a somewhat higher statistical occurrence in association with a given outcome does not mean that it is reasonable or cost-effective to alter the patient care plan. On balance, there might be more potential deleterious outcomes from performing additional procedures on incorrectly labeled high-risk patients than actual fetal problems identified.

The single, most important conceptual advance in the prenatal diagnosis of DS in the past 2 to 3 decades has been the understanding that the US visualization of fetal nuchal translucency (NT) was a very powerful marker of DS, when performed correctly.[11] Because the technology assessment literature is replete with failures to expand the use of successfully piloted techniques into routine clinical practice as the technology emerges,[12] organizations such as the Fetal Medicine Foundation in London and later the Nuchal Translucency Quality Review program of the Society for Maternal-Fetal Medicine began quality assessment programs and credentialing.[11] These programs were designed to minimize the likelihood of poor-quality US measurements impacting the accuracy of the algorithm for risk assessment and, thus, lowering the sensitivity and specificity of the US test. Credentialed training has improved the outcomes of US testing to some degree, and emerging concepts such as "Performance Adjusted Risks," which incorporates the individual provider's performance into the calculation of a "likelihood ratio" for the patient, can improve detection by as much as 3%, which at the national level is significant, translating in the United States to more than 100 additional cases detected per year.[3]

The mainstay of screening for the past 15 years has been "combined" first-trimester screening, which includes free β-hCG, PAPP-A, and the US screening for NT. Experience with more than one million patients has shown that when the biochemical parameters are measured appropriately and the US is performed and interpreted with proper quality control and assessment measures, combined screening can identify about 85% of DS pregnancies. Recent experience in Denmark has shown detection near 90% with ever decreasing requirements for procedures.[7]

Pregnancies with increased NT measurements and normal karyotypes represent a distinct risk group. More than 100 genetic conditions have been found in such cases — the most common of which are cardiac anomalies and Noonan syndrome.[13] The authors think that all patients with NT measurements greater than 3 mm (some say 3.5 mm) should be offered a fetal echocardiogram to search for cardiac anomalies, even if the 20-week anatomy scan is normal. With increased utilization of chromosomal microarray (CMA) analysis, some cases with increased NT will be shown to have previously unrecognized deletions or duplications.[14]

Noninvasive Prenatal Screening with Cell-Free Fetal DNA

The "holy grail" of prenatal screening was for decades the concept that fetal cells could be obtained from a maternal blood sample and thus need and risk of an invasive, diagnostic procedure for aneuploidy would be avoided.[15] In the 1990s, the focus was on methods to separate out the rare fetal cells (perhaps 1 in 10,000,000) in the circulation. Numerous articles and a large National Institutes of Health–sponsored trial (NIFTY) explored various separation strategies (fluorescent-activated and magnetic-activated cell sorting), but ultimately the technologies were not substantive enough to permit fetal cells in maternal blood to emerge as a viable screening approach.[15]

In 1997, Lo and colleagues[16] patented and published a method for taking paternal DNA, amplifying it, and using it for the diagnosis of fetal gender. Over the years, there have been many approaches attempted, for example, using digital polymerized chain reaction of DNA and RNA, as well as methylation differences. These approaches attempted, with inadequate success, to reliably investigate free fetal DNA (ffDNA).[17] Since 2011, the main approach has been using next-generation sequencing (NGS), also called massively parallel shotgun sequencing (MPSS), in which DNA amplification is performed millions of times simultaneously using probes of approximately 36 base-pairs, which provides enough specificity to accurately identify from which chromosome the excess fragments derive. Overall, the genome is interrogated more than 100 times so that there is enough power to reliably determine the relative concentrations of DNA fragments for a given chromosomal region compared with the expected concentrations.[18–20] For example, chromosome 21 normally encompasses approximately 1.32% of the genome DNA. If one were to observe approximately 2%, then it could readily be concluded that there was a trisomy for chromosome 21. Obviously, however, it is not realistically possible to obtain a noninvasive specimen that is exclusively fetal. Thus, the number of chromosome probes from the fetus is figuratively drowned in maternal DNA, such that the actual percentage increase is about 0.1%. However, by counting the genome more than 100 times using the MPSS approach, the reliability is significantly improved.

With any parameter, there is always a bell-shaped curve of counts that is amenable to being treated as a parametric measurement. As such, the algorithm looks at the standard deviation (SD) of the counts and considers values beyond 3 + SD as being abnormal. With MPSS, this is done for all chromosomes.

Some companies use targeted probes or targeted sequencing in which only the chromosomes of interest are interrogated.[19] Proponents argue that by limiting their focus, their tests are cheaper. However, such an approach is short-sighted. The future of cell-free DNA is not DS. It is an expansion of disorders including Mendelian diseases. For the MPSS technology, only the bioinformatics are needed. For targeted probes and sequencing, one has to go back to the beginning and repeat everything. Ultimately, the "expensive" test today is the cheaper one tomorrow.

These techniques can produce both false positives and false negatives. US imaging may or may not be consistent with the abnormality. It is important to recognize that, despite a literature reporting sensitivities approaching 99% for DS, a 99% sensitivity is *not* a 99% positive predictive value.[21] Of those cases "at risk," diagnostic procedures such as amniocentesis or chorionic villus sampling (CVS) must then be offered for confirmation.

It is well-appreciated statistical dogma that although sensitivity and specificity do not vary with prevalence, the predictive values do.[22] Thus, although in a 40 year old with a DS + ffDNA screen the likelihood of actually having a fetus with DS may be 70% or greater, in younger women the likelihood is much lower. For example, if there is a 99% sensitivity and a 99% specificity (1% false positives) in a 26 year old, the actual positive predictive value can be as low as 11%. That would be comparable to a 3-mm NT measurement on US. After several years of concern after NT measurements were introduced, it is now reasonably well understood that NT is only an indicator of odds, and not a definitive answer. The same is true of non invasive prenatal screening (NIPS).

Public health policy debates over the introduction of ffDNA screening methods will be very harsh because the costs for these methods approach the total reimbursements from Medicaid in many jurisdictions for 9 months' worth of care, including labor and delivery.[23] Blunt cost assessments, including the savings from pregnancies with serious problems that are terminated, will be necessary to determine a true financial cost/benefit ratio. Recent data show that the marginal cost for finding 1 additional case of DS beyond those already found by combined screening in the low-risk population is greater than $3 million. It will not be until the cost of NIPS is reduced to the $400 range that the costs will even begin to break even. Ultimately, only a contingent protocol with a few cases "on the bubble," which reflex to NIPS, might be cost-effective.[24,25] Those cases at high risk should go directly to diagnostic procedures rather than just "kicking the can" down the road for 2 more weeks before an answer is then sought.

PRENATAL DIAGNOSTIC PROCEDURES
Overview

Invasive procedures for prenatal diagnosis of fetal disease are available throughout gestation from conception. Prenatal diagnosis requires direct assessment of fetal tissue. Since the late 1960s, this has been possible by the aspiration of amniotic fluid. Beginning in the 1980s, chorionic villi have been obtained either transcervically or transabdominally. Other tissues, such as skin, muscle, liver, and fetal blood, have been obtained occasionally for those diagnoses that cannot be accomplished by sampling amniotic fluid or villi. Assisted reproduction technologies enable diagnosis (or exclusion) of several disorders on the 4-cell to 8-cell embryo before implantation. These procedures have come to be known as a continuum of approaches, rather than distinct entities that are independent of one another.

Amniocentesis

Invasive procedures for diagnosis of fetal genetic disorders have been available since techniques for culturing and karyotyping of amniotic fluid fibroblasts were developed[12] in the late 1960s to early 1970s. It has been the mainstay for 40 years, but a major disadvantage of amniocentesis, however, is that results are usually not available until late in the second trimester, generally 17 to 20 weeks of gestation, by which time the pregnancy is very visible, the mother has felt the baby moving, the bonding process is accelerated, and consideration of termination is more emotionally and physically onerous than earlier in gestation.[26] Improvements in US and increasing expertise in US-guided procedures enabled physicians in the 1980s to move to the first trimester, introducing CVS and then early amniocentesis (EA).

EA, performed between 10 and 14 weeks of gestation, was offered as a "safer" alternative to CVS, but this technique has been almost completely abandoned because[27] it was associated with amniotic fluid leakage that led to talipes.[28] Ironically, the "safe" procedure had far more risk than the "risky" one.

Multiple Gestations

With infertility treatments, multiple births in the United States have tripled to about 3% of births, and multiples constitute an even higher percentage of patients presenting for prenatal diagnosis.[6] One-third of naturally occurring multiple gestations are monozygotic, and with infertility therapies, approximately 20% of twins are monozygotic. Thus, in most cases separate sampling of amniotic fluid from both sacs is required to assess correctly the karyotype of each fetus. In general, the chance that at least one dizygotic twin has an abnormal karyotype is essentially twice the age-related risk.[1] However, the risks of procedures in multiples do not appear to be increased significantly, probably because such procedures are disproportionately performed by subspecialists (perinatologists and geneticists) who typically have more experience and expertise.[1] When the anatomic relationship of the sacs and the chorioamniotic membrane between them are clearly discernible, it is generally straightforward to sample both sacs with continuous US guidance.

Historically, injection of a dye into the first sac after aspiration of AF was considered a helpful marker.[29] The authors have long ago abandoned this. Their technique is, after obtaining the specimen from a sac, to use the aspiration syringe to withdraw another 5 cc of AF and then immediately eject it back into the cavity (**Fig. 1**). The fluid injected

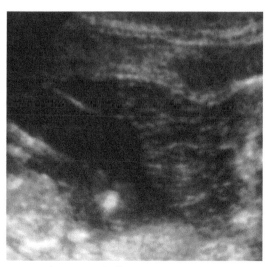

Fig. 1. Twin amniotic sacs. After removal of specimen, 5 cc of AF is aspirated into syringe and then immediately reinjected, which produces a "snowstorm" of particulate matter already in cavity. Left side is now clear for second aspiration.

dredges up sludge in the cavity and creates a "snowstorm," which demarcates the different sacs.

Abnormally elevated amniotic fluid AFP (AF AFP) when there is no obvious cause, such as US-visualized spina bifida, indicates the need to test for acetylcholinesterase (AChE). The combination of an abnormally elevated AF AFP and a positive AChE is associated in most cases with fetal malformations or with fetal death. Transfer of these materials across the membranes may confuse clinical interpretation of AF AFP and AChE results in twin pregnancies. Discordant AF AFP results are more common in dizygotic twins, perhaps because of the dichorionic diamniotic membrane between the sacs. AChE diffuses readily across the membranes and cannot be used to determine which twin is abnormal.[30]

Safety and Complications of Amniocentesis

Multiple studies over the past 4 decades have investigated the risks of amniocentesis.[31] As with all prenatal procedures, there is a constellation of factors developing concurrently that render definitive assessment difficult. Most importantly, there is a well-understood background rate of fetal loss that diminishes with advancing gestational ages, and there is a dramatic correlation between maternal age and the risk of spontaneous loss. If the data are limited to those fetuses known to be euploid, the correlation persists but is less dramatic.

The only randomized trial of amniocentesis versus no amniocentesis in low-risk patients was done in the mid 1980s by Tabor and colleagues[32] in Copenhagen, who found nearly a 1% increase in pregnancy loss following amniocentesis. Numerous more recent studies have suggested a much lower complication rate, with the general consensus being that in experienced hands fetal loss after amniocentesis is approximately 1 in 400 greater than background rates. One often-quoted study from the FASTER trial suggested that the risk was as low as 1 in 1600, but this estimate resulted from an error in statistical analysis.[33] In reality, their loss rate was 1 in 350.

Maternal complications such as sepsis and death are also very rare, but never zero.

Trauma to the fetus during amniocentesis has been reported, including central nervous system injury and amniotic band syndrome.[34] However, fetal injury caused by the amniocentesis needle was never very common and should now be very rare with US-guided procedures.

Chorionic Villus Sampling

Since the introduction of amniocentesis into high-risk obstetrics in the 1970s, there has been a constant desire to move prenatal diagnoses as early in gestation as possible.[1] In the mid 1980s, the combination of increasingly sophisticated US imaging and laboratory cytogenetic advances made first-trimester sampling of chorionic villi possible.

Indications

With the rare exception of those patients whose primary risk is for a neural tube defect, virtually any patient seen in the first trimester who would be considered a candidate for amniocentesis is also a candidate for CVS.[1] CVS has the advantage of earlier diagnosis, allowing earlier intervention when chosen, and increased privacy in patients' reproductive choices. Developments in screening, principally the first trimester, combined protocol of free β-hCG, PAPP-A, and NT, meaning that most DS pregnancies, for example, can be identified in the first trimester. The authors think that it is not reasonable to routinely identify high-risk patients in the first trimester and then force the patient to wait a month for an amniocentesis when a CVS could provide the answer much sooner.

In the 1980s, CVS patients were generally scheduled to be seen at about 10 weeks after their last menstrual period (LMP). With the development of

1. NT screening that cannot be reliably performed until nearly 12 weeks' gestation and
2. To a minor degree the concern about limb reduction defects (LRD), which proved to be unfounded

CVS is now routinely performed at about 12 weeks. If an abnormality is found, the patient may choose to terminate by the safer, easier, quicker, and cheaper suction method that can be used in the first trimester. Second-trimester termination techniques are more expensive, have higher complication rates, and are without privacy because the pregnant status of the patient has usually become obvious by this time.[1]

Multiple gestations
The authors routinely perform CVS on multiple gestations because they believe strongly that CVS has significant advantages over amniocentesis. When patients choose fetal reduction (FR), either because of a diagnosed fetal abnormality or because of the increased risks of abnormality associated with multiples, FR has much better morbidity and mortality statistics in the first trimester than later on in the pregnancy. The authors now perform CVS with fluorescent in situ hybridization (FISH) analysis overnight, followed by FR the next afternoon in about 85% to 90% of their reduction cases.[35]

Placental and fetal locations must be meticulously noted to avoid sampling one twin twice and the other not at all (**Fig. 2**). Nevertheless, there is always the small risk of cross-contamination of samples. Operators must be facile with both the transabdominal (TA) and the transcervical (TC) approach to maximize the ability to obtain specimens and to minimize the chance of cross-contamination (**Fig. 3**). Furthermore, the operators must make sure they are actually getting the specimens from the placenta and not the placenta of a "vanishing twin,"s which may occur in up to 3% of pregnancies and is more likely to show chromosomal abnormalities.[36]

In general, placental location determines whether the approach will be TC or TA. For most cases, this decision will be straightforward. If the placenta is low-lying, posterior, or previa, a TC approach is appropriate (see **Fig. 3**).[36] CVS is relatively easy to perform in these cases and may be attempted by trainees under supervision. As placental position moves upward or lateral, if the uterus is retroverted, or there are fibroids, for example, TC CVS is more technically challenging. The placenta can often be maneuvered into a more horizontal (TC) or vertical (TA) configuration by judicious manipulation of bladder volume and using the speculum handle to alter the angle of

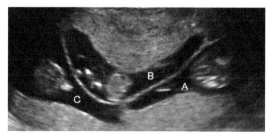

Fig. 2. Triplet gestation in transverse scan show 2 posterior placentas and one anterior placenta.

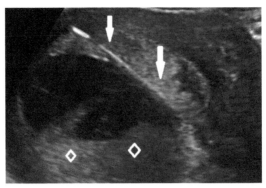

Fig. 3. Same patient as **Fig. 2,** but scan now longitudinal show CVS catheter pathway (*arrows*) of anterior placenta by TC approach. Posterior placenta (*diamonds*) is also reached transcervically.

the cervical canal. If the placenta is anterior and fundal, an abdominal approach is usually indicated. Large subchorionic hematomas and fibroids should be avoided if possible and sometimes dictate the approach. Overall, the TC approach requires more experience than TA. In the authors' experience, either TA or TC is clearly indicated in about 40% of cases; in the remaining 60%, either approach can be used.[36]

It is the authors' experience that most patients from "western" cultures would rather have a "Pap smear"-like experience than a TA needle procedure. Only patients from very conservative cultures, for whom examination of a woman by a male physician is problematic, automatically prefer the abdominal approach. In multiple gestations, sampling using both approaches is routine.

Other factors must be considered before attempting CVS. For patients with a history of genital herpes simplex or a recent group B streptococcus (GBS) infection, such cases should be individualized; the small or theoretic risk of introducing an infection into the fetal-placental tissues should be discussed with the patient. Although routine culturing is not warranted, TA CVS and amniocentesis are usually offered when a significant risk of active GBS is present.[37]

TA-CVS also has been applied successfully in the second and third trimesters for prenatal diagnosis, with results comparable with amniocentesis and probably associated with a smaller risk of pregnancy loss than cordocentesis. The major advantage of late CVS is the possibility of obtaining rapid results in situations where such information is needed for decisions about mode and timing of delivery, pregnancy termination, or fetal therapy. Such situations include the ultrasonographic diagnosis of fetal anomalies late in the second trimester, close to the legal limit in gestational age, after which termination of pregnancy is no longer possible. Late CVS also offers a distinct advantage over cordocentesis in cases complicated by oligohydramnios. Prenatal availability of fetal karyotype in pregnancies complicated by severe intrauterine growth restriction or fetal anomalies may influence the mode of delivery, the management of intrapartum fetal distress, which is a common phenomenon in fetuses with chromosome anomalies, or the decision for surgical intervention within the first few hours after birth.[36]

Safety of Chorionic Villus Samplings

For first-trimester diagnosis, either TA-CVS or TC-CVS is the preferred method of choice, whereas EA carries a significant risk for fetal loss and fetal malformations.

Both TC and TA methods are necessary to have the most complete, practical, and safe approach to first trimester diagnosis.

In the early 1990s, it was suggested that CVS may be associated with specific fetal malformations, particularly LRDs.[37,38] Today, based on the published data, it is clear that there is no increased risk for LRDs or any other birth defect when CVS is performed at greater than 70 days of gestation. There is a minimal risk between 8 and 9 weeks, and about a 1% risk of LRD, if the procedure is performed between 24 and 42 days after fertilization (6–7 weeks LMP).[36]

Recent data suggest that CVS is in fact safer in experienced hands than mid trimester amniocentesis.[39] A meta-analysis by Mujezinovic and Alfirevic[31] has shown that the loss rates from amniocentesis and CVS were equivalent. More recent data from Denmark suggest that the procedure risks of CVS and amniocentesis are the same, and that the incidence of late-term complications is actually lower in the CVS group than in those who have amniocentesis.[39]

Accuracy of chorionic villus sampling cytogenetic results
A major concern with all prenatal diagnostic procedures is the possibility of discordance between the prenatal cytogenetic diagnosis and the actual fetal karyotype. With CVS, these discrepancies can occur from either maternal tissue contamination or from true biologic differences between the extra embryonic tissue (ie, placenta) and the fetus. Fortunately, it was demonstrated in the 1980s that genetic evaluation of chorionic villi provides a high level of accuracy, particularly in regard to the diagnosis of common trisomies.[40] Clinical errors and misinterpretation are rare, and the need for repeat testing continues to decrease as more knowledge about the characteristics of chorionic villi is obtained. Today, approximately 0.5% of CVS cases have an ambiguous finding that requires further confirmation by amniocentesis.[1] Overall, CVS is associated with a low rate of maternal cell contamination or chromosomal abnormalities confined to the placenta.

Confined placental mosaicism
Mosaicism occurs in about 0.5% to 2% of all CVS samples,[41] and it is confirmed in the fetus in 10% to 40% of these cases. In contrast, amniotic fluid cell mosaicism is observed in only 0.1% to 0.3% of cultures, but, when found, is confirmed in the fetus in ~70% of cases.[41] Feto-placental discrepancies are known to occur because the chorionic villi consist of a combination of extra embryonic tissue of different sources that become separated and distinct from those of the embryo in early developmental stages. Specifically, at the 32-celled to 64-celled blastocyst, only 3 to 4 blastomeres differentiate into the inner cell mass, which forms the embryo, mesenchymal core of the chorionic villi, the amnion, yolk sac, and chorion, whereas the rest of the cells become the precursors of the extra embryonic tissues.[41]

When discordances between CVS and AF cell karyotypes were first appreciated in the 1980s, they were interpreted as a "problem" of CVS. It is now realized that in fact they represent an opportunity to identify real issues, such as uniparental disomy (UPD), that can have significant clinical impact that otherwise would not be detectable.

LABORATORY ANALYSES

Metaphase karyotyping, usually with G banding, has been the "gold standard" for cytogenetics for 30 years. It will not be elaborated on further here. In addition to the standard cytogenetic techniques, several methods have originated from the interface between cytogenetics and molecular biology, commonly referred to as "molecular cytogenetics." In general, these techniques use fluorescently labeled DNA probes that bind to a specific chromosomal region and thus allow assessment of the presence and number of specific genomic loci within a cell.

FISH was first introduced in the early 1990s. FISH functions as a bridge between conventional cytogenetics and molecular DNA testing and enables sensitive and relatively fast evaluation of the number and location of large pieces of chromosomes by direct visualization of specific regions under the microscope.[42]

One of the major advantages of FISH over the standard banding methods is its ability to recognize subtle chromosomal changes such as deletions or duplications, which result in an alteration of normal gene dosage.[42] Specific commercial FISH probes are available to recognize specific microdeletions (eg, DiGeorge/velo-cardio-facial syndrome that most often results from a 3-Mb deletion on chromosomal region 22q11.2). Unlike standard cytogenetic techniques, which require dividing cells in metaphase, FISH may be applied to interphase nuclei of nondividing cells[43] obviating cell culture, which usually requires 10 to 14 days. Use of FISH significantly shortens the procedure time for analysis of chromosomal numeric aberrations in prenatal diagnosis and preimplantation genetic diagnosis (PGD).[44]

The fundamental limitation of using FISH in the clinical setting is that in most cases the clinician must have a prior knowledge of or a high index of suspicion for the specific chromosome aberration in question. Thus, a genome-wide molecular cytogenetic approach for detecting copy number imbalances at a higher resolution is needed. In the past few years, advances in molecular cytogenetic techniques enabled the detection of small genomic alterations (eg, deletions and duplications) generally termed "submicroscopic alterations" (ie, under the 5–10 Mb resolution for conventional karyotyping), on a genome-wide scale. Some of these microdeletions or microduplications are associated with well-described clinical syndromes and others may have significant clinical implications. These conditions result from changes in the amount of genetic material along the chromosome and thus are termed copy number variants (CNVs). These CNVs include deletions and duplications in the range of thousands to millions of base-pairs. CNVs can be either benign or pathogenic, depending on their location and genetic content.

CMA enables the simultaneous analysis of the entire genome to identify deletions and duplications 100 to 1000 times smaller than those identified by karyotype, without the need to preselect the target. A variety of different probes are in clinical usage, including large ones derived from bacterial artificial chromosomes (BAC array), small ones consisting of oligonucleotide sequences (oligo-array), and even smaller single-nucleotide polymorphisms (SNP arrays). Newer technology was based on hundreds of thousands of smaller and denser oligonucleotide probes, providing resolution to 50 to 100 kb, allowing detection of duplications and deletions that may affect only a single gene. Recently, there is increasing use of SNP arrays that are able to detect loss of heterozygosity (LOH), characteristic of UPD. Currently, there are array designs that incorporate high-quality nonpolymorphic copy number probes along with sufficient SNP probes to identify CNVs as well as LOH and UPD.

Performing genome-wide analysis is not flawless. It has long been known that there are significant CNVs in the human genome that have no apparent phenotypic effects.[1] Given the large degree of cytogenetically visible polymorphism in the human karyotype, it is not surprising that there would be even more variation within normal individuals at a submicroscopic level. When used as a clinical diagnostic tool, it is not desirable to detect a large number of CNVs that either are benign or represent *variants of uncertain clinical significance* (VOUS). For this reason, clinical array designs disperse their probes on those regions of the genome containing single-copy sequence and most known coding sequences and functional genes, attempting to maximize the yield of pathogenic CNVs but minimizing the detection of benign CNVs found in the normal population.

Pediatricians have largely abandoned the karyotype as the primary cytogenetic in analysis in favor of CMA. Some authorities (including the authors of this article) think that CMA should replace standard cytogenetic analysis in prenatal diagnosis. Obviously the detection rate is increased, but there is a tradeoff. Balanced chromosomal rearrangements (translocations and inversions) are not detected with CMA because there is no gain or loss of genetic material. Thus, de novo, apparently balanced rearrangements identified by standard karyotyping will be missed; these may be associated with some risk of congenital abnormalities,[45] such as by interruption of genes at the breakpoints.

In cases of an anomaly diagnosed on ultrasonography, additional clinically relevant information from CMA is gained in 6.0% to 6.5% of patients.[14,46,47] The overall incidence of VOUSs is 1.1% to 1.5% for all indications.[14,46]

Many studies have found that, at a minimum, there is a 0.5% baseline risk for the identification of a significant microdeletion or microduplication, even in women with an uneventful prenatal examination.[14,46] VOUS prenatally can also create challenges in counseling expectant parents. Ultimately, the true incidence of finding significant abnormalities on CMA that cannot be detected by traditional karyotype or US will be at least 1%,[14,46] which is a far higher threshold than the 0.5% seen with maternal age 35. As such, the authors routinely now offer all patients, regardless of maternal age, a diagnostic test (preferably CVS in the first trimester) with CMA analysis. This diagnostic testing represents a major culture change. Acceptance seems to be following a classic "red" state versus "blue" state dichotomy. It will take several years for the dust to settle.

Preimplantation Genetic Diagnosis

For couples at risk of transmitting a genetic disease or a chromosomal aberration to their offspring, PGD and transfer of unaffected embryos offer an alternative to prenatal diagnosis by CVS or amniocentesis, followed by termination of pregnancy of an affected fetus. Molecular PGD was initially used for embryo sexing in couples at risk for X-linked diseases. During the last 2 decades, the range of genetic abnormalities that can be detected by PGD has increased exponentially and the only prerequisite for PGD is that the disease-causing mutation is known. Even if the mutation is not specified, molecular analysis can be made by using linked polymorphic markers based on haplotype analysis of family members. Initially, PGD has traditionally been used for early-onset severe conditions (such as cystic fibrosis, fragile X). However, PGD can also be used to prevent late-onset conditions such as in carriers of cancer predisposition genes (eg, Huntington disease or BRCA for breast and ovarian cancer and other late-onset conditions). Increasingly, it is also used to have children whose stem cells can be used to treat siblings who need bone marrow transplants to cure genetic disorders or malignancies. (However, the authors always recommend diagnostic testing by CVS or amniocentesis to confirm PGD results because, even with the newest methods, there is still about a 1% discordancy between PGD and analyses on much higher number of cells. PGD need to be viewed as an excellent screening test but it is not diagnostic.)

SUMMARY

There have been tremendous advances in the ability to screen for the "odds" of having a genetic disorder (both Mendelian and chromosomal). At the same time, diagnostic capabilities have in parallel logarithmically increased as genetics research moves from cytogenetic to molecular techniques for both chromosomes and Mendelian disorders. With microarray analyses on fetal tissue now showing a minimum risk for any pregnancy being at least 1 in 150 and ultimately greater than 1%, it is thought that all patients, regardless of age, should be offered CVS/amniocentesis and microarray analysis. Ultimately, as sequencing techniques replace other laboratory methods, the only question will be whether these tests are performed on villi, amniotic fluid cells, or maternal blood.

REFERENCES

1. Evans MI, Johnson MP, Yaron Y, et al, editors. Prenatal diagnosis: genetics, reproductive risks, testing, and management. New York: McGraw Hill Publishing Co; 2006.
2. Ashkenazi Jewish carrier screening: integrated genetics. Available at: https://www.labcorp.com/wps/portal/!ut/p/c1/04_SB8K8xLLM9MSSzPy8xBz9CP0os3h_U2cv30B_IwN_f3MDA88APyM_byN_Q3cfA30_j_zcVP2CbEdFAPxk0Is!/dl2/d1/L0lDU0lKSWdrbUEhIS9JRFJBQUlppQ2dBek15cXchL1lCSkoxTkExTkk1MC01RncvN19PNUNKTVFPMjBPTzcwMEIQTjJOSzJPMUdENS9JX19fXzE!/?WCM_PORTLET=PC_7_O5CJMQO20OO700IPN2NK2O1GD5_WCM&WCM_GLOBAL_CONTEXT=/wps/wcm/connect/IntGeneticsLib/integratedgenetics/home/our+services/reproductive+testing/aj-carrier-test. Accessed February, 2015.
3. Evans MI, Cuckle HS. Performance adjusted risks (PAR): a method to improve the quality of algorithm performance while allowing all to play. Prenat Diagn 2011;31:797–801.
4. Srinivasan BS, Evans EA, Flannick J, et al. A universal carrier test for the long tail of Mendelian disease. Reprod Biomed Online 2010;4:537–51.
5. National Human Genome Research Institute. Regulation of genetic tests. Available at: http://www.genome.gov/10002335. Accessed February, 2015.
6. Martin JA, Hamilton BE, Osterman MJ, et al. Births: final data for 2012. Natl Vital Stat Rep 2015;64(1):1–68.
7. Evans MI, Hallahan TW, Krantz D, et al. Meta-analysis of first trimester Down syndrome screening studies: free beta-human chorionic gonadotropin significantly outperforms intact human chorionic gonadotropin in a multimarker protocol. Am J Obstet Gynecol 2007;196:198–205.
8. Hassan S, Romero R, Vidyadhari D, et al. Vaginal progesterone reduces the rate of preterm birth in women with a sonographic short cervix: a multicenter, randomized, double-blind, placebo-controlled trial. Ultrasound Obstet Gynecol 2011;38:18–31.
9. Benacerraf BR, Nadel A, Bromley B. Identification of second trimester fetuses with autosomal trisomy by use of a sonographic scoring index. Radiology 1994;193:135–40.
10. Lau TK, Evans MI. Second trimester sonographic soft markers: what can we learn from the experience of first trimester nuchal translucency screening? Ultrasound Obstet Gynecol 2008;32:123–5.
11. Wright D, Syngelaki A, Bradbury D, et al. First trimester screening for Trisomies 21, 18, and13 by ultrasound and biochemical testing. Fetal Diagn Ther 2014;35:118–26.
12. Jacobson JB, Barter RH. Intrauterine diagnosis and management of genetic defects. Am J Obstet Gynecol 1967;99:795–801.
13. Souka AP, Von Kaisenberg CS, Hyett JA, et al. Increased nuchal translucency with normal karyotype. Am J Obstet Gynecol 2005;192:1005–21.

14. Wapner RJ, Martin CL, Levy B, et al. Chromosomal microarray versus karyotyping for prenatal diagnosis. N Engl J Med 2012;367:2175–84.
15. Bianchi DW, Simpson JL, Jackson LG, et al. Fetal gender and aneuploidy detection using fetal cells in maternal blood: analysis of NIFTY I data. Prenat Diagn 2002;22:609–15.
16. Lo YM, Corbetta N, Chamberlain PF, et al. Presence of fetal DNA in maternal plasma and serum. Lancet 1997;350:485–7.
17. Lo YM. Noninvasive prenatal detection of fetal chromosomal aneuploidies by maternal plasma nucleic acid analysis: a review of the current state of the art. BJOG 2009;116:152–7.
18. Ehrich M, Deciu C, Zwiefelhofer T, et al. Noninvasive detection of fetal trisomy 21 by sequencing of DNA in maternal blood: a study in a clinical setting. Am J Obstet Gynecol 2011;204:205.e1–11.
19. Sparks AB, Wang ET, Struble CA, et al. Selective analysis of cell free DNA in maternal blood for evaluation of fetal trisomy. Prenat Diagn 2012;32:3–9.
20. Bianchi DW, Wilkins-Haug L. Integration of noninvasive DNA testing for aneuploidy into prenatal care: what has happened since the rubber met the road? Clin Chem 2014;60:78–87.
21. Chitty LS, Bianchi DW. Noninvasive prenatal testing: the paradigm is shifting rapidly. Prenat Diagn 2013;33:511–3.
22. Galen RS, Gambino SR. Beyond normality: the predictive value and efficacy of medical diagnoses. Baltimore (MD): MD John Wiley and Sons; 1975.
23. Krantz DA, Hallahan TW, Carmichael JB, et al. Utilization of a 1/1000 cutoff in combined screening for Down Syndrome in younger women AMA patients provides cost advantages compared with NIPS. Am J Obstet Gynecol 2014;210:S111.
24. Cuckle HS, Benn P, Pergament E. Maternal cfDNA screening for Down syndrome – a cost sensitivity analysis. Prenat Diagn 2013;33:636–42.
25. Evans MI, Sonek J, Hallahan T, et al. Cell-free fetal DNA screening in the USAnited States: a cost analysis of screening strategies. Ultrasound Obstet Gynecol 2015;45:74–83.
26. Fletcher JC, Evans MI. Maternal bonding in early fetal ultrasound examinations. N Engl J Med 1983;308:392–3.
27. Hanson FW, Happ RL, Tennant FR, et al. Ultrasonography-guided early amniocentesis in singleton pregnancies. Am J Obstet Gynecol 1990;162:1376–81.
28. Wilson RD. Early amniocentesis: a clinical review. Prenat Diagn 1995;15:1259–73.
29. Van der Pol JS, Wolf H, Boer K, et al. Jejunal atresia related to the use of methylene blue in genetic amniocentesis in twins. Br J Obstet Gynaecol 1992;99:141–3.
30. Drugan A, Sokol RJ, Syner FN, et al. Clinical implications of amniotic fluid AFP in twin pregnancies. J Reprod Med 1989;34:977–81.
31. Mujezinovic F, Alfirevic Z. Procedure-related complications of amniocentesis and chorionic villus sampling: a systematic review. Obstet Gynecol 2007;110:687–94.
32. Tabor A, Phillip J, Masden M, et al. Randomized controlled trial of genetic amniocentesis in 4606 low-risk women. Lancet 1986;1:1287–93.
33. Eddleman KA, Malone FD, Sullivan L, et al. Pregnancy loss rates after midtrimester amniocentesis. Obstet Gynecol 2006;108:1067–72.
34. Squier M, Chamberlain P, Zaiwalla Z, et al. Five cases of brain injury following amniocentesis in mid-term pregnancy. Dev Med Child Neurol 2000;42(8):554–60.
35. Rosner M, Pergament E, Andriole S, et al. Detection of genetic abnormalities using CVS and FISH prior to fetal reduction in sonographically normal appearing fetuses. Prenat Diagn 2013;33:940–4.

36. Evans MI, Rozner G, Yaron Y, et al. CVS in Evans MI. In: Johnson MP, Yaron Y, editors. Prenatal diagnosis: genetics, reproductive risks, testing, and management. New York: McGraw Hill Publishing Co; 2006. p. 433–42.
37. Silverman NS, Sullivan MW, Jungkind DL, et al. Incidence of bacteremia associated with chorionic villus sampling. Obstet Gynecol 1994;84(6):1021–4.
38. Akolekar R, Beta J, Picciarelli G, et al. Procedure related risk of misscarriage following amniocentesis and chorionic villus sampling: a systematic review and meta-analysis. Ultrasound Obstet Gynecol 2015;45:16–26.
39. Wulff R, Tabor A. Risk of fetal loss from invasive testing. Presented at the meeting of Fetal Medicine Foundation. 2013.
40. Rhoads GG, Jackson LG, Schlesselman SE, et al. The safety and efficacy of chorionic villus sampling for early prenatal diagnosis of cytogenetic abnormalities. N Engl J Med 1989;320:609.
41. Ledbetter DH, Zachary JL, Simpson MS, et al. Cytogenetic results from the US collaborative study on CVS. Prenat Diagn 1992;12(5):317.
42. van Ommen GJ, Breuning MH, Raap AK. FISH in genome research and molecular diagnostics. Curr Opin Genet Dev 1995;5(3):304.
43. Evans MI, Klinger KW, Isada NB, et al. Rapid prenatal diagnosis by fluorescent in situ hybridization of chorionic villi: an adjunct to long-term culture and karyotype. Am J Obstet Gynecol 1992;167:1522.
44. Verlinsky Y, Cieslak J, Freidine M, et al. Polar body diagnosis of common aneuploidies by FISH. J Assist Reprod Genet 1996;13:157–62, 100.
45. Manning M. Hudgins L Array-based technology and recommendations for utilization in medical genetics practice for detection of chromosomal abnormalities. Genet Med 2010;12(11):742–5.
46. Shaffer LG, Dabell MP, Fisher AJ, et al. Experience with microarray-based comparative genomic hybridization for prenatal diagnosis in over 5000 pregnancies. Prenat Diagn 2012;32(10):976–85.
47. Handyside AH, Robinson MD, Simpson RJ, et al. Isothermal whole genome amplification from single and small numbers of cells: a new era for preimplantation genetic diagnosis of inherited disease. Mol Hum Reprod 2004;10(10): 767–72.

Screening for Congenital Heart Disease During Anatomical Survey Ultrasonography

Mert Ozan Bahtiyar, MD[a],*, Joshua A. Copel, MD[a,b]

KEYWORDS

- Congenital heart disease • Prenatal ultrasound screening • Neonatal outcome

KEY POINTS

- A systematic approach to fetal heart examination, regular feedback, and implementation of training programs could improve detection rates and in turn neonatal outcome.
- In utero detection of congenital heart disease (CHD) allows possible prenatal interventions.
- In utero detection of CHD improves postnatal outcome.

INTRODUCTION

Congenital heart disease (CHD) is among the most common congenital abnormalities. The prevalence of CHD ranges between 0.6% and 1.2% of live births.[1,2] Despite its high prevalence, CHD is also among the most commonly missed fetal abnormalities.[3] Experience of the operator, choice of transducer, maternal body habitus, previous abdominal surgery, gestational age, fetal position, and amount of amniotic fluid are some of the factors that can affect prenatal diagnosis rates.[4] A systematic approach to fetal heart examination (**Box 1**), regular feedback, and implementation of training programs could improve detection rates and, in turn, neonatal outcome.[5]

Early detection of major CHD is important for prenatal counseling, for determining appropriate prenatal care, and for possible therapeutic interventions. Prenatal

The authors have nothing to disclose.
[a] Maternal-Fetal Medicine, Department of Obstetrics, Gynecology & Reproductive Science, Yale Fetal Cardiovascular Center, Yale Fetal Care Center, Yale School of Medicine, 333 Cedar Street, New Haven, CT 06520, USA; [b] Department of Pediatrics, Yale School of Medicine, 333 Cedar Street, New Haven, CT 06520, USA
* Corresponding author. Department of Obstetrics, Gynecology & Reproductive Sciences, Yale School of Medicine, 333 Cedar Street, P.O. Box 208063, New Haven, CT 06520-8063.
E-mail address: mert.bahtiyar@yale.edu

Box 1
Cardiac examination check list

Situs

Size

Location

Axis

Heart rate and rhythm

Four chamber

  LA = RA

  LV = RV

  RV has moderator band, anterior

  AV valves

    Two distinct AV valves

    Tricuspid slightly apically displaced

  Interventricular septum intact

  Foramen ovale present

  Foraminal flap opens in to LA

LVOT

RVOT

3-VV/3-VTV

Abbreviations: AV, atrioventricular; LA, left atrium; LV, left ventricle; LVOT, left ventricular outflow tract; RA, right atrium; RV, right ventricle; RVOT, right ventricular outflow tract; 3-VTV, 3-vessel trachea view; 3-VV, 3-vessel view.

---

detection of specific types of CHD has been repeatedly shown to improve neonatal outcomes.[6–10]

Most women have at least 1 ultrasound examination during pregnancy.[11] For most examiners performing transabdominal ultrasonography, 18 to 22 weeks of gestation is the optimal time for fetal anatomic assessment,[11,12] although others advocate earlier transvaginal scans.[13,14]

The American College of Obstetricians and Gynecologists,[11] the American Institute of Ultrasound in Medicine,[15] and the International Society of Ultrasound in Obstetrics and Gynecology[16] offer extensive recommendations and guidelines on prenatal screening for congenital heart defects. The minimal elements of a standard examination of the fetal heart include the 4-chamber view, left outflow tract, and right outflow tract. This article emphasizes practical aspects of these guidelines.

INITIAL ASSESSMENT

The basic assessment of the fetal heart should include confirming abdominal situs, situs of the heart, and the axis, size, and location of the heart within the fetal chest. It is crucial that fetal laterality is determined based on fetal position. There is a natural tendency to assign the situs based on the fetal heart and stomach being on the same site of the body, but one must be certain of which side is left and which is right (**Fig. 1**).

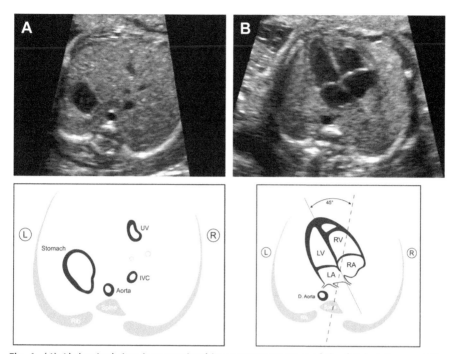

Fig. 1. (*A*) Abdominal situs is ascertained in a transverse view of the fetal abdomen. After determining fetal laterality from position of the fetus in utero, the stomach should be identified on the fetal left side with the descending aorta (D. Aorta) and inferior vena cava (IVC) to the left and right sides of the spine, respectively. A short segment of the umbilical vein (UV) is seen. (*B*) Cardiac position and axis: the heart is mainly on the left (L) side. The cardiac apex points to the left by 45 ± 20° in relation to the anteroposterior axis of the chest. LA, left atrium; LV, left ventricle; R, right; RA, right atrium; RV, right ventricle. (*From* International Society of Ultrasound in Obstetrics and Gynecology, Carvalho JS, Allan LD, et al. ISUOG practice guidelines (updated): sonographic screening examination of the fetal heart. Ultrasound Obstet Gynecol 2013;41(3):350; with permission.)

On a cross section of the fetal chest, the fetal heart is mostly located in the left hemithorax. If an imaginary line is drawn between the fetal spine and the sternum, only part of the right atrium (RA) is located to the right of this line.

The axis of the fetal interventricular septum creates an angle of 45 ± 20° with the anterior-posterior line (see **Fig. 1**).[17] Although it is not diagnostic, significant left axis deviation (>75°) is frequently associated with CHD, which are mostly conotruncal anomalies.[18,19] The fetal heart should occupy less than one-third of the fetal chest area in a cross-sectional view of the thorax at the level of 4-chamber view. Similarly, the circumference of the fetal heart should be no more than one-third of the circumference of the fetal chest. However, subjective assessment of the fetal heart is equally adequate. This assessment can easily be accomplished when the operator answers the question "Can I place 2 more hearts in this chest?" The fetal heart rate should be assessed. Rhythm abnormalities that are present can usually be noted during heart rate assessment.

General assessment of the fetal heart provides significant information. Abnormalities suspected or noted during general assessment of the heart should prompt careful evaluation of the fetal anatomy, as they are often associated with significant concurrent congenital anomalies (**Box 2**).

Box 2
Anomalies can be identified due to concerns during initial fetal heart assessment

1. Situs inversus
2. Abnormal location (shift of the heart with or without axis change)
   a. CDH
   b. Agenesis of fetal lung
   c. Congenital lung abnormalities
3. Axis deviation (extreme left or right axis deviation)
   a. CDH
   b. Outflow abnormalities
4. Cardiomegaly
5. Rate and rhythm
   a. Bradycardia
   b. Tachycardia
   c. Irregular rhythm

BASIC ASSESSMENT
Four-Chamber View

The 4-chamber view can be obtained in a cross section of the fetal chest directly superior to the diaphragm (**Fig. 2**) and can be obtained more than 95% of fetuses at 18 weeks.[20] Once the situs, axis, location, and size of the fetal heart are assessed, attention should be directed to the other details.

- First, the number of chambers should be noted. In a normal heart, there are 4 chambers: 2 atria and 2 ventricles.
- The left atrium (LA) is similar in size to RA. The LA can be identified via the flap of the foramen ovale, which should open into the LA. The posterior surface of the LA is irregular because of the entry of the pulmonary veins.
- The left ventricle (LV) is similar in size to the right ventricle (RV), although often there is a slight dominance of the right side, which has a slightly higher cardiac output than does the left.
- The morphologic RV is trabeculated compared with the smooth-looking endocardial surface of the LV, and the RV contains the moderator band, which is a distinct muscular band near the apex of the RV.
- The RV should be anterior to the LV.
- The basal portion of the interatrial septum (septum primum), upper portion of the interventricular septum, and atrioventricular (AV) valves form the cardiac crux.
- Two distinct and separate AV valves should be documented. It should be noted that the tricuspid valve is located anteriorly and slightly displaced apically.
- On the other hand, if there is no offset, an atrioventricular septal defect (AVSD) should be suspected (**Fig. 3**). If an AVSD is seen, there is a high risk of trisomy 21. Approximately one-third of fetuses with AVSD have trisomy 21. Conversely, 15% to 20% of newborns with Down syndrome have AVSDs.[21]

As part of the 4-chamber view the interventricular septum should be assessed. The interventricular septum can be assessed in 2 different planes, long axis and short axis.

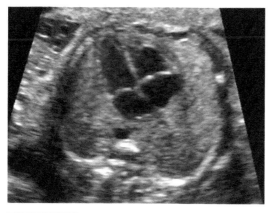

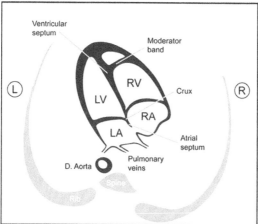

Fig. 2. Four-chamber view. The key elements of the normal mid-trimester 4-chamber view include heart area no more than one-third of chest area, right- and left-sided structures approximately equal (chamber size and wall thickness), a patent foramen ovale with its valve in the left atrium, an intact cardiac crux with normal offset of the 2 atrioventricular valves and intact ventricular septum. The morphologic right ventricle (RV) is identified by the presence of the moderator band and tricuspid valve, this valve inserting more apically in the septum than does the mitral valve (normal offset). D. Aorta, descending aorta; L, left; LA, left atrium; LV, left ventricle; R, right; RA, right atrium. (*From* International Society of Ultrasound in Obstetrics and Gynecology, Carvalho JS, Allan LD, et al. ISUOG practice guidelines (updated): sonographic screening examination of the fetal heart. Ultrasound Obstet Gynecol 2013;41(3):351; with permission.)

Most commonly the long-axis view of the septum is used for assessment. Large septal defects can be visualized with 2-dimensional gray-scale ultrasonography. However, small defects might only be seen with color Doppler assessment. While visualizing an apical 4-chamber view, there might be drop-out artifacts at the thin membranous portion of the septum, which might be mistaken for a ventricular septal defect (**Fig. 4**). If color Doppler is used to assess the interventricular septum, velocity scale and gain should be adjusted appropriately to avoid aliasing. Isolated, small interventricular septal defects are among the most difficult lesions to detect.[22]

Finally, the location of the descending aorta should be noted. Normally, the aorta is located to the left of the spinal column. If the aorta is seen more medially or on the right side of the spinal column, right-sided aortic arch should be suspected and

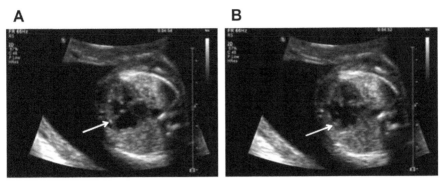

Fig. 3. Complete atrioventricular septal defect (CAVSD). Four-chamber heart visualized during systole (*A*) and diastole (*B*). This case is a known trisomy 21 fetus with CAVSD. In this case, there is a single common atrioventricular valve (*arrow*).

attention should be paid at visualization of the three-vessel view (3-VV) (see later discussion).

The 4-chamber view alone has a low sensitivity in detecting CHD.[23] Although early retrospective studies suggested a potential detection rate as high as 80% to 90%,[23,24] later prospective studies have shown lower detection rates. Overall when used as a screening tool in the general population, the 4-chamber view can be expected to detect 30% to 40% of cases of CHD.[22,24–26] However, it is not adequate for detecting all types of CHD, such as outflow ventricular septal defects, coarctation, tetralogy of Fallot, transposition of the great arteries, double outlet RV, and truncus arteriosus. Additional views of the fetal heart should be carefully evaluated for a more comprehensive assessment.

Defects expected to be associated with an abnormal 4-chamber view include hypoplasia of the RV or LV, AVSD, double-inlet ventricle, Ebstein anomaly, single ventricle, and large ventricular septal defects (**Box 3**). Screening with the 4-chamber view should also identify dextrocardia, situs inversus, ectopia cordis, cardiomyopathies, pericardial effusion, cardiac tumors, tricuspid or mitral atresia, and stenosis.

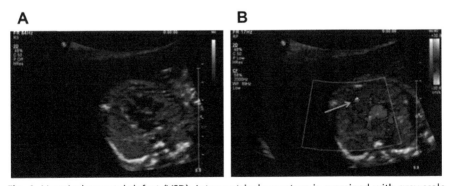

Fig. 4. Ventricular septal defect (VSD). Interventricular septum is examined with gray scale (*A*) and color Doppler (*B*) ultrasound. Although the interventricular septum appeared normal during gray-scale examination, color Doppler showed an isolated muscular VSD. Arrow points the turbulent blood flow across the VSD.

Box 3
Anomalies can be identified through basic cardiac examination

Four-chamber view

1. AVSD
2. Hypoplastic left heart syndrome
3. Mitral stenosis
4. Tricuspid atresia
5. Epstein anomaly
6. Hypertrophy
7. Pericardial effusion
8. Intracardiac masses

LVOT

1. Overriding aorta
2. Double outlet RV
3. Aortic valve stenosis
4. Transposition of great arteries
5. Truncus
6. Ventricular septal defect

RVOT

1. Pulmonary valve stenosis
2. Transposition of great arteries
3. Truncus arteriosus

3-VV

1. Vascular ring
2. Right-sided aortic arch

Hypoplastic ventricles and AVSDs are the defects most often detected prenatally by the 4-chamber view.[22,27,28]

Outflow Tracts (Left and Right Ventricular Outflow Tracts)

Many conotruncal abnormalities are missed if only a 4-chamber view is used for CHD screening, as only approximately 30% of conotruncal abnormalities are associated with an abnormal 4-chamber view.[29] Aortic and pulmonary outflow tracts, the left and right ventricular outflow tracts, respectively, are a standard part of the comprehensive cardiac evaluation and should be included in every ultrasound examination.[11,12]

The left ventricular outflow tract (LVOT) is evaluated in 5-chamber, long-axis view (**Fig. 5**). To obtain this, the long axis of the heart is placed as perpendicular as possible to the ultrasound beam and the ultrasound transducer is rotated at its central axis until the LVOT is visualized. Often a slight tilt of the transducer cephalad from a 4-chamber view accomplishes the same effect in terms of visualizing the LVOT. Continuity between the interventricular septum and the aortic valve and ascending aorta should

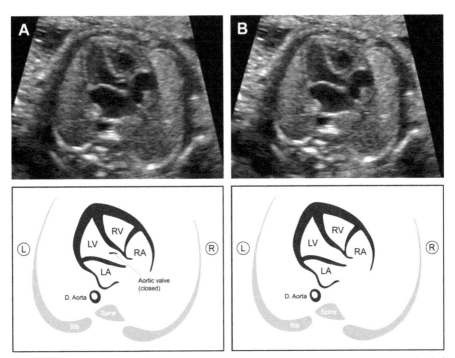

Fig. 5. Left ventricular outflow tract view. This view shows a vessel connected to the left ventricle (LV). It is important to demonstrate continuity between the interventricular septum and the anterior wall of this vessel, which in the normal heart corresponds to the aorta. The aortic valve should not be thickened and should be shown to open freely. The aortic valve is closed in (*A*) and open in (*B*). D. Aorta, descending aorta; L, left; LA, left atrium; R, right; RA, right atrium; RV, right ventricle. (*From* International Society of Ultrasound in Obstetrics and Gynecology, Carvalho JS, Allan LD, et al. ISUOG practice guidelines (updated): sonographic screening examination of the fetal heart. Ultrasound Obstet Gynecol 2013;41(3):354; with permission.)

be carefully sought, along with continuity between the anterior leaflet of the mitral valve and the posterior wall of the aorta. The aortic valve should move freely without thickening. If there is visible dilation of the ascending aorta immediately superior to the aortic valve, valvular stenosis should be suspected.

The right ventricular outflow tract (RVOT) is typically visualized in the short axis view of the heart; this can be achieved by tilting the ultrasound probe toward the fetal head from the 4-chamber view, slightly beyond the position used to see the LVOT. The main pulmonary artery, which originates from the RV and is anterior to the LVOT, should be documented. The pulmonary artery bifurcates, with the main pulmonary artery directed posteriorly toward the ductus arteriosus and the right pulmonary artery wrapping around the aortic root. The main pulmonary artery is slightly bigger in caliber than the aortic root. If a major difference in caliber is suspected, the patient should be referred for a fetal echocardiogram, as this could be a sign of aortic or pulmonary stenosis (**Fig. 6**).

While the outflow tracts are being evaluated it is crucial to document ventriculoarterial concordance; this means that the anterior chamber is the RV and the main artery originating from the RV is the pulmonary artery. Similarly, the posterior ventricle is confirmed as the LV and the main artery originating from the LV is the

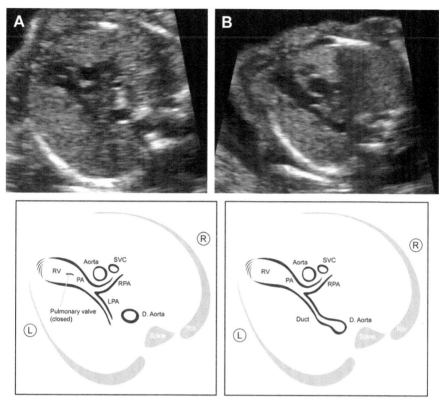

Fig. 6. Right ventricular outflow tract view. This view shows a vessel connected to the right ventricle (RV). In the normal heart this vessel crosses over the aorta, which helps in identifying it as the main pulmonary artery (PA). The pulmonary valve should not be thickened and should open freely. In (A), the bifurcation of the PA into both pulmonary branches can be seen. The pulmonary valve is closed. In (B), the plane of insonation is slightly more cephalad. The PA, right pulmonary artery (RPA), and arterial duct are seen. D. Aorta, descending aorta; L, left; LPA, left pulmonary artery; R, right; SVC, superior vena cava. (*From* International Society of Ultrasound in Obstetrics and Gynecology, Carvalho JS, Allan LD, et al. ISUOG practice guidelines (updated): sonographic screening examination of the fetal heart. Ultrasound Obstet Gynecol 2013;41(3):355; with permission.)

aorta. It is equally important to document, in real time, that 2 great arteries, pulmonary artery and aorta, cross each other and the pulmonary artery is located anteriorly.

The 3-Vessel View and 3-Vessel Trachea View

The 3-VV is a transverse view of the fetal upper mediastinum where normally the oblique section of the main pulmonary artery, the transverse aortic arch, and a cross section of the superior vena cava are arranged in a straight line (**Fig. 7**).[30] When the ultrasound transducer is angled further toward the fetal head, the 3-vessel trachea view (3-VTV) is obtained (**Fig. 8**). The normal 3-VTV view includes a V-shaped vascular confluence in which one arm is the ductus arteriosus and the other is the transverse aortic arch. In fetuses with vascular ring, this view is distorted, and it

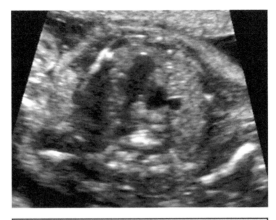

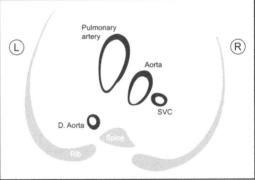

Fig. 7. Three-vessel view. This view best demonstrates the relationship between the pulmonary artery, aorta, and superior vena cava (SVC) in the upper mediastinum. The correct position and alignment of the 3 vessels as well as their relative size should be noted. The pulmonary artery, to the left, is the largest of the 3 and the most anterior, whereas the SVC is the smallest and most posterior. D. Aorta, descending aorta. (*From* International Society of Ultrasound in Obstetrics and Gynecology, Carvalho JS, Allan LD, et al. ISUOG practice guidelines (updated): sonographic screening examination of the fetal heart. Ultrasound Obstet Gynecol 2013;41(3):356; with permission.)

appears like a U, with the ductus arteriosus and aortic arch confluent behind the trachea (**Fig. 9**).

If a 3-VV or 3-VTV cannot be confidently obtained, then right-sided aortic arch, interrupted aortic arch, coarctation of the aorta, RVOT abnormalities, and pulmonary stenosis should be suspected.

FETAL ECHOCARDIOGRAM

Several researchers have suggested that one approach to improving detection of fetal cardiac anomalies lies in offering universal fetal echocardiography, with detection rates of 80% or more depending on gestational age.[31,32] However, universal fetal echocardiography is not practical and cost-effective at this time.[33] A fetal echocardiography examination may be necessary if an abnormality or suspected abnormality is found on the standard examination. Otherwise, fetal echocardiography should be offered to patients with appropriate indications (**Box 4**).[34,35]

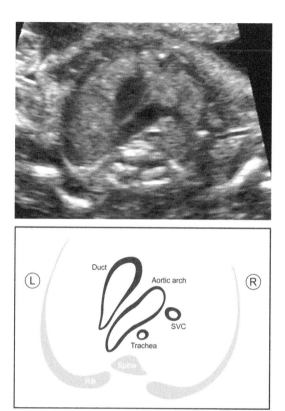

Fig. 8. Three-vessel and trachea view. This view best demonstrates the transverse aortic arch and its relationship with the trachea. In the normal heart, both the aortic arch and the ductal arch are located to the left of the trachea in a V-shaped configuration. L, left; R, right; SVC, superior vena cava. (*From* International Society of Ultrasound in Obstetrics and Gynecology, Carvalho JS, Allan LD, et al. ISUOG practice guidelines (updated): sonographic screening examination of the fetal heart. Ultrasound Obstet Gynecol 2013;41(3):356; with permission.)

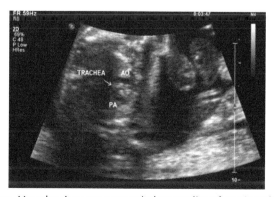

Fig. 9. Vascular ring. Vascular rings are congenital anomalies of aortic arch development. In this case aorta and abnormal vessel converge behind the trachea.

Box 4
Indications for fetal echocardiogram

Indications with higher risk profile (estimated >2% absolute risk)

Maternal pregestational diabetes mellitus

Diabetes mellitus diagnosed in the first trimester

Maternal phenylketonuria (uncontrolled)

Maternal autoantibodies (SSA/SSB+)

Maternal medications

ACE inhibitors

Retinoic acid

NSAIDs in third trimester

Maternal first-trimester rubella infection

Maternal infection with suspicion of fetal myocarditis

Assisted reproduction technology

CHD in first-degree relative of fetus (maternal, paternal, or sibling with CHD)

First- or second-degree relative with disorder with mendelian inheritance with CHD association

Fetal cardiac abnormality suspected on obstetric ultrasound examination

Fetal extracardiac abnormality suspected on obstetric ultrasound examination

Fetal karyotype abnormality

Fetal tachycardia or bradycardia or frequent or persistent irregular heart rhythm

Fetal increased NT greater than 95% ($\geq$3 mm)

Monochorionic twinning

Fetal hydrops or effusions

Indications with lower risk profile (estimated >1% but <2% absolute risk)

Maternal medications

Anticonvulsants

Lithium

Vitamin A

SSRIs (only paroxetine)

NSAIDs in first/second trimester

CHD in second-degree relative of fetus

Fetal abnormality of the umbilical cord or placenta

Fetal intra-abdominal venous anomaly

Not indicated ($\leq$1% risk)

Maternal gestational diabetes mellitus with HbA1c <6%

Maternal medications

SSRIs (other than paroxetine)

Vitamin K agonists warfarin (Coumadin), although fetal survey is recommended

Maternal infection other than rubella with seroconversion only

Isolated CHD in a relative other than first or second degree

Abbreviations: ACE, angiotensin-converting enzyme; HbA1c, hemoglobin A1c; NSAID, nonsteroidal anti-inflammatory drug; NT, nuchal translucency; SSRI, selective serotonin reuptake inhibitor.

From Donofrio MT, Moon-Grady AJ, Hornberger LK, et al. Diagnosis and treatment of fetal cardiac disease: a scientific statement from the American Heart Association. Circulation 2014;129(21):2183–242; with permission.

SUMMARY

CHD are among the most common congenital defects. Second-trimester ultrasound surveillance provides a unique opportunity for detection of CHD. Although prenatal ultrasonography is not a perfect tool, every effort should be made to examine the fetal heart in detail. Four-chamber, LVOT, and RVOT are standard views, which should be included in every prenatal ultrasound examination. The authors also propose that 3-VV should be included in standard fetal cardiac evaluation. A systematic approach to fetal heart examination (see **Box 1**), regular feedback, and implementation of training programs could improve detection rates and, in turn, neonatal outcome. There is no routine ultrasound examination. Every fetal heart should be accepted to be abnormal until otherwise proven. It is crucial to examine fetal heart meticulously, as early detection of major CHD is important for prenatal counseling, for determining appropriate prenatal care, and for possible therapeutic interventions. Finally, it has been repeatedly shown that prenatal detection of specific types of CHD improves neonatal outcomes.

REFERENCES

1. Ferencz C, Rubin JD, McCarter RJ, et al. Congenital heart disease: prevalence at live birth. The Baltimore-Washington Infant Study. Am J Epidemiol 1985; 121(1):31–6.
2. Hoffman JI. Congenital heart disease: incidence and inheritance. Pediatr Clin North Am 1990;37(1):25–43.
3. Crane JP, LeFevre ML, Winborn RC, et al. A randomized trial of prenatal ultrasonographic screening: impact on the detection, management, and outcome of anomalous fetuses. The RADIUS Study Group. Am J Obstet Gynecol 1994; 171(2):392–9.
4. DeVore GR, Medearis AL, Bear MB, et al. Fetal echocardiography: factors that influence imaging of the fetal heart during the second trimester of pregnancy. J Ultrasound Med 1993;12(11):659–63.
5. Hunter S, Heads A, Wyllie J, et al. Prenatal diagnosis of congenital heart disease in the northern region of England: benefits of a training programme for obstetric ultrasonographers. Heart 2000;84(3):294–8.
6. Bonnet D, Coltri A, Butera G, et al. Detection of transposition of the great arteries in fetuses reduces neonatal morbidity and mortality. Circulation 1999;99(7): 916–8.
7. Tworetzky W, McElhinney D, Reddy V, et al. Improved surgical outcome after fetal diagnosis of hypoplastic left heart syndrome. Circulation 2001;103(9): 1269–73.

8. Andrews R, Tulloh R, Sharland G, et al. Outcome of staged reconstructive surgery for hypoplastic left heart syndrome following antenatal diagnosis. Arch Dis Child 2001;85(6):474–7.

9. Franklin O, Burch M, Manning N, et al. Prenatal diagnosis of coarctation of the aorta improves survival and reduces morbidity. Heart 2002;87(1):67–9.

10. Copel J, Tan A, Kleinman C. Does a prenatal diagnosis of congenital heart disease alter short-term outcome? Ultrasound Obstet Gynecol 1997;10(4):237–41.

11. American College of Obstetricians and Gynecologists. ACOG Practice Bulletin No. 101: Ultrasonography in pregnancy. Obstet Gynecol 2009;113(2 Pt 1):451–61.

12. American Institute of Ultrasound in Medicine. AIUM practice guideline for the performance of an ultrasound examination for detection and assessment of developmental dysplasia of the hip. J Ultrasound Med 2013;32(7):1307–17.

13. Benacerraf B. Advancing further the sonographic estimation of Down syndrome risk–how early can we go? Ultrasound Obstet Gynecol 2008;31(2):129–31.

14. Timor-Tritsch IE, Fuchs KM, Monteagudo A, et al. Performing a fetal anatomy scan at the time of first-trimester screening. Obstet Gynecol 2009;113(2 Pt 1):402–7.

15. American Institute of Ultrasound in Medicine. AIUM practice guideline for the performance of obstetric ultrasound examinations. J Ultrasound Med 2013;32(6):1083–101.

16. International Society of Ultrasound in Obstetrics and Gynecology, Carvalho JS, Allan LD, et al. ISUOG Practice Guidelines (updated): sonographic screening examination of the fetal heart. Ultrasound Obstet Gynecol 2013;41(3):348–59.

17. Comstock CH. Normal fetal heart axis and position. Obstet Gynecol 1987;70(2):255–9.

18. Smith RS, Comstock CH, Kirk JS, et al. Ultrasonographic left cardiac axis deviation: a marker for fetal anomalies. Obstet Gynecol 1995;85(2):187–91.

19. Shipp TD, Bromley B, Hornberger LK, et al. Levorotation of the fetal cardiac axis: a clue for the presence of congenital heart disease. Obstet Gynecol 1995;85(1):97–102.

20. Tegnander E, Eik-Nes SH, Linker DT. Incorporating the four-chamber view of the fetal heart into the second-trimester routine fetal examination. Ultrasound Obstet Gynecol 1994;4(1):24–8.

21. Al-Hay AA, MacNeill SJ, Yacoub M, et al. Complete atrioventricular septal defect, Down syndrome, and surgical outcome: risk factors. Ann Thorac Surg 2003;75(2):412–21.

22. Kirk JS, Comstock CH, Lee W, et al. Sonographic screening to detect fetal cardiac anomalies: a 5-year experience with 111 abnormal cases. Obstet Gynecol 1997;89(2):227–32.

23. Copel J, Pilu G, Green J, et al. Fetal echocardiographic screening for congenital heart disease: the importance of the four-chamber view. Am J Obstet Gynecol 1987;157(3):648–55.

24. Allan LD, Crawford DC, Chita SK, et al. Prenatal screening for congenital heart disease. Br Med J (Clin Res Ed) 1986;292(6537):1717–9.

25. Todros T, Capuzzo E, Gaglioti P. Prenatal diagnosis of congenital anomalies. Images Paediatr Cardiol 2001;3(2):3–18.

26. Stoll C, Garne E, Clementi M, et al. Evaluation of prenatal diagnosis of associated congenital heart diseases by fetal ultrasonographic examination in Europe. Prenat Diagn 2001;21(4):243–52.

27. Allan LD, Sharland GK, Milburn A, et al. Prospective diagnosis of 1,006 consecutive cases of congenital heart disease in the fetus. J Am Coll Cardiol 1994;23(6): 1452–8.
28. Sharland GK, Allan LD. Screening for congenital heart disease prenatally. Results of a 2 1/2-year study in the South East Thames Region. Br J Obstet Gynaecol 1992;99(3):220–5.
29. Paladini D, Rustico M, Todros T, et al. Conotruncal anomalies in prenatal life. Ultrasound Obstet Gynecol 1996;8(4):241–6.
30. Yoo SJ, Lee YH, Kim ES, et al. Three-vessel view of the fetal upper mediastinum: an easy means of detecting abnormalities of the ventricular outflow tracts and great arteries during obstetric screening. Ultrasound Obstet Gynecol 1997; 9(3):173–82.
31. Acherman RJ, Evans WN, Luna CF, et al. Prenatal detection of congenital heart disease in southern Nevada: the need for universal fetal cardiac evaluation. J Ultrasound Med 2007;26(12):1715–9 [quiz: 1720–1].
32. Stumpflen I, Stumpflen A, Wimmer M, et al. Effect of detailed fetal echocardiography as part of routine prenatal ultrasonographic screening on detection of congenital heart disease. Lancet 1996;348(9031):854–7.
33. Bahtiyar MO, Copel JA. Improving detection of fetal cardiac anomalies: a fetal echocardiogram for every fetus? J Ultrasound Med 2007;26(12):1639–41.
34. Donofrio MT, Moon-Grady AJ, Hornberger LK, et al. Diagnosis and treatment of fetal cardiac disease: a scientific statement from the American Heart Association. Circulation 2014;129(21):2183–242.
35. American Institute of Ultrasound in Medicine. AIUM practice guideline for the performance of fetal echocardiography. J Ultrasound Med 2013;32(6):1067–82.

What You Need to Know When Managing Twins

10 Key Facts

Lynn L. Simpson, MSc, MD

KEYWORDS

- Twins • Chorionicity • Anomalies • Fetal echocardiography • Discordant growth
- Twin-twin transfusion syndrome • Twin delivery

KEY POINTS

- Accurate dating and determination of chorionicity is critical in the management of twin pregnancies.
- Structural anomalies, placental abnormalities, cervical shortening, and fetal growth disturbances are all more common in twins.
- Because of the unique complications related to monochorionicity, serial surveillance is recommended throughout gestation to optimize outcomes.

10 KEY FACTS

1. Twins Are Common

A twin pregnancy is no longer a novel occurrence. Twins now compromise more than 3% of all live births in the United States.[1] Advances in reproductive technologies have been the main driver of this increase, but practitioners need to maintain a high level of suspicion when certain clinical characteristics are detected. Before the routine use of ultrasound, more than half of twin gestations were undiagnosed until the intrapartum period.[2] In contemporary obstetrics, timely detection is expected by patients and provides the best opportunity to optimize care of these potentially complicated pregnancies (**Box 1**).

2. Establish Due Date Early

Correct dating is of paramount importance for the proper management of twin pregnancies. Correct dating is highlighted by recent reviews that recommend that uncomplicated dichorionic twins be delivered at 38 weeks, monochorionic twins at 36 weeks,

The author has nothing to disclose.
Department of Obstetrics and Gynecology, Columbia University Medical Center, 622 West 168th Street, PH-16, New York, NY 10032, USA
E-mail address: ls731@cumc.columbia.edu

Obstet Gynecol Clin N Am 42 (2015) 225–239
http://dx.doi.org/10.1016/j.ogc.2015.01.002
0889-8545/15/$ – see front matter © 2015 Elsevier Inc. All rights reserved.

Box 1
Clinical suspicion of twins

- Larger than expected uterine size
- Strong family history of fraternal twins
- Severe hyperemesis gravidarum
- Elevated serum β-HCG
- Use of assisted reproductive technologies

---

and monoamniotic twins at 34 weeks compared with 41 weeks for singletons.[3] For both twins and singletons, pregnancy dating is best performed in the first trimester using the crown-rump length (CRL) (**Box 2**).[4]

Accuracy of the CRL to predict the due date before 14 weeks is ±5 to 7 days.[5] In the second and third trimesters, multiple biometric measurements are used to calculate gestational age, but this approach is less precise. In patients that present late for care with uncertain menstrual dates, a repeat ultrasound in 3 to 4 weeks to assess interval growth can be useful to confirm the assigned due date. For twins conceived by means of in vitro fertilization (IVF), the due date should be calculated from the age of the embryo and date of transfer.[5] Regardless of how a pregnancy was conceived, dating can be ambiguous if there is a significant size discrepancy between the twins. In these cases, dating using the larger twin decreases the risk of overlooking early intrauterine fetal growth restriction (IUGR), but the smaller CRL has been shown to be more accurate in the estimation of gestational age in twins.[6,7] Serial evaluation of twin growth may help to clarify pregnancy dating when early ambiguity exists.

3. Chorionicity Is Critical

Chorionicity has a significant impact on obstetric management and risks for complications. Unlike dizygotic twins that are always dichorionic, monozygotic twins may be dichorionic or monochorionic depending on when the embryo split (**Table 1**). Correct assignment of chorionicity is close to 100% when carried out in the first trimester but decreases to 90% in the second trimester.[8,9] A recent study found that before 20 weeks, ultrasound incorrectly assigned chorionicity in 6.4% of twins overall with 4% of dichorionic twins and 19% of monochorionic twins misclassified.[10] Thus, chorionicity should be established at the time of the initial ultrasound, optimally in the first trimester.

Early in the first trimester, the number of gestational sacs equals the number of chorions, and a few weeks later, the visualization of 2 separate placentas can be used to establish dichorionicity. In twins with a single or fused placenta, characteristics of the intervening membrane can help distinguish between dichorionic and monochorionic placentation. Membrane thickness, number of layers, and the presence of either the λ or the T-sign can be evaluated by early ultrasound. In dichorionic twins, the

---

Box 2
Importance of accurate dating in twins

- Correct timing for screening and diagnostic testing
- Accurate interpretation of twin growth
- Appropriate initiation of antenatal testing
- Optimal scheduling of twin deliveries

Table 1
Types of placentation in monozygotic twins

Timing of Embryo Splitting in Monozygotic Twins (d)	Frequency (%)	Placentation
2–3	30	Dichorionic, diamniotic
3–8	70	Monochorionic, diamniotic
8–13	<1	Monochorionic, monoamniotic

separating membrane is thicker because it is composed of 2 amnions and 2 chorions, compared with only 2 layers of amnion in monochorionic twins. Although a membrane thickness of 2 mm has been suggested as a threshold to distinguish between dichorionic and monochorionic twins, it does not perform reliably as a single diagnostic test.[11] The λ sign, consisting of placental tissue observed between the layers of the intervening membrane at its base, is diagnostic of dichorionicity (**Fig. 1**).[12] The T-sign, which is composed of the 2 opposing amnions at the base of the separating membrane, is characteristic of monochorionic placentation (**Fig. 2**). Although gender

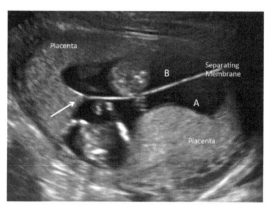

Fig. 1. Two placentas with twin peak sign (*arrow*) diagnostic of dichorionic placentation. A, twin A; B, twin B.

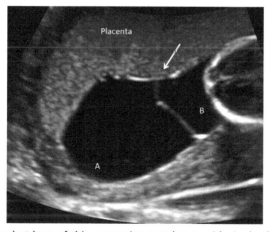

Fig. 2. T-sign (*arrow*) at base of thin separating membrane with single placenta diagnostic of monochorionic diamniotic placentation. A, twin A; B, twin B.

is not useful if both twins are the same, different phenotypic genders imply dichorionicity except in rare cases.

Establishing amnionicity is also important in monochorionic twins because monoamniotic twins have increased risks and are managed differently than diamniotic twins. The presence of a separating membrane ensures the presence of 2 amnions in both dichorionic and monochorionic gestations. In some cases, the intervening membrane in monochorionic twins can be extremely thin and difficult to visualize early in gestation, leading to an incorrect assignment of monoamnionicity. Transvaginal ultrasound and repeat imaging may be necessary to distinguish between twins with monochorionic diamniotic and monoamniotic placentation. The number of yolks sacs is not a reliable diagnostic criterion for amnionicity.

4. Trisomy 21 Screening Is Similar

As in singleton pregnancies, nuchal translucency (NT) is important for the assessment of risk for aneuploidy and anomalies in twins. The sensitivity of NT combined with maternal age for trisomy 21 is similar in twins and singletons, but the screen-positive rate is higher, particularly in monochorionic twins.[13] Even in the absence of trisomy 21, twins with monochorionic placentation have increased NT measurements compared with dichorionic twins.[14] These increased NT measurements may reflect the higher likelihood of structural abnormalities in identical twins as well as the potential for complications related to intertwin anastomoses within a shared placenta. The detection rate for Down syndrome in twins can be increased by combining maternal age and NT with serum levels of free β-human chorionic gonadotropin (β-HCG) and pregnancy-associated plasma protein A (PAPP-A), but chorionicity must be taken into consideration (**Table 2**).[15,16]

A cystic hygroma may be unexpectedly observed at the time of NT screening. Although an assortment of chromosomal and structural abnormalities have been associated with large NT and first-trimester cystic hygroma, both are risk factors for congenital cardiac anomalies.[17,18] Functional as well as structural heart disease occurs more frequently in monochorionic twins. An additional benefit of assessing the NT in twins with monochorionic placentation is that a 20% intertwin difference has more than a 30% risk of fetal death or the subsequent development of severe twin-twin transfusion syndrome (TTTS), thereby identifying cases that require increased scrutiny during follow-up surveillance.[19]

Maternal serum screening in the second trimester with the quadruple test may be used for patients presenting late for care as long as the presence of twins is taken into consideration when interpreting the results. Although cell-free fetal DNA testing is not yet endorsed by the American College of Obstetricians and Gynecologists for

Table 2 Performance of first-trimester risk assessment in twins		
Trisomy 21 Screening	Nuchal Translucency (%)	Combined with Free β-HCG and PAPP-A (%)
Monochorionic twins	73	84
Dichorionic twins	68	70
All twins	69	72
All singletons	73	85

Adapted from Cleary-Goldman J, Berkowitz RL. First trimester screening for down syndrome in multiple pregnancy. Semin Perinatol 2005;29:399; with permission.

multiple gestations, it is already being offered and used for trisomy 21 screening in patients with twins.[20]

5. Malformations Not Rare

The purpose of the second-trimester anatomic survey in twins is the same as for singletons: to provide reassurance that the fetuses are developing normally with no suspected structural anomalies. Patient preparation before ultrasound is essential because twins have a higher background risk for major malformations than the 2% reported in singletons.[21] Although the rate per fetus remains roughly the same in dizygotic twins, this amounts to an overall rate of 3% to 4% for the pregnancy. For patients with monochorionic twins, the frequency of congenital anomalies is nearly twice that in twins with dichorionic placentation.[22] Furthermore, in about 90% of twin pregnancies with a congenital anomaly, only one twin is affected, and when both twins have an anomaly, only 10% of dichorionic and 20% of monochorionic twins have the same structural defect.[21] As a result of these risks, a high level of suspicion for abnormalities is warranted when scanning twins.

In singleton pregnancies, only one-third to one-half of all congenital anomalies are diagnosed prenatally, and the detection rate is expected to be even lower in multiple gestations.[23] Certain malformations, such as those involving the central nervous system, are usually detected during routine ultrasound, whereas major heart defects are frequently missed in twins.[23] This finding is of clinical importance because congenital heart disease is more common in monochorionic twins, with a prevalence of 7.5%.[24] Although controversial, there are some data to suggest that twins conceived by IVF are also at increased risk for cardiac anomalies irrespective of chorionicity.[25,26] The cardiac screening examination, consisting of the 4-chamber view and views of the outflow tracts, detects about one-third of congenital heart defects prenatally.[27,28] Fetal echocardiography, when done in experienced centers, can detect close to 100% of major cardiac anomalies so twins at increased risk should undergo fetal echocardiographic evaluation.[29] Given the challenge of imaging multiple fetuses in variable positions in mid gestation, repeat ultrasound examinations may be necessary to complete the twin anatomic surveys and ensure the absence of major malformations. The management of discordant twin anomalies will depend on the gestational age at diagnosis, placentation, type of defect, and potential for associated pregnancy complications (**Box 3**).

6. Confirm Placental Location

The evaluation of each placenta is an important component of the ultrasound examination of multiple gestations. Placenta previa is 40% higher in twins, likely related to the larger placental mass.[30] Vasa previa is also more common due to velamentous cord insertions, found in 10% of twins compared with 1% of singletons.[31] A transvaginal ultrasound with color flow imaging can easily eliminate the presence of a placenta or fetal vessels overlying the cervix (**Fig. 3**). Given the high rate of perinatal

---

Box 3
Indications for fetal echocardiography specific to twins

- Spontaneous monochorionic twins

- All IVF conceived twins

- Complicated monochorionic twins (conjoined twins, TRAP syndrome, TTTS, TAPS)

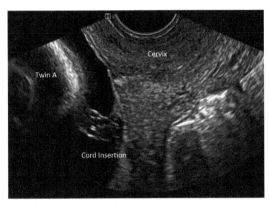

Fig. 3. Velamentous cord insertion of twin A near cervix.

mortality associated with undiagnosed vasa previa, routine transvaginal ultrasound with color is recommended in twins.

The placental cord insertion (PCI) of each twin should also be routinely evaluated with color flow imaging. In addition to diagnosing vasa previa, velamentous PCIs are more frequent in monochorionic diamniotic twins and are associated with an increased likelihood of TTTS, unequal placental sharing with discordant twin growth, and selective IUGR.[32,33] Furthermore, perinatal mortality is increased 3-fold in monochorionic twins found to have a velamentous PCI.[32] Routine PCI determination can help identify monochorionic diamniotic twins that warrant increased sonographic surveillance for TTTS and disturbances in twin growth.[34] The early detection of these conditions should trigger adjustments in management that may help to reduce the risk of perinatal death.

7. Check Cervical Length

Although universal screening is controversial, cervical length assessment is informative when caring for patients with preexisting risk factors for preterm delivery. Given more than one-half of all twins deliver before term, an awareness of cervical length tends to impact patient counseling and obstetric care.[35] The transvaginal approach is optimal for the determination of cervical length and the response to Valsalva or fundal pressure. In the second trimester, a cervical length of 20 to 25 mm or less is found in 5% to 10% of twins and increases the likelihood of a preterm birth 3-fold to 5-fold (**Table 3**).[36] The negative predictive value of a mid trimester cervical length of greater than 35 mm is more than 90%, which provides reassurance to patients with twins.[37] Although the optimal cervical length threshold and the frequency of follow-up cervical

Table 3 Prediction of preterm delivery in twins				
Cervix ≤20 mm at 20–24 wk	Sensitivity (%)	Specificity (%)	Positive LR	Negative LR
Preterm birth <28 wk	35	93	5.2	0.69
Preterm birth <32 wk	39	96	10.1	0.64
Preterm birth <34 wk	29	97	9.0	0.74

Abbreviation: LR, likelihood ratio.

Adapted from Conde-Agudelo A, Romero R, Hassan SS, et al. Transvaginal sonographic cervical length for the prediction of spontaneous preterm birth in twin pregnancies: a systematic review and metaanalysis. Am J Obstet Gynecol 2010;203:128.e1–12; with permission.

assessments are uncertain, a baseline measurement in the mid trimester and serial assessments at the time of subsequent growth studies in the second trimester and early third trimester can identify those at highest risk for spontaneous preterm birth.

8. Follow Twin Growth

The traditional approach to estimating fetal weight in singletons, using abdominal palpation and symphysis fundal height, is unreliable in twins. Because the assessment of fetal growth is of critical importance when managing twins, serial sonographic evaluation of fetal biometry is warranted.[38] Sequential growth scans can detect early growth restriction or discordance that might otherwise be missed and identify those cases that require increased fetal surveillance.

Singletons and twins tend to follow similar growth patterns until the third trimester, at which time twin growth begins to lag.[39] IUGR, defined as an estimated fetal weight of 10th percentile or less for gestational age, can be assigned using singleton or twin growth curves. A conservative approach for following twin growth is to use singleton curves so that cases of poor growth are not overlooked. Although there are different definitions of growth discordance, the most commonly used is a variance of 20% or more, calculated as the difference in the estimated fetal weights of the twins divided by the estimated fetal weight of the larger twin. An early sonographic clue of developing discordant growth is disparate abdominal circumferences (**Fig. 4**). An intertwin abdominal circumference difference of 20 mm or more or a ratio of less than 0.93 is predictive of discordant birth weights.[40] Both IUGR and twin discordance are associated with a higher likelihood of fetal and perinatal death compared with normally grown and concordant twins.[41,42] Following twin growth every 4 weeks is recommended for the early detection of growth abnormalities and timely initiation of antenatal fetal testing.[38]

Amniotic fluid abnormalities, such as oligohydramnios and polyhydramnios, may also be identified incidentally during routine growth studies. Although there are different methods to assess amniotic fluid volume in twins, a popular approach is to measure the maximal vertical pocket (MVP) in each sac. Using this method, oligohydramnios is defined as an MVP less than 2 cm, and polyhydramnios is defined as an MVP of greater than 8 cm.[12,34] As in singletons, cases of oligohydramnios and polyhydramnios require additional investigations to determine the underlying cause as well as ongoing antenatal testing to ensure twin well-being. TTTS should be considered when both conditions, or oligohydramnios-polyhydramnios sequence, are

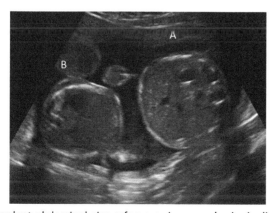

Fig. 4. Early discordant abdominal circumferences in monochorionic diamniotic twins. A, twin A; B, twin B.

detected in a monochorionic pair.[34] In the third trimester, twin presentation should also be determined during ultrasound to aid in delivery planning, particularly when growth abnormalities are present. As skills in breech delivery decline, planned cesarean delivery is increasing for all twin pregnancies to avoid combined vaginal-cesarean births.

9. Monochorionic Twins at Risk Until Birth

Although serial surveillance is justified in all twin pregnancies with anomalies, cervical shortening, fetal growth disturbances, and amniotic fluid abnormalities, monochorionic twins require extra scrutiny for several unique problems. Certain conditions associated with monochorionicity, such as monoamniotic twins, conjoined twins, and twin reversed arterial perfusion (TRAP) syndrome, tend to be recognized in the first trimester. In these rare cases, referral to a specialist with experience in complicated monochorionic twins is recommended for patient counseling and advice about subsequent care (**Box 4**).

Unequal placental sharing with discordant twin growth and/or selective intrauterine fetal growth restriction

Beyond the first trimester, seemingly uncomplicated monochorionic twins may yet face life-threatening situations because of the sharing of a single placenta. Although discordant twin growth and IUGR may complicate twins with dichorionic placentation, the cause and implications tend to differ in monochorionic twins. Discordant growth occurs in 15% to 25% of twins with monochorionic placentation.[43,44] When compared with monochorionic twins with concordant growth, velamentous PCIs and unequally shared placentas are more common in cases with growth abnormalities.[45] Selective IUGR in monochorionic twins has been classified into 3 clinical groups based on Doppler studies of the umbilical artery: type I has positive Doppler flow; type II has persistent absent or reversed end diastolic velocity flow; and type III has intermittent absent or reversed end diastolic flow.[44] Early disturbances in twin growth, particularly when associated with abnormal diastolic flow in the umbilical artery, have the poorest prognosis with a 15% to 20% risk of intrauterine fetal demise.[44] TTTS can coexist with unequal placental sharing, complicating the diagnosis and management of the pregnancy. Overall, the latency between the development of abnormal diastolic flow in the umbilical artery and fetal deterioration necessitating delivery tends to be longer in monochorionic twins compared with singletons with IUGR, but frequent surveillance is still warranted once fetal viability is reached.[46]

Twin-twin transfusion syndrome

TTTS affects about 10% of monozygotic twins and develops, in part, because of placental anastomoses that link the circulations of the twins.[34] In affected pregnancies, blood flow in these anastomoses is unbalanced with one twin, the donor, transferring a net volume to its co-twin, the recipient. Factors associated with the

---

Box 4
High-risk conditions associated with monochorionicity

- Unequal placental sharing with discordant twin growth or selective IUGR
- TTTS
- TAPS
- Single-twin demise

subsequent development of TTTS include velamentous PCIs and twin differences in NT and amniotic fluid volume.[34,47] The diagnosis of TTTS is made by ultrasound so serial sonographic surveillance of monochorionic twins is necessary to detect this condition in its earliest stages. Oligohydramnios-polyhydramnios sequence, the finding of low fluid in one sac and high fluid in the other sac, is essential for the diagnosis of TTTS (**Table 4**).[34,48] Doppler velocimetry of the middle cerebral arteries may demonstrate elevated peak systolic velocities in the donor twin, suggesting fetal anemia and reduced peak systolic velocities in the recipient twin, implying polycythemia consistent with coexisting twin anemia-polycythemia sequence (TAPS).[49] Both fetal echocardiography and fetal MRI are ancillary studies that may provide additional information about the impact of TTTS on the twins. Cardiac dysfunction, biventricular hypertrophy, and functional or structural right ventricular outflow obstruction may develop in the recipient twin over time.[34] Central nervous system abnormalities, such as hemorrhagic or ischemic changes, have been detected in cases of TTTS, which carries a less favorable prognosis.[50]

Given the risk of TTTS in monochorionic twins, serial sonographic surveillance is recommended every 2 weeks beginning in the second trimester.[34] Management options for TTTS vary depending on gestational age and stage at time of diagnosis. These options may include pregnancy termination, selective reduction of an anomalous, growth restricted, or hydropic co-twin, fetoscopic laser photocoagulation of intertwin placental anastomoses, amnioreduction, expectant observation, or delivery. Most cases of TTTS are detected in the second trimester, and, in advanced stages (II–IV), fetoscopic laser photocoagulation is currently considered the best treatment approach to improve perinatal survival.[34] This procedure tends to be used between 16 and 26 weeks' gestation and is performed in conjunction with an amnioreduction to normalize the fluid in the recipient's sac immediately after laser completion. The management of stage I TTTS is controversial because only 10% to 30% of cases progress, whereas most cases remain stable, resolve spontaneously, or do not recur after a single amnioreduction.[51,52]

Following laser therapy for advanced TTTS, serial sonographic surveillance is required to assess the twins' response to treatment. When successful, TTTS resolves with normalization of amniotic fluid volume in both sacs, visualization of the donor's bladder, and improvement in the recipient's twin cardiac function.[53] Umbilical artery Doppler studies may remain abnormal in the presence of coexisting unequal placental sharing with discordant twin growth and, in these cases, antenatal fetal testing should be incorporated into third-trimester management. Serial ultrasound evaluation for recurrent TTTS, reversed TTTS, TAPS, and unequal placental sharing is also recommended until delivery.[34]

Table 4
Sonographic staging of twin-twin transfusion syndrome

Quintero TTTS Stage	Features
I	MVP fluid <2 cm in the donor sac and >8 cm in the recipient sac
II	Nonvisualization of the fetal bladder in donor twin for >60 min
III	Absent or reversed umbilical artery diastolic flow, reversed ductus venosus a-wave flow, or pulsatile umbilical vein flow
IV	Fetal hydrops in 1 or both twins
V	Fetal demise in 1 or both twins

Data from Quintero RA, Morales WJ, Allen MH, et al. Staging of twin-twin transfusion syndrome. J Perinatol 1999;19:550–55.

The prognosis of TTTS depends on the gestational age at diagnosis, clinical stage, and progression of disease. Early-stage TTTS that presents beyond 26 weeks and does not progress tends to have a favorable outcome for both twins. However, most advanced TTTS presents in the second trimester, and the overall expected perinatal survival after laser therapy in these cases is 50% to 70%.[34] Without treatment, perinatal mortality is 70% to 100% in advanced stages of TTTS.[34,54] Of pregnancies treated with fetoscopic laser, both twins survive in 50% of cases; a single twin survives in 30% of cases, and there are no surviving twins in 20% of cases.[34] Although procedure-related twin loss is a recognized complication of fetoscopic laser photocoagulation, survival with neurologic handicap is a serious long-term sequela of TTTS, with or without treatment. Interventricular hemorrhage, cystic periventricular leukomalacia, and subsequent diagnosis of neurodevelopmental delay and cerebral palsy remain risks for survivors of TTTS. Overall, rates of long-term neurologic sequelae in laser-treated TTTS are 5% to 20%.[34] Additional risks related to preterm delivery and prematurity may impact the long-term outcomes for the surviving twins of these complicated monochorionic diamniotic pregnancies.

Twin anemia-polycythemia sequence

Spontaneous TAPS occurs in 5% of monochorionic diamniotic twins and is usually not diagnosed until after birth.[49] At delivery, one twin is pale and the other plethoric, and the twins are found to have discordant hemoglobins. Like TTTS, intertwin anastomoses in the monochorionic placenta result in a chronic imbalance of blood flow from donor to recipient; however, in TAPS the flow is presumably low and slow through small anastomoses so significant amniotic fluid abnormalities do not develop. Iatrogenic TAPS, observed in up to 10% of TTTS cases treated with fetoscopic laser photocoagulation, is more likely to be recognized before birth because of increased sonographic surveillance after laser.[49] Incomplete coagulation of all pathologic anastomoses, particularly small unidirectional connections, can result in the development of TAPS.[55]

Serial surveillance for iatrogenic TAPS should be routine after laser photocoagulation. Diagnosis is made by an elevated peak systolic velocity in the middle cerebral artery of greater than 1.5 MoM in one twin and less than 0.8 MoM in the other twin.[49] Screening for spontaneous TAPS in otherwise uncomplicated monochorionic twins is not routine but should be considered when minor variances in amniotic fluid are detected during serial ultrasounds. Without the utilization of Doppler velocimetry, this may be the only sonographic clue of TAPS in otherwise uncomplicated twins with monochorionic diamniotic placentation. TAPS and TTTS can coexist, but the oligohydramnios-polyhydramnios sequence will be absent in TAPS. The management of TAPS is controversial, but options may include termination, observation, repeat laser, fetal transfusion, or delivery depending on gestational age. The perinatal outcome of TAPS is also uncertain, ranging from double twin demise to newborn twins with no obvious long-term sequelae.[49] At the present time, prevention of iatrogenic TAPS is perhaps the best strategy to decrease the frequency of this condition and its adverse consequences.

Single-twin demise

Overall, it is expected that only 50% of spontaneous twin pregnancies identified in the first trimester will result in 2 live-born infants.[56] The finding of a vanishing twin early in gestation is associated with a favorable prognosis of the surviving twin, similar to that of a singleton pregnancy. However, unlike the death of a dichorionic twin, the death of one monochorionic twin has potential risks to the well-being of its co-twin, because of

Table 5	
Recommended delivery of twin pregnancies	
Twin Characteristics	**Recommended Timing of Delivery**
Dichorionic, diamniotic	38 wk
Dichorionic, diamniotic with IUGR	36–37 wk
Monochorionic, diamniotic	34–37 wk
Monochorionic, diamniotic with IUGR or oligohydramnios, abnormal Doppler studies	32–34 wk
Diamniotic with single fetal death	If ≥34 wk, consider delivery If <34 wk, individualize
Monoamniotic with single fetal death	Consider delivery, individualize
Monoamniotic	32–34 wk

Data from Spong CY, Mercer BM, D'Alton M, et al. Timing of indicated late-preterm and early-term birth. Obstet Gynecol 2011;118:323–33.

the shared placenta and intertwine anastomoses. Cases of neurologic injury and co-twin demise have been reported following the death of a monochorionic twin as early as 14 weeks' gestation.[57] Beyond the first trimester, intrauterine demise of one fetus occurs in about 5% of twin gestations.[58] Twins with structural malformations are more likely to die in utero than their anatomically normal co-twins. The smaller twin of a discordant twin pair or a twin with early-onset IUGR is also more likely to die before birth.[44] It is estimated that there is a 3-fold to 4-fold increase in intrauterine death in monochorionic twins compared with dichorionic twins.[59] Complications unique to monochorionic twins that contribute to a higher likelihood of single-twin demise include cord entanglement in monoamniotic twins, conjoined twins, TRAP, TTTS, unequal placental sharing, and TAPS. Intrauterine death of one monochorionic twin is associated with a 10% risk of double fetal demise and a 10% to 30% risk of neurologic injury in the surviving co-twin.[59] Immediate delivery of a monochorionic twin after demise of its co-twin does not eliminate the risk of neurologic handicap. Clinical management of these pregnancies depends on the gestational age and the detection of fetal or maternal complications.

10. Individualize Delivery of Twins

There are many different factors that influence the timing of twin deliveries. Active preterm labor, premature rupture of membranes, hemorrhage from placenta previa or abruption, as well as serious maternal conditions may require prompt preterm delivery. Once viability is reached and antenatal surveillance is initiated, expeditious delivery of twins is recommended regardless of gestational age if testing implies impending harm.[60] General guidelines have been developed to assist the clinician with the scheduling of both complicated and uncomplicated twins, allowing some latitude for individualization (**Table 5**).[60]

SUMMARY

Key points in managing twins, such as dating, determination of chorionicity, prenatal screening for chromosomal and structural abnormalities, and placental evaluation, should be standard practice. Cervical length measurements and fetal growth studies are recommended in twins, but the optimal timing and frequency of these assessments remain unclear. However, it is evident that monochorionic twins require serial surveillance for a multitude of potential complications that are unique to twins sharing a single placenta. Although favorable outcomes can be attained for most twins, these pregnancies should never be considered low risk.

REFERENCES

1. Martin JA, Hamilton BE, Osterman MJ. Three decades of twin births in the United States, 1980-2009. NCHS Data Brief 2012;80:1–8.
2. Kurtz GR, Keating WJ, Loftus JB. Twin pregnancy and delivery: analysis of 500 twin pregnancies. Obstet Gynecol 1995;6:370–8.
3. Lee YM. Delivery of twins. Semin Perinatol 2012;36:195–200.
4. Morin L, Lim K. Ultrasound in twin pregnancies. J Obstet Gynaecol Can 2011;33: 643–56.
5. American College of Obstetricians and Gynecologists. Committee Opinion, Number 611. Method for estimating due date. Obstet Gynecol 2014;124:863–6.
6. Chaudhuri K, Su LL, Wong PC, et al. Determination of gestational age in twin pregnancy: which fetal crown-rump length should be used? J Obstet Gynaecol Res 2013;39:761–5.
7. Salomon LJ, Cavicchioni O, Bernard JP, et al. Growth discrepancy in twins in the first trimester of pregnancy. Ultrasound Obstet Gynecol 2005;26:512–6.
8. Carroll SG, Soothill PW, Abdel-Fattah SA, et al. Prediction of chorionicity in twin pregnancies at 10-14 weeks gestation. BJOG 2002;109:182–6.
9. Lee YM, Cleary-Goldman J, Thanker HM, et al. Antenatal sonographic prediction of twin chorionicity. Am J Obstet Gynecol 2006;195:863–7.
10. Blumenfeld YJ, Momirova V, Rouse DJ, et al. Accuracy of sonographic chorionicity classification in twin gestations. J Ultrasound Med 2014;33:2187–92.
11. Bracero LA, Byrne DW. Ultrasound determination of chorionicity and perinatal outcome in twin pregnancies using dividing membrane thickness. Gynecol Obstet Invest 2003;55:50–7.
12. DeJesus Allison SO, Javitt MC, Glanc P, et al. ACR Appropriateness Criteria® Multiple gestations. Ultrasound Q 2012;28:149–55.
13. Sebire NJ, Snijders RJ, Hughes K, et al. Screening for trisomy 21 in twin pregnancies by maternal age and fetal translucency at 10-14 weeks of gestation. BJOG 1996;103:999–1003.
14. Cheng PJ, Huang SY, Shaw SW, et al. Difference in nuchal translucency between monozygotic and dizygotic spontaneously conceived twins. Prenat Diagn 2010; 30:247–50.
15. Madsen HN, Ball S, Wright D, et al. A reassessment of biochemical marker distributions in trisomy 21-affected and unaffected twin pregnancies in the first trimester. Ultrasound Obstet Gynecol 2011;37:38–47.
16. Cleary-Goldman J, Berkowitz RL. First trimester screening for Down syndrome in multiple pregnancy. Semin Perinatol 2005;29:395–400.
17. Simpson LL, Malone FD, Bianchi DW, et al. Nuchal translucency and the risk of congenital heart disease. Obstet Gynecol 2007;109:376–83.
18. Malone FD, Ball RH, Nyberg DA, et al. First-trimester septated cystic hygroma: prevalence, natural history, and pediatric outcome. Obstet Gynecol 2005;106: 288–94.
19. Kagan KO, Gazzoni A, Sepulveda-Gonzalez G, et al. Discordance in nuchal translucency thickness in the prediction of severe twin-to-twin transfusion syndrome. Ultrasound Obstet Gynecol 2007;29:527–32.

20. American College of Obstetricians and Gynecologists. Committee Opinion, Number 545. Noninvasive prenatal testing for fetal aneuploidy. Obstet Gynecol 2012; 120:1532–4.

21. Boyle B, McConkey R, Garne E, et al. Trends in the prevalence, risk and pregnancy outcome of multiple births with congenital anomaly: a registry-based study in 14 European countries 1984-2007. BJOG 2013;120:707–16.

22. Glinianaia SV, Rankin J, Wright C. Congenital anomalies in twins: a register-based study. Hum Reprod 2008;23:1306–11.

23. Zhang XH, Qiu LQ, Huang JP. Risk of birth defects increased in multiple births. Birth Defects Res A Clin Mol Teratol 2011;91:34–8.

24. Pettit KE, Merchant M, Machin GA, et al. Congenital heart defects in a large, unselected cohort of monochorionic twins. J Perinatol 2013;33:457–61.

25. Reefhuis J, Honein MA, Schieve LA, et al. Assisted reproductive technology and major structural birth defects in the United States. Hum Reprod 2009;24:360–6.

26. Bahtiyar MO, Campbell K, Dulay AT, et al. Is the rate of congenital heart defects detected by fetal echocardiography among pregnancies conceived by in vitro fertilization really increased? A case-historical control study. J Ultrasound Med 2010;29:917–22.

27. Acherman RJ, Evans WN, Luna CF, et al. Prenatal detection of congenital heart disease in southern Nevada: the need for universal fetal cardiac evaluation. J Ultrasound Med 2007;26:1715–9.

28. Friedberg MK, Silverman NH, Moon-Grady AJ, et al. Prenatal detection of congenital heart disease. J Pediatr 2009;155:26–31.

29. Fetal Echocardiography Task Force, American Institute of Ultrasound in Medicine Clinical Standards Committee, American College of Obstetricians and Gynecologists, et al. AIUM practice guideline for the performance of fetal echocardiography. J Ultrasound Med 2011;30:127–36.

30. Ananth CV, Demissie K, Smulian JC, et al. Placenta previa in singleton and twin births in the United States, 1989 through 1998: a comparison of risk factor profiles and associated conditions. Am J Obstet Gynecol 2003;188:275–81.

31. Gandhi M, Cleary-Goldman J, Ferrara L, et al. The association between vasa previa, multiple gestations, and assisted reproductive technology. Am J Perinatol 2008;25:587–9.

32. Hack KE, Nikkels PG, Koopman-Esseboom C, et al. Placental characteristics of monochorionic diamniotic twin pregnancies in relation to perinatal outcome. Placenta 2008;29:976–81.

33. De Paepe ME, Shapiro S, Young L, et al. Placental characteristics of selective birth weight discordance in diamniotic-monochorionic twin gestations. Placenta 2010;31:380–6.

34. Society for Maternal-Fetal Medicine, Simpson LL. Twin-twin transfusion syndrome. Am J Obstet Gynecol 2013;208:3–18.

35. To MS, Fonseca EB, Molina FS, et al. Maternal characteristics and cervical length in the prediction of spontaneous early preterm delivery in twins. Am J Obstet Gynecol 2006;194:1360–5.

36. Conde-Agudelo A, Romero R, Hassan SS, et al. Transvaginal sonographic cervical length for the prediction of spontaneous preterm birth in twin pregnancies: a systematic review and metaanalysis. Am J Obstet Gynecol 2010;203:128.e1–12.

37. Schwartz R, Prieto J. Shortened cervical length as a predictor of preterm delivery in twin gestations. J Reprod Med 2010;55:147–50.

38. Reddy UM, Abuhamad AZ, Levine D, et al. Fetal imaging: executive summary of a Joint Eunice Kennedy Shriver National Institute of Child Health and Human

Development, Society for Maternal-Fetal Medicine, American Institute of Ultrasound in Medicine, American College of Obstetricians and Gynecologists, American College of Radiology, Society for Pediatric Radiology, and Society of Radiologists in Ultrasound Fetal Imaging Workshop. Am J Obstet Gynecol 2014;210:387–97.

39. Papageorghiou AT, Bakoulas V, Sebire NJ, et al. Intrauterine growth in multiple pregnancies in relation to fetal number, chorionicity and gestational age. Ultrasound Obstet Gynecol 2008;32:890–3.

40. Klam SL, Rinfret D, Leduc L. Prediction of growth discordance in twins with the use of abdominal circumference ratios. Am J Obstet Gynecol 2005;192:247–51.

41. Odibo AO, McDonald RE, Stamilio DM, et al. Perinatal outcomes in growth-restricted twins compared with age-matched growth-restricted singletons. Am J Perinatol 2005;22:269–73.

42. Wen SW, Fung KF, Huang L, et al. Fetal and neonatal mortality among twin gestations in a Canadian population: the effect of intrapair birthweight discordance. Am J Perinatol 2005;22:279–86.

43. Gratacos E, Ortiz JU, Martinez JM. A systemic approach to the differential diagnosis and management of the complications of monochorionic twin pregnancies. Fetal Diagn Ther 2012;32:145–55.

44. Gratacos E, Lewi L, Munoz B, et al. A classification system for selective intrauterine growth restriction in monochorionic pregnancies according to umbilical artery Doppler flow in the smaller twin. Ultrasound Obstet Gynecol 2007;30:28–34.

45. Lopriore E, Pasman SA, Klumper FJ, et al. Placental characteristics in growth-discordant monochorionic twins: a matched case-control study. Placenta 2012;33:171–4.

46. Vanderheyden TM, Fichera A, Pasquini L, et al. Increased latency of absent end-diastolic flow in the umbilical artery of monochorionic twin fetuses. Ultrasound Obstet Gynecol 2005;26:44–9.

47. De Paepe ME, Shapiro S, Greco D, et al. Placental markers of twin-to-twin transfusion syndrome in diamniotic-monochorionic twins: a morphometric analysis of deep artery-to-vein anastomoses. Placenta 2010;31:269–76.

48. Quintero RA, Morales WJ, Allen MH, et al. Staging of twin-twin transfusion syndrome. J Perinatol 1999;19:550–5.

49. Slaghekke F, Kist WJ, Oepkes D, et al. Twin anemia-polycythemia sequence: diagnostic criteria, classification, perinatal management and outcome. Fetal Diagn Ther 2010;27:181–90.

50. Quarello E, Molho M, Ville Y. Incidence, mechanisms, and patterns of fetal cerebral lesions in twin-to-twin transfusion syndrome. J Matern Fetal Neonatal Med 2007;20:589–97.

51. Bebbington MW, Tiblad E, Huesler-Charles M, et al. Outcomes in a cohort of patients with stage I twin-to-twin transfusion syndrome. Ultrasound Obstet Gynecol 2010;36:48–51.

52. Rossi C, D'Addario V. Survival outcomes of twin-twin transfusion syndrome in stage I: a systemic review of the literature. Am J Perinatol 2013;30:5–10.

53. Van Mieghem T, Klaritsch P, Done E, et al. Assessment of fetal cardiac function before and after therapy for twin-to-twin transfusion syndrome. Am J Obstet Gynecol 2009;200:400.e1–7.

54. Berghella V, Kaufmann M. Natural history of twin-twin transfusion syndrome. J Reprod Med 2001;46:480–4.

55. Chmait RH, Assaf SA, Benirschke K. Residual vascular communications in twin-twin transfusion syndrome treated with sequential laser surgery: frequency and clinical implications. Placenta 2010;31:611–4.

56. Samuels P. Ultrasound in the management of the twin gestation. Clin Obstet Gynecol 1988;31:110–22.
57. Weiss JL, Cleary-Goldman J, Tanji K, et al. Multicystic encephalomalacia after first-trimester intrauterine fetal death in monochorionic twins. Am J Obstet Gynecol 2004;190:563–5.
58. Kilby MD, Govind A, O'Brien PM. Outcome of twin pregnancies complicated by a single intrauterine death: a comparison with viable twin pregnancies. Obstet Gynecol 1994;84:107–9.
59. Ong SS, Zamora J, Khan KS, et al. Prognosis for the co-twin following single-twin death: a systematic review. BJOG 2006;113:992–8.
60. Spong CY, Mercer BM, D'Alton M, et al. Timing of indicated late-preterm and early-term birth. Obstet Gynecol 2011;118:323–33.

Short Cervical Length Dilemma

 CrossMark

Anju Suhag, MD, Vincenzo Berghella, MD*

KEYWORDS

- Short cervix • Preterm birth • Progesterone • Cerclage • Pessary • Cervical length

KEY POINTS

- Preterm birth (PTB) is the leading cause of neonatal mortality and accounts for approximately 70% of neonatal deaths and 36% of infant deaths.
- Transvaginal ultrasound (TVU) cervical length (CL) screening is the gold standard CL screening for prediction of PTB.
- TVU CL should be done properly using The Cervical Length Education and Review (CLEAR) criteria.
- In singleton pregnancies without prior spontaneous preterm birth but with a short cervix less than or equal to 20 mm before 24 weeks, vaginal progesterone is indicated from the time of diagnosis to 36 weeks.
- In singleton pregnancies with prior spontaneous PTB, serial CL screening is indicated between 16 and 23 weeks 6 days, in addition to weekly 17-hydroxyprogesterone caproate (from 16–36 weeks). Should the cervix shorten to less than 25 mm, ultrasound-indicated cerclage is recommended.
- Routine CL screening is not yet recommended for twins because no intervention (eg, cerclage, progesterone) has been definitively proven to be beneficial in this population.
- In symptomatic women with preterm labor, TVU CL is recommended for management, and FFN for borderline CL 20 to 29 mm.

 Video of TVU CL screening accompanies this article at http://www.obgyn.theclinics.com/

INTRODUCTION: INDICATIONS FOR TRANSVAGINAL ULTRASOUND CERVICAL LENGTH SCREENING

Preterm birth (PTB) is the leading cause of neonatal mortality and the most common reason for antenatal hospitalization.[1,2] In the United States, 1 in 9 babies are born

The authors have nothing to disclose.
Division of Maternal-Fetal Medicine, Department of Obstetrics and Gynecology, Sidney Kimmel Medical College, Thomas Jefferson University, 833 Chestnut Street, First Floor, Philadelphia, PA 19107, USA
* Corresponding author.
E-mail address: vincenzo.berghella@jefferson.edu

Obstet Gynecol Clin N Am 42 (2015) 241–254
http://dx.doi.org/10.1016/j.ogc.2015.01.003
0889-8545/15/$ – see front matter © 2015 Elsevier Inc. All rights reserved.

prematurely. Worldwide, 15 million babies are born too soon each year, and more than 1 million of those infants die as a result of their early births.[3] PTBs account for approximately 70% of neonatal deaths and 36% of infant deaths, as well as 25% to 50% of cases of long-term neurologic impairment in children.[2,4–6] A 2006 report from the Institute of Medicine estimated the annual cost of PTB in the United States to be $26.2 billion or more than $51,000 per premature infant.[2,7]

Nearly half a million babies are born too soon in the United States each year, which ranked 131 out of 184 countries according to a May 2012 global report on premature birth issued by the March of Dimes[8] and several partners. With tremendous research efforts, the rate of PTB has decreased over decades. The rate of PTB in the United States peaked in 2006 at 12.8%. The US rate of PTB dropped to 11.4% in 2013. The ultimate goal of March of Dimes is a prematurity rate of 9.6% by 2020.[8] A March of Dimes report card is maintained for the national rate of PTB. It compares the rate of PTB in different states in the United States (available at: marchofdimes.org/reportcard). The goal of 9.6% was determined by using published research to estimate the maximum achievable benefits of applying known strategies to prevent PTB, including smoking cessation programs, progesterone treatments for medically eligible women, lowering the number of pregnancies from infertility treatments that result in multiples, and preventing medically unnecessary cesarean sections and inductions before 39 weeks of pregnancy. This goal also expects that more women will have insurance coverage in the future, and that continued research will yield new medical advances in the next decade. March of Dimes partners with various organizations, such as the US Department of Health and Human Services, the American Congress of Obstetricians and Gynecologists (ACOG), and the Society for Maternal-Fetal medicine (SMFM), for various campaigns, including "Healthy Babies are Worth the Wait," "Strong Start," and so forth.

HOW TO USE CERVICAL LENGTH SCREENING CLINICALLY

More than 2 decades ago, transvaginal ultrasound (TVU) began to be used to measure maternal cervical length (CL) during pregnancy and to predict the risk of PTB.[9–12] CL can be measured with any of these techniques: transvaginal, transabdominal, or translabial ultrasound. TVU is the gold standard for CL measurement. Transabdominal ultrasound (TAU) CL measurement is less sensitive in detection of short CL, noted to overestimate CL and underdiagnose short CL,[13] and has several limitations (eg, need for full bladder, cervix obscured by the fetal parts, lower quality image due to distance from abdominal probe to the cervix).[14] TVU CL screening has been shown to have superior cost-effectiveness compared with TAU, with TVU associated with better prevention of PTB.[14,15] All major guidelines that have described CL screening have clearly recommended TVU, including SMFM,[16] ACOG,[17] Royal College of Obstetrics and Gynecology,[18] and Society of Obstetricians and Gynecologists of Canada.[19] Given all this evidence, TAU should not be used for CL screening.

TVU CL is used at the authors' institution for CL screening. The recommendations for CL screening technique have been described by the Cervical Length Education and Review (CLEAR) program,[20] provided by the SMFM through its Perinatal Quality Foundation (available at: www.perinatalquality.org/clear). The CLEAR program provides an official education program on the CL screening technique, examination, and continuing image review to certify perinatologists, obstetric physicians, residents or fellows in training, and sonographers to accurately perform TVU CL screening. TVU CL screening should be performed clinically only after this program has been completed.

TVU CL screening is done after the patient empties her bladder (**Fig. 1**, Video 1). Then, a sterile transvaginal probe is inserted into the anterior vaginal fornix. Next, withdraw the probe until the image blurs to reduce compression from the transducer, then reapply just enough pressure to create the best image. The transvaginal of cervix should occupy 75% of the screen and the lower tip of the bladder area (empty) should also be visible. The anterior width of cervical thickness should be equal to the posterior cervical thickness and there should be no increased echogenicity in the cervix due to excessive pressure. Before measurement, the internal os, external os, and the entire endocervical canal should be identified. The calipers should be correctly placed to measure the distance from the internal os to the external os. Three measurements of CL are usually obtained. Then, mild fundal pressure is applied for about 15 seconds to watch for funneling or cervical shortening. It is advised to reduce probe pressure while fundal or suprapubic pressure is applied. The total time for TVU CL screening is approximately 5 minutes. TVU screening is a safe, acceptable, and reliable screening test, which is now widely used to screen women for their risk for PTB.[21] With proper technique, the intraobserver and interobserver variabilities are less than 10%.[22] Compared with abdominal and transperineal ultrasound, TVU for CL screening is more reliable.[14,21,23]

WHO AND WHEN TO SCREEN, AND WHAT TO DO IF TRANSVAGINAL ULTRASOUND CERVICAL LENGTH IS SHORT

TVU CL screening could be considered in the in following population categories[21]:

- Asymptomatic singleton pregnancies without prior PTB
- Asymptomatic singleton pregnancies with prior PTB
- Asymptomatic multiple pregnancies
- Symptomatic singleton pregnancies.

There are various population characteristics that can affect the performance of CL screening. These population characteristics include singleton versus multiple gestation, symptomatic versus asymptomatic women, intact membranes versus ruptured membranes, prior PTB versus no prior PTB, prior cervical surgery versus no prior cervical surgery, and many others.[21,24–33] For example, the sensitivity and positive predictive value of a short cervix is very different in women with or without prior PTB. In singletons without prior spontaneous PTB (sPTB), the sensitivity of short CL for subsequent PTB is approximately 35 to 45%,[24,25] and the positive predictive

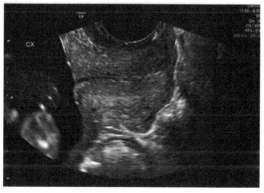

Fig. 1. CL 30 mm at 18 weeks gestational age by TVU CL screening.

value is approximately 20 to 30%, which means that most women with short CL will deliver at or greater than 35 weeks.[22,34] Sensitivity of TVU CL is also about 35% in twins.[27] The sensitivity for PTB of short CL in singletons with prior sPTB is much higher, about 70%.[26]

ASYMPTOMATIC SINGLETON PREGNANCIES WITHOUT PRIOR SPONTANEOUS PRETERM BIRTH (UNIVERSAL TRANSVAGINAL ULTRASOUND CERVICAL LENGTH SCREENING)

The role of universal TVU CL screening in the low-risk population of singletons without prior sPTB is still being debated (**Fig. 2**). In general, this population represents more than 90% of the pregnant population and is the group in which most PTBs occur. Currently, neither SMFM nor ACOG mandate universal TVU CL screening in every practice; however, both state it may be considered in this population.[16,17] If TVU CL is offered to these women, both SMFM and ACOG stress that TVU CL should be done properly. Quality should be enhanced with CLEAR criteria (www.perinatalquality.org/clear), strict guidelines followed (ie, the ones reviewed in this article), and scope creep offering interventions not based on evidence should be avoided.

The authors started universal TVU CL screening in January 2012 at our institution, Thomas Jefferson University. We never did TAU screening. Universal TVU CL screening required changes in our ultrasound appointment schedule, education of staff and patients, and completion of CLEAR certification by all full-time sonographers. We developed handouts for patients, making TVU CL an opt-out option. TVU CL at 18 to 23 weeks 6 days, the time when anatomy ultrasound is usually done, is our routine, which patients can opt out of. In 2012 and 2013, there was over 75% acceptance of TVU CL screening in low-risk women without prior PTB, with rates approaching 90% in 2014.[35] Women with prior term births, those with a language barrier (for us, mostly Chinese), and those with a male sonographer, were the 3 groups with the lowest acceptance rates.[35] The incidence of TVU CL 20 mm or less was about 1.1% in women with

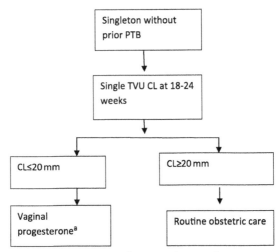

Fig. 2. Algorithm for asymptomatic singleton without prior spontaneous PTB. [a] Daily 200 mg suppository or 90 mg gel from time of diagnosis of short CL to 36 weeks. (*Adapted from* Society for Maternal-Fetal Medicine. Berghella V. Progesterone and preterm birth prevention: translating clinical trials data into clinical practice. Am J Obstet Gynecol 2012;206(5):377–8; with permission.)

singleton gestations without prior sPTB undergoing universal TVU CL screening between 18 and 23 weeks 6 days.[36] This is similar to rates near 1% found by other investigators.[37] The incidence of TVU CL less than 25 mm in this population of only singletons without prior sPTB at this early gestational age of about 20 weeks was only about 1.5%.[36]

SMFM and ACOG recommend that if TVU CL less than or equal to 20 mm is detected by TVU before 24 weeks, vaginal progesterone should be offered.[16,17] This is based on evidence from at least 2 randomized controlled trials (RCTs), which showed that vaginal progesterone decreased the incidence of PTB before 34 weeks in these women by about 45% compared with placebo[25,38] (**Table 1**) and improved neonatal outcomes.[25] This intervention has been found to be cost-effective and, in fact, saves costs up to $13 billion per year.[15,39] In women with prior term births, the incidence of CL less than or equal to 20 mm is slightly lower (0.8%) compared with nulliparous women (1.4%), therefore, universal screening may also be helpful in this population.[40]

Cerclage has not been shown to be of benefit in singleton pregnancies without sPTB. The lack of benefit of cerclage in these patients is supported by a meta-analysis of 4 randomized trials in which singleton pregnancies were screened with TVU CL and randomly assigned to cerclage or no cerclage if the cervix was less than 25 mm before 24 weeks.[41] Cerclage did not lead to a significant reduction in PTB less than 35 weeks (26% compared with 33%) compared to no cerclage (relative risk [RR] 0.76, 95% CI 0.52–1.15) if the patients had no risk factors for PTB.[41] Therefore, cervical cerclage is not currently recommended for women with singleton gestations without prior PTB but with short CL before 24 weeks. Given the 24% nonsignificant decrease in PTB associated with cerclage in this population, larger RCTs are needed to conclusively answer this important clinical question.

A pessary is a potential noninvasive intervention in a woman with a short cervix. A pessary seems to change the angle of the cervix in relation to the uterus, reduces both pressure on the cervix and contact between the fetal membranes and vaginal bacteria, and, therefore, can potentially decrease rate of PTB. In 2012, a multicenter trial randomly assigned 385 pregnant women with CL less than or equal to 25 mm at 20 to 23 weeks to use of a cervical pessary or no pessary.[42] Most of these patients (89%) had no history of PTB, and none were treated with progesterone or cerclage. The pessary group had a significantly lower rate of sPTB than the expectant management group (see **Table 1**). No adverse events were noted. A subsequent trial by Hui and colleagues[43] failed to confirm benefit of pessaries in this population (see **Table 1**). With current evidence, pessaries cannot yet be recommended in this or other populations for prevention of PTB. Several other RCTs are ongoing to assess efficacy of pessaries in prevention of PTB.

ASYMPTOMATIC SINGLETON PREGNANCIES WITH PRIOR SPONTANEOUS PRETERM BIRTH

Women with prior PTB, which usually represent about up to 10% of the pregnant population, are at risk for recurrent PTB (**Fig. 3**).[44] Some of these women may also have cervical insufficiency as suggested by painless cervical dilation leading to second trimester loss or PTB. These women should be screened with serial TVU CL about every 2 weeks, starting at 16 weeks, and ending before 24 weeks.[26] Some of these high-risk women, such as those with very early (eg, <24 weeks) prior PTB or second trimester loss, or those with large or multiple cone biopsies, could also start CL screening at 14 weeks or even earlier.[45] If women with prior PTB have TVU CL less than 25 mm, ultrasound indicated cerclage is indicated.

Table 1
Selected randomized controlled trials using transvaginal ultrasound cervical length screening

RCT	Study Population	Intervention	Primary Outcome	Results
Ultrasound-indicated Cerclage				
Althuisius et al,[46] 2001	Singleton with risk factors of PTB and prior PTB, 14–27 wk, CL<25 mm (N = 35)	Cerclage vs no cerclage	PTB <34 wk	0% vs 44% (P = .002)
Rust et al,[47] 2001	Singleton and multiple gestations, 16–24 wk, CL<25 mm or funneling >25% (N = 113)	Cerclage vs no cerclage	PTB <34 wk	35% vs 36% (P = .8)
To et al,[48] 2004	Singleton, 22–24 wk, CL≤15 mm (N = 243)	Cerclage vs no cerclage	PTB <33 wk	22% vs 26% (P = .44)
Berghella et al,[49] 2004	Singleton with risk factors of PTB and twins, 14–24 wk, CL<25 mm or funneling >25% (N = 61)	Cerclage vs no cerclage	PTB <35 wk	45% vs 47% (P = .91)
Owen et al,[50] 2009	Singleton with prior PTB, 16–23 wk, CL<25 mm (N = 302)	Cerclage vs no cerclage	PTB <35 wk	32% vs 42% (P = .09)
Vaginal Progesterone				
Fonseca et al,[38] 2007	Singleton and multiple gestations, 20–25 wk, CL≤15 mm (N = 250)	Vaginal progesterone vs placebo	PTB <34 wk	19% vs 34% (RR 0.56, 95% CI 0.36–0.86, P = .02)
Hassan et al,[25] 2011	Singleton, 19–23 wk, CL 10–20 mm (N = 458)	Vaginal progesterone vs placebo	PTB <33 wk	9% vs 16% (RR 0.55, 95% CI 0.33–0.92, P = .02)
Pessary				
Goya et al,[42] 2012	Singleton, 20–23 wk, CL≤25 mm (N = 385)	Pessary (arabin) vs no pessary	PTB <34 wk	6% vs 27% (odds ratio 0.18, 0.08–0.37, P<.0001)
Hui et al,[43] 2013	Singleton, 20–24 wk, CL<25 mm (N = 108)	Pessary (arabin) vs no pessary	PTB <34 wk	9% vs 6% (RR 1.04, 0.94–1.12, P = .46)

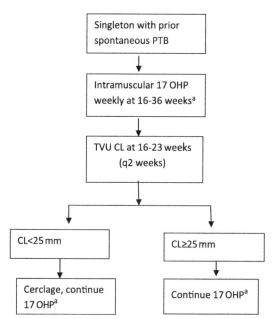

Fig. 3. Algorithm for asymptomatic singleton with prior PTB. 17OHP, 17-hydroxyprogesterone acetate. [a] 250 mg intramuscular from 16-20 weeks to 36 weeks; vaginal progesterone can be used in alternative. (*Adapted from* Society for Maternal-Fetal Medicine. Berghella V. Progesterone and preterm birth prevention: translating clinical trials data into clinical practice. Am J Obstet Gynecol 2012;206(5):380; with permission.)

There have been 5 published randomized trials to assess the efficacy of cervical cerclage in women with prior history of sPTB and short CL less than 25 mm (see **Table 1**).[46–50] Althuisius and colleagues[46] published a 2-tiered, randomized trial of 35 high-risk women who were thought to have cervical insufficiency based on obstetric risk factors. Study subjects were randomized to history-indicated cerclage (HIC) and CL surveillance. Women who developed short cervix were randomized to ultrasound-indicated cerclage (UIC) versus no cerclage. The outcomes were similar in those women who randomly underwent HIC versus UIC. Interestingly, none of the women with CL 25 mm or more experienced any PTB; however, the rate of PTB less than 34 weeks in women with a short cervix who received cerclage was 0% versus 44% in the no cerclage group ($P = .002$). Rust and colleagues[47] performed a randomized trial of 138 women with singleton pregnancies who had risk factors for PTB and who developed CL less than 25 mm or funneling more than 25%. They were randomized to cerclage versus no cerclage. The rate of PTB less than 34 weeks gestation in the cerclage group was 35% versus 36% in the no cerclage group ($P = .8$). To and colleagues[48] performed a randomized trial in women with short cervix less than 15 mm, and 253 women were randomized to cerclage versus no cerclage. The rate of PTB less than 33 weeks was 22% in women with cerclage versus 26% in women with no cerclage ($P = .44$). The study by Berghella and colleagues[49] randomized women at high risk for PTB with short cervix less than 25 mm or funneling more than 25% to cerclage versus no cerclage. The rate of PTB less than 35 weeks was similar (45% in cerclage and 47% in no cerclage group, $P = .91$). The fifth trial was a multicenter randomized trial by Owen and colleagues.[50] They screened women with prior PTB with TVU CL. Women with short cervix less than 25 mm were randomized to cerclage versus no cerclage. The rate of PTB less than 35 weeks was 32% in cerclage group and 42% in no cerclage group ($P = .09$). In planned analyses, the rates of PTB less than 37 weeks (45% in cerclage and 60% in no cerclage group, $P = .01$), PTB less than 24 weeks (6% in cerclage and 14% in the no cerclage group, $P = .03$), and perinatal mortality (9% in cerclage and 16% in no cerclage group, P = .046) were noted to be significantly less frequent in cerclage group.[50]

In 2011, a patient-level meta-analysis of these 5 trials[51] evaluated cerclage for women with previous sPTB, singleton gestations, and short CL less than 25 mm before 24 weeks of gestation. The meta-analysis showed a 30% reduction in recurrent PTB at less than 35 weeks of gestation (28.4% in cerclage and 41.3% in no cerclage group, RR 0.70, CI 0.55–0.89) and 36% decrease in composite perinatal mortality and morbidity[51] (15.6% in cerclage and 24.8% in no cerclage group, RR 0.64, CI 0.45–0.91). Previable PTB less than 24 weeks and perinatal mortality were also significantly decreased. The investigators estimated that 6500 newborns could be saved from perinatal death and 23,100 PTBs would be prevented by this management in the United States. In this clinical scenario, it would take approximately 20 cerclage procedures to prevent one perinatal death.[51]

ASYMPTOMATIC MULTIPLE GESTATIONS

For women with multiple gestations, the authors do not currently suggest TVU CL screening. Although multiple pregnancies are at high risk for PTB, CL measurement is not a sensitive screening test for prediction of PTB in this population. No intervention (eg, progesterone supplementation, cerclage, pessary) has been definitively proven beneficial in preventing PTB in women with multiple gestation and short CL in trials focused on this population.[52] Vaginal progesterone has been studied in a limited number of twin pregnancies with short CL and shows some benefit, deserving further study.[53] In twin gestations with short cervix, cerclage may increase the risk of PTB.[41] A pessary has been noted to decrease the rate of PTB less than 28 weeks and less than 32 weeks in twin pregnancies with TVU CL less than 38 mm before 23 weeks gestational age in one trial,[54] with further level 1 data needed to confirm these findings.

SYMPTOMATIC SINGLETON PREGNANCIES WITH PRETERM LABOR

Preterm labor (PTL) is traditionally defined as regular contractions and documented cervical change by manual examination between 20 and 36 weeks gestational age (**Fig. 4**). PTB is usually preceded by cervical changes at the internal os. Manual cervical examination has been historically the method of diagnosing PTL. Manual examination of cervix is subjective, not very reproducible, and is noted to have about 52% interobserver variability.[55] Compared with manual examination, TVU has been noted to be a better predictor of PTB.[22,56–59] About 75% of women with an asymptomatic short cervix on ultrasound have no appreciable changes by manual examination. TVU CL is the gold standard in assessment of cervix because it is safe, well accepted by women, most reproducible, and has low (<10%) interobserver and intraobserver variability.[22,23] It is important for clinicians to identify women who would benefit from interventions for PTL. Many pregnant women who complain of regular preterm contractions are actually not in true PTL. About 70% to 80% of women diagnosed with PTL do not deliver preterm, and more than half of these women will continue pregnancy until term.[60] The screening of women with symptomatic PTL should mostly be done using TVU CL and fetal fibronectin (FFN) testing.[61–64] With these screening tests, clinicians can identify women at high risk for PTB who might need corticosteroids, tocolytics, and transfer

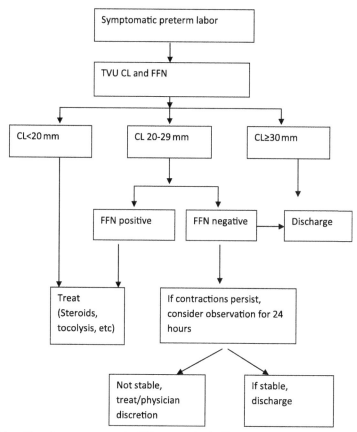

Fig. 4. Algorithm for symptomatic PTL. FFN, fetal fibronectin. (*Adapted from* Ness A, Visintine J, Ricci E, et al. Does knowledge of cervical length and fetal fibronectin affect management of women with threatened preterm labor? A randomized trial. Am J Obstet Gynecol 2007;197(4):426.e1–7; with permission.)

to a level III neonatal intensive care unit. On the other hand, a negative screening test would avoid expense associated with interventions.

FFN is a basement membrane protein that promotes cellular adhesion at uterine-placental and decidual-chorionic interfaces, and is released into cervicovaginal secretions when the extracellular matrix of the chorionic-decidual interface is disrupted in women with preterm contractions. FFN is normally present in the cervicovaginal discharge before 20 to 22 weeks and is always present in the amniotic fluid.[65] The knowledge of TVU CL[66] and FFN[67] is associated with decrease in rate of PTB. FFN testing should not routinely be used in asymptomatic women at low risk for PTB.[68] Cervicovaginal FFN test is most accurate in predicting sPTB within 7 to 10 days of testing among women with symptoms of threatened PTB before advanced cervical dilatation.[69] The accuracy of FFN testing is limited to within 7 days of symptomatic PTL, with a sensitivity and specificity of 76% (95% CI 69–82), and 82% (95% CI 79–85).[65,70] FFN testing alone is less than optimal in predicting PTB because of the low positive predictive value of less than 30%[65,71] and high false-positive rate. Due to the limitation of FFN alone, it is suggested that the women with preterm contractions be screened with TVU CL screening first and, if the cervix is borderline

(20–29 mm), FFN testing is suggested to improve screening of women who are at risk for PTB within 1 to 2 weeks of presentation.[62–64] Women with preterm contractions but TVU CL greater than 30 mm represent about 50% of women presenting with threatened PTL. These women have a less than 2% chance of delivering within 1 week and a greater than 95% chance of delivering equal to or greater than 35 weeks without therapy.[62] They should, therefore, be reassured and discharged without any interventions, and can be followed as outpatients with PTL precautions.

The authors suggest the following management of symptomatic PTL (see **Fig. 4**). This approach uses high sensitivity and negative predictive value of CL greater than 30 mm, and high positive predictive value of CL of less than or equal to 20 mm, and specificity of FFN.[59,63] In women with threatened PTL between 24 to 34 weeks with intact membrane and cervical dilation less than 3 cm, the authors suggest obtaining FFN testing, followed by TVU CL screening. Before obtaining an FFN sample, avoid bimanual examination, TVU, introduction of intravaginal lubricants or medications, and also avoid FFN testing in women with vaginal bleeding or sexual intercourse in the previous 24 hrs. An FFN is obtained using sterile speculum examination and a Dacron swab is used to obtain the sample from vaginal secretions in the posterior fornix. The FFN swab is held until TVU CL screening is completed. Women with TVU CL greater than 30 mm are much less likely to deliver preterm because CL greater than 30 mm has a close to 100% negative predictive value for PTB between 34 and 37 weeks. A TVU CL less than or equal to 20 mm has about 70% positive predictive value for PTB and these women are at high risk for PTB. In women with CL greater than 30 mm or less than 20 mm, FFN testing can be avoided. If FFN is positive in women with TVU CL between 20 and 29 mm, then treatment is suggested as in women with TVU CL less than or equal to 20 mm. If FFN is negative in women with CL 20 to 29 mm, management can be determined based on presence or absence of symptomatic preterm contractions, but usually no intervention is suggested.

SUMMARY: DISCUSSION

Short CL is no longer a dilemma. Several randomized trials have shown efficacy of interventions that reduce PTB when CL is short. In asymptomatic singletons without prior sPTB, TVU CL should be done at 18 to 23 weeks. In the 1% with CL less than or equal to 20 mm at that time, vaginal progesterone should be given (see **Fig. 2**). In asymptomatic singletons with prior sPTB, progesterone weekly and TVU CL every 2 weeks should be started at 16 weeks. If TVU CL shortens to less than 25 mm, which occurs in about 40% of these women, cerclage should be recommended (see **Fig. 3**). In twins, the authors do not yet recommend TVU CL screening; however, promising data on vaginal progesterone and pessary may soon change this recommendation. In symptomatic women with PTL, the authors recommend generally using TVU CL, and FFN as indicated, as per **Fig. 4**.

SUPPLEMENTARY DATA

Video related to this article can be found online at http://dx.doi.org/10.1016/j.ogc. 2015.01.003.

REFERENCES

1. Martin JA, Hamilton BE, Sutton PD, et al. Births: final data for 2008. Natl Vital Stat Rep 2010;59(1):1–72. Available at: http://www.cdc.gov/nchs/data/nvsr/nvsr59/ nvsr59_01.pdf. Accessed November 24, 2014.

2. Committee on Practice Bulletins—Obstetrics, The American College of Obstetricians and Gynecologists. ACOG practice bulletin Number 127, June 2012. Management of preterm labor. Obstet Gynecol 2012;119(6):1308–17.
3. March of Dimes May 2012 global report. Available at: http://www.marchofdimes.org/mission/the-global-problem-of-premature-birth.aspx. Accessed November 24, 2014.
4. Volpe JJ. Overview: perinatal and neonatal brain injury. Ment Retard Dev Disabil Res Rev 1997;3:1–2.
5. Mathews TJ, MacDorman MF. Infant mortality statistics from the 2006 period linked birth/infant death data set. Natl Vital Stat Rep 2010;58(17):1–31.
6. MacDorman MF, Callaghan WM, Mathews TJ, et al. Trends in preterm-related infant mortality by race and ethnicity: United States, 1999—2004. NCHS Health E-Stat. Hyattsville (MD): National Center for Health Statistics; 2007. Available at: http://www.cdc.gov/nchs/data/hestat/infantmort99-04/infantmort99-04.htm. Accessed November 24, 2014.
7. Institute of Medicine. Preterm birth: causes, consequences, and prevention. Washington, DC: National Academies Press; 2007.
8. March of Dimes report card. Available at: http://www.marchofdimes.org/mission/prematurity-reportcard.aspx. Accessed November 24, 2014.
9. Andersen HF, Nugent CE, Wanty SD, et al. Prediction of risk for preterm delivery by ultrasonographic measurement of cervical length. Am J Obstet Gynecol 1990;163:859–67.
10. Andersen HF. Transvaginal and transabdominal ultrasonography of the uterine cervix during pregnancy. J Clin Ultrasound 1991;19:77–83.
11. Smith CV, Anderson JC, Matamoros A, et al. Transvaginal sonography of cervical width and length during pregnancy. J Ultrasound Med 1992;11:465–7.
12. Parry S, Elovitz M. Pros and cons of maternal cervical length screening to identify women at risk of spontaneous preterm delivery. Clin Obstet Gynecol 2014;57(3):537–46.
13. Hernandez-Andrade E, Romero R, Ahn H, et al. Transabdominal evaluation of uterine cervical length during pregnancy fails to identify a substantial number of women with a short cervix. J Matern Fetal Neonatal Med 2012;25(9):1682–9.
14. Berghella V, Bega G. Ultrasound evaluation of the cervix. In: Callen PW, editor. Ultrasonography in obstetrics and gynecology. 5th edition. Philadelphia: Saunders Elsevier; 2008. p. 698–720.
15. Cahill AG, Odibo AO, Caughey AB, et al. Universal cervical length screening and treatment with vaginal progesterone to prevent preterm birth: a decision and economic analysis. Am J Obstet Gynecol 2010;202(6):548.e1–8.
16. Society for Maternal-Fetal Medicine Publications Committee, with assistance of Vincenzo Berghella. Progesterone and preterm birth prevention: translating clinical trials data into clinical practice. Am J Obstet Gynecol 2012;206(5):376–86.
17. Committee on Practice Bulletins—Obstetrics, The American College of Obstetricians and Gynecologists. Practice bulletin no. 130: prediction and prevention of preterm birth. Obstet Gynecol 2012;120(4):964–73.
18. Royal College of Obstetricians and Gynaecologists (RCOG). Cervical cerclage. London: Royal College of Obstetricians and Gynaecologists (RCOG); 2011. p. 21 (Green-top guideline; no. 60).
19. Lim K, Butt K, Crane JM. Ultrasonographic cervical length assessment in predicting preterm birth in singleton pregnancies. J Obstet Gynaecol Can 2011;33(5):486–99.
20. CLEAR guidelines. Available at: https://clear.perinatalquality.org/. Accessed November 24, 2014.

21. Berghella V. Transvaginal ultrasound assessment of the cervix and prediction of spontaneous preterm birth. Available at: www.uptodate.com. Accessed November 24, 2014.
22. Berghella V, Tolosa JE, Kuhlman KA, et al. Cervical ultrasonography compared to manual examination as a predictor of preterm delivery. Am J Obstet Gynecol 1997;177:723–30.
23. Mella MT, Berghella V. Prediction of preterm birth: cervical sonography. Semin Perinatol 2009;33(5):317–24.
24. Iams JD, Goldenberg RL, Meis PJ, et al. The length of the cervix and the risk of spontaneous premature delivery. National Institute of Child Health and Human Development Maternal Fetal Medicine Unit Network. N Engl J Med 1996;334:567.
25. Hassan SS, Romero R, Vidyadhari D, et al, PREGNANT Trial. Vaginal progesterone reduces the rate of preterm birth in women with a sonographic short cervix: a multicenter, randomized, double-blind, placebo-controlled trial. Ultrasound Obstet Gynecol 2011;38(1):18–31.
26. Owen J, Yost N, Berghella V, et al. Mid-trimester endovaginal sonography in women at high risk for spontaneous preterm birth. JAMA 2001;286:1340–8.
27. Goldenberg RL, Iams JD, Miodovnik M, et al. The preterm prediction study: risk factors in twin gestations. National Institute of Child Health and Human Development Maternal-Fetal Medicine Units Network. Am J Obstet Gynecol 1996;175:1047–53.
28. Vendittelli F, Mamelle N, Munoz F, et al. Transvaginal ultrasonography of the uterine cervix in hospitalized women with preterm labor. Int J Gynaecol Obstet 2001; 72:117–25.
29. Visintine J, Berghella V, Henning D, et al. Cervical length for prediction of preterm birth in women with multiple prior induced abortions. Ultrasound Obstet Gynecol 2008;31:198–200.
30. Airoldi J, Berghella V, Sehdev H, et al. Transvaginal ultrasonography of the cervix to predict preterm birth in women with uterine anomalies. Obstet Gynecol 2005; 106:553–6.
31. Berghella V, Pereira L, Gariepy A, et al. Prior cone biopsy: prediction of preterm birth by cervical ultrasound. Am J Obstet Gynecol 2004;191:1393–7.
32. Rafael TJ. Short cervical length. In: Berghella V, editor. Preterm birth: prevention and management. New York: Wiley-Blackwell; 2010. p. 130–48.
33. Guzman ER, Walters C, O'Reilly-Green C, et al. Use of cervical ultrasonography in prediction of spontaneous preterm birth in triplet gestations. Am J Obstet Gynecol 2000;183:1108–13.
34. Iams JD, Goldenberg RL, Mercer BM, et al. The preterm prediction study: can low-risk women destined for spontaneous preterm birth be identified? Am J Obstet Gynecol 2001;184:652–5.
35. Orzechowski KM, Nicholas SS, Baxter JK, et al. Implementation of a universal cervical length screening program for the prevention of preterm birth. Am J Perinatol 2014;31(12):1057–62.
36. Orzechowski KM, Boelig RC, Baxter JK, et al. A universal transvaginal cervical length screening program for preterm birth prevention. Obstet Gynecol 2014; 124(3):520–5.
37. Facco FL, Simhan HN. Short ultrasonographic cervical length in women with low-risk obstetric history. Obstet Gynecol 2013;122(4):858–62.
38. Fonseca EB, Celik E, Parra M, et al, Fetal Medicine Foundation Second Trimester Screening Group. Progesterone and the risk of preterm birth among women with a short cervix. N Engl J Med 2007;357(5):462–9.

39. Werner EF, Han CS, Pettker CM, et al. Universal cervical-length screening to prevent preterm birth: a cost-effectiveness analysis. Ultrasound Obstet Gynecol 2011;38:32–7.

40. Orzechowski KM, Boelig R, Nicholas SS, et al. Is universal cervical length screening indicated in women with prior term birth. Am J Obstet Gynecol 2015; 212(2):234.

41. Berghella V, Odibo AO, To MS, et al. Cerclage for short cervix on ultrasonography: meta-analysis of trials using individual patient-level data. Obstet Gynecol 2005;106(1):181–9.

42. Goya M, Pratcorona L, Merced C, et al, Pesario Cervical para Evitar Prematuridad (PECEP) Trial Group. Cervical pessary in pregnant women with a short cervix (PECEP): an open-label randomised controlled trial. Lancet 2012;379(9828):1800–6.

43. Hui SY, Chor CM, Lau TK, et al. Cerclage pessary for preventing preterm birth in women with a singleton pregnancy and a short cervix at 20 to 24 weeks: a randomized controlled trial. Am J Perinatol 2013;30(4):283–8.

44. Iams JD, Berghella V. Care for women with prior preterm birth. Am J Obstet Gynecol 2010;203(2):89–100.

45. Berghella V, Talucci M, Desai A. Does transvaginal sonographic measurement of cervical length before 14 weeks predict preterm delivery in high-risk pregnancies? Ultrasound Obstet Gynecol 2003;21:140–4.

46. Althuisius SM, Dekker GA, Hummel P, et al. Final results of the cervical incompetence prevention randomized cerclage trial (CIPRACT): therapeutic cerclage with bed rest versus bed rest alone. Am J Obstet Gynecol 2001;185:1106–12.

47. Rust OA, Atlas RO, Reed J, et al. Revisiting the short cervix detected by transvaginal ultrasound in the second trimester: why cerclage therapy may not help. Am J Obstet Gynecol 2001;185:1098–105.

48. To MS, Alfirevic Z, Heath VC, et al. Cervical cerclage for prevention of preterm delivery in women with short cervix: randomized controlled trial. Lancet 2004; 363:1849–53.

49. Berghella V, Odibo AO, Tolosa JE. Cerclage for prevention of preterm birth in women with a short cervix found on transvaginal ultrasound examination: a randomized trial. Am J Obstet Gynecol 2004;191:1311–7.

50. Owen J, Hankins G, Iams JD, et al. Multicenter randomized trial of cerclage for preterm birth prevention in high-risk women with shortened mid-trimester CL. Am J Obstet Gynecol 2009;201:375.e1–8.

51. Berghella V, Rafael T, Szychowski J, et al. Cerclage for short cervix on ultrasound in singleton gestations with prior preterm birth: meta-analysis of trials using individual patient-level data. Obstet Gynecol 2011;117:663–71.

52. Roman AS, Rebarber A, Pereira L, et al. Efficacy of ultrasound indicated cerclage in multiple gestations. J Ultrasound Med 2005;24:763–8.

53. Romero R, Nicolaides K, Conde-Agudelo A, et al. Vaginal progesterone in women with an asymptomatic sonographic short cervix in the midtrimester decreases preterm delivery and neonatal morbidity: a systematic review and metaanlysis of individual patient data. Am J Obstet Gynecol 2012;206(2):124.e1–19.

54. Liem S, Schuit E, Hegeman M, et al. Cervical pessaries for prevention of preterm birth in women with a multiple pregnancy (ProTWIN): a multicentre, open-label randomised controlled trial. Lancet 2013;382(9901):1341–9.

55. Phelps YJ, Higby K, Smyth MH, et al. Accuracy and intraobserver variability of simulated cervical dilatation measurements. Am J Obstet Gynecol 1995;173:942–5.

56. Gomez R, Galasso M, Romero R, et al. Ultrasonographic examination of the uterine cervix is better than cervical digital examination as a predictor of the

likelihood of premature delivery in patients with preterm labor and intact membranes. Am J Obstet Gynecol 1994;171:956–64.

57. Okitsu O, Miruma T, Nakayama T, et al. Early prediction of preterm delivery by transvaginal ultrasonography. Ultrasound Obstet Gynecol 1992;2:402–9.

58. Crane JM, Van Den Hof M, Armson BA, et al. Transvaginal ultrasound in the prediction of preterm delivery: singleton and twin gestations. Obstet Gynecol 1997;90:357–63.

59. Berghella V, Ness A, Bega G, et al. Cervical sonography in women with symptoms of preterm labor. Obstet Gynecol Clin North Am 2005;32(3):383–96.

60. Guinn DA, Goepfert AR, Owen J, et al. Management options in women with preterm uterine contractions: a randomized clinical trial. Am J Obstet Gynecol 1997;177:814–8.

61. DeFranco EA, Lewis DF, Odibo AO. Improving the screening accuracy for preterm labor: is the combination of fetal fibronectin and cervical length in symptomatic patients a useful predictor of preterm birth? A systematic review. Am J Obstet Gynecol 2013;208(3):233.e1–6.

62. Gomez R, Romero R, Medina L, et al. Cervicovaginal fibronectin improves the prediction of preterm delivery based on sonographic cervical length in patients with preterm uterine contractions and intact membranes. Am J Obstet Gynecol 2005;192:350–9.

63. Ness A, Visintine J, Ricci E, et al. Does knowledge of cervical length and fetal fibronectin affect management of women with threatened preterm labor? A randomized trial. Am J Obstet Gynecol 2007;197(4):426.e1–7.

64. van Baaren GJ, Vis JY, Wilms FF, et al. Predictive value of cervical length measurement and fibronectin testing in threatened preterm labor. Obstet Gynecol 2014;123(6):1185–92.

65. Lockwood CJ. Fetal fibronectin for prediction of preterm labor and delivery. Available at: www.uptodate.com. Accessed November 24, 2014.

66. Berghella V, Baxter JK, Hendrix NW. Cervical assessment by ultrasound for preventing preterm delivery. Cochrane Database Syst Rev 2009;(3): CD007235.

67. Berghella V, Hayes E, Visintine J, et al. Fetal fibronectin testing for reducing the risk of preterm birth. Cochrane Database Syst Rev 2008;(4):CD006843.

68. American College of Obstetricians and Gynecologists. ACOG Practice Bulletin. Assessment of risk factors for preterm birth. Clinical management guidelines for obstetrician-gynecologists. Number 31, October 2001. (Replaces Technical Bulletin number 206, June 1995; Committee Opinion number 172, May 1996; Committee Opinion number 187, September 1997; Committee Opinion number 198, February 1998; and Committee Opinion number 251, January 2001). Obstet Gynecol 2001;98:709–16.

69. Honest H, Bachmann LM, Gupta JK, et al. Accuracy of cervicovaginal fetal fibronectin test in predicting risk of spontaneous preterm birth: systematic review. BMJ 2002;325:301–11.

70. Sanchez-Ramos L, Delke I, Zamora J, et al. Fetal fibronectin as a short-term predictor of preterm birth in symptomatic patients: a meta-analysis. Obstet Gynecol 2009;114(3):631–40.

71. Lockwood CJ. Predicting premature delivery—no easy task. N Engl J Med 2002; 346(4):282–4.

Preterm Labor

Approach to Decreasing Complications of Prematurity

Anna Locatelli, MD[a], Sara Consonni, MD[a],
Alessandro Ghidini, MD[b],*

KEYWORDS

- Prematurity • Tocolysis • Antibiotics • Corticosteroids • In utero transfer
- Magnesium sulfate • Mode of delivery • Delayed cord clamping

KEY POINTS

- Implementation of certain obstetric practices in women in preterm labor can significantly improve the prognosis for the premature neonate.
- Tocolytic agents can delay preterm birth for at least 2 days, thus allowing the administration of antenatal corticosteroid and in utero transfer to appropriate neonatal health care settings; these two interventions reduce perinatal mortality.
- Antepartum administration of magnesium sulfate in preterm delivery reduces the risk of cerebral palsy.
- In preterm birth, cesarean delivery offers survival advantage in nonvertex presentation.
- In preterm infants, delayed cord clamping is associated with a reduced risk of blood transfusion, intraventricular hemorrhage, necrotizing enterocolitis, and mortality (<32 weeks).

INTRODUCTION

The rate of mortality and sequelae in preterm neonates has been decreasing over the years worldwide. In great part, this is caused by improvements in neonatal care. However, the obstetricians also play a relevant role, as implementation of certain procedures in women in preterm labor (PTL) can significantly affect the prognosis for the premature neonate. The authors review the best-evaluated practices and, whenever possible, assess them in terms of effect on clinically relevant outcomes (eg, neonatal mortality or morbidity) rather than surrogate outcomes (eg, pregnancy prolongation).

The authors have nothing to disclose.
[a] Department Obstetrics and Gynecology, University of Milano-Bicocca, Carate-Giussano, Milano-Bicocca 20841, Italy; [b] Inova Alexandria Hospital, Alexandria, VA 22304, USA
* Corresponding author. Antenatal Testing Center, 4320 Seminary Road, Alexandria, VA 22304.
E-mail address: Alessandro.Ghidini@Inova.org

TOCOLYTICS

The pathophysiology leading to PTL is multifactorial, with initiating factors including intrauterine infection, inflammation, ischemia, uterine overdistension, and hemorrhage. Contractions are not the starting point of most preterm births, as they are usually preceded by cervical ripening and decidual activation; this is important to understand why therapy for PTL targeting only contractions has been modestly effective and it has not been shown to reduce the incidence of preterm birth.[1]

The methodology of many randomized clinical trials (RCTs) on tocolytics is limited by the lack of sufficient numbers of patients enrolled and lack of comparison with a placebo. Such limitations in the individual studies make it difficult to evaluate the efficacy of classes of tocolytics using meta-analysis.

The current evidence suggests that tocolytic agents can delay preterm birth for at least 2 days, thus allowing the administration of antenatal corticosteroid (ACS) and in utero transfer to appropriate neonatal health care settings. There is no convincing evidence that tocolytic agents improve substantive perinatal outcomes (such as rates of perinatal death or neonatal morbidities associated with prematurity, like respiratory distress syndrome or intraventricular hemorrhage) or provide long-term benefits compared with no tocolytic therapy.

Several tocolytic agents can inhibit uterine contractility (**Table 1**).[2–7] The decision as to which tocolytic agent should be used as first-line therapy for an individual patient should be based on multiple factors, including efficacy, gestational age, presence of maternal comorbidities, and the frequency and severity of side effects.

Betamimetics, Cox inhibitors, and calcium channel blockers seem beneficial in delaying birth for more than 48 hours when compared with no tocolytic treatment, whereas for other tocolytics there is no evidence of benefit for pregnancy prolongation. Most tocolytics are associated with side effects that often depend on their class and mechanism of action. Such side effects can be very frequent and serious, such as with betamimetics, but they can be considerable also for calcium channel blockers, oxytocin receptor antagonists, and nitric oxide donors. The Food and Drug Administration has issued a warning against prolonged maintenance tocolysis (beyond 48–72 hours) for betamimetics.

Some trials have compared different types of tocolytics among themselves. **Table 2** displays the results of the meta-analyses of such trials.[3–7]

Type of Tocolytic

The best tocolytic should maximize safety and efficacy. Calcium channel blockers, oxytocin receptor antagonists, and Cox inhibitors are all associated with fewer maternal side effects compared with betamimetics and magnesium sulfate, which have significantly higher rates of side effects requiring a change of medication. Moreover magnesium sulfate administered for longer than 5 to 7 days can lead to fetal and neonatal bone demineralization and fractures; thus only short-term (usually <48 hours) use of magnesium sulfate is advocated in obstetric care.[8]

In terms of pregnancy prolongation for at least 48 hours, it is highest with prostaglandin inhibitors compared with placebo (odds ratio [OR] 5.39), followed by calcium channel blockers (OR 2.71) and the oxytocin receptor blocker atosiban (OR 2.02).[9]

In terms of reduction of neonatal morbidity, particularly respiratory distress syndrome, no class of tocolytic has been significantly superior to placebo, with the limitation that larger studies were conducted at a time when steroids were not routinely administered to patients.

Cox inhibitors and calcium channel blockers may, thus, be the best tocolytics in terms of pregnancy prolongation, improvement of neonatal outcome, and risk of

Table 1
Tocolytic drug versus placebo or no treatment

Drug	Patients	Pregnancy Outcomes	Adverse Drug Reactions	Neonatal Outcomes	Source
Betamimetics vs placebo or no treatment	1367	Reduced risk of birth <48 h (RR 0.68) No reduced risk of delivery <37 wk	Palpitation, chest pain, headache, hyperglycemia, hypokalemia, dyspnea, nausea or vomiting, tremor, nasal stuffiness, cessation of treatment	No benefit	Neilson et al,[2] 2014
Calcium channel blocker vs placebo or no treatment	173	Reduced risk of birth <48 h (RR 0.30) No reduced risk of delivery <37 wk	Flushing, headache, and vertigo	Not reported	Flenady et al,[3] 2014
Cox inhibitors vs placebo or no treatment	36	Reduced risk of delivery <37 wk (RR 0.21)	Could not be adequately assessed because of insufficient data	No benefit	King et al,[4] 2005
Magnesium sulfate vs placebo or no treatment	449	No differences for birth <48 h	No significant differences for maternal adverse events severe enough to stop treatment	Borderline increased risk of perinatal death (RR 4.56, 95% CI 1.00–20.9)	Crowther et al,[5] 2014
Oxytocin receptor antagonists vs placebo or no treatment	854	No reduced delivery <48 h	Increased side effects requiring cessation of treatment (RR 4.02)	No benefit	Flenady et al,[6] 2014
Nitric oxide donors vs placebo or no treatment	336	No reduced delivery <48 h	Increased adverse reactions (RR 1.49) and headache (RR 1.95)	No benefit	Duckitt et al,[7] 2014

Abbreviations: CI, confidence interval; RR, relative risk.
Data from Refs.[2–7]

Table 2
Comparisons among classes of tocolytics

Drug	Patients	Pregnancy Prolongation	Adverse Drug Reactions	Neonatal Outcomes	Source
Calcium channel blockers vs betamimetics	1926	Reduced birth <34 wk in the calcium channel blockers group (RR 0.78) Reduced birth <37 wk (RR 0.89)	Lower risk of discontinued treatment caused by side effects (RR 0.22) and adverse reactions in general (RR 0.36) in the calcium channel blockers group	No differences for perinatal mortality Reduced RDS, necrotizing enterocolitis, and IVH in the calcium channel blockers group	Flenady et al,[3] 2014
Calcium channel blockers vs oxytocin receptor antagonists	226	No differences for preterm birth <28 or <34 wk or birth within 48 h Women receiving atosiban had increased rates of preterm birth <37 wk (RR 1.56)	No difference in discontinuation of therapy because of side effects	No differences for perinatal mortality, serious infant morbidity, or NICU admission	Flenady et al,[3] 2014
Calcium channel blockers vs magnesium sulfate	943	No differences in preterm birth <34 or 37 wk or birth within 48 h	Maternal side effects less frequent for calcium channel blockers	No differences for perinatal mortality or infant morbidity	Flenady et al,[3] 2014
Calcium blockers vs Cox inhibitors	301	Reduced birth within 48 h in calcium blockers (RR 0.42)	No differences in maternal adverse drug reactions	No differences for mortality or serious infant morbidity	Flenady et al,[3] 2014
Oxytocin receptor antagonists vs betamimetics	1402	No differences for birth <28 wk, birth within 48 h	Atosiban: fewer adverse drug reactions requiring cessation of treatment	No differences for mortality or serious infant morbidity	Flenady et al,[6] 2014

Cox inhibitors vs any other tocolytic	168	Reduced birth <37 wk (RR 0.53)	Cox inhibitors: less risk of adverse effects leading to treatment cessation or any adverse drug reaction	No differences in infant mortality and morbidity but insufficient data	King et al,[4] 2005
Magnesium sulfate vs betamimetics	1375	No differences for preterm birth <37 wk, birth within 48 h	Magnesium was more likely to lead to treatment discontinuation than betamimetics	No differences in infant mortality and morbidity	Crowther et al,[5] 2014
Nitric oxide donors vs betamimetics	691	No reduced preterm birth <32, 34 37 wk, birth within 24 and 48 h and 7 d	Betamimetics were associated with increased rates of side effects: tachycardia, chest pain, palpitations, shortness of breath, and nausea	No differences in infant mortality and morbidity	Duckitt et al,[7] 2014

Abbreviations: IVH, intraventricular hemorrhage; NICU, neonatal intensive care unit; RDS, respiratory distress syndrome; RR, relative risk. Data from Refs.[3–7]

maternal side effects. In patients at less than 32 weeks' gestation, indomethacin may be a reasonable first choice based on its efficacy, ease of administration, and minimal side effects. At 32 to 34 weeks, nifedipine may be a reasonable first choice because it does not carry the risks of oligohydramnios and premature closure of ductus arteriosus observed with indomethacin.

The use of maintenance therapy with a tocolytic agent following an initial treatment of threatened PTL is not recommended. The use of a combination of tocolytic agents for delaying preterm birth is not recommended.

Optimal Dosage

Little evidence is available on the optimal dosage. For calcium channel blockers, one small study compared 20 mg/L repeated in 30 minutes followed by 120 to 160 mg slow-release nifedipine daily for 48 hours versus lower doses (10 mg repeated every 15 minutes for a maximum of 4 doses, followed by 60–80 mg slow release daily for 48 hours). There were no significant differences between groups for birth within 48 hours, before 28, 34, or 37 weeks, in mean interval from trial entry to delivery, maternal side effects, perinatal mortality, and morbidity.[10]

ANTIBIOTICS

Given the known association of PTL with increased frequency of subclinical intra-amniotic infection, several RCTs have evaluated the benefit of antibiotics in PTL. A variety of antibiotics have been studied (including ampicillin or amoxicillin with or without sulbactam or clavulanic acid; erythromycin, clindamycin, mezlocillin, ceftizoxime, or metronidazole) for durations ranging from 3 to 10 days. Compared with placebo, there is no clear neonatal benefit from prophylactic antibiotic treatment of PTL with intact membranes. Evidence from a Cochrane systematic review of 14 RCTs involving more than 7800 women with PTL and no clinical signs of infection revealed some maternal benefit in terms of lower risk of infection but increased risk of neonatal death (**Table 3**).[11]

At 7 years of age, there was no significant difference between children whose mothers had received antibiotics compared with those who received placebo with respect to moderate or severe functional impairment (relative risk [RR] 1.07, 95%

Table 3 Antibiotics for PTL		
Outcome	Benefit (RR)	Significance (95% CI)
Maternal infection	0.74	0.63–0.86
Birth within 48 h	1.04	0.89–1.23
Birth before 36 or 37 wk	0.98	0.92–1.05
Perinatal death	1.22	0.88–1.69
Stillbirth	0.73	0.43–1.26
Neonatal death	1.57	1.03–2.40
Infant death after 28 d	1.06	0.68–1.67
Infant respiratory distress syndrome	0.99	0.84–1.16
Necrotizing enterocolitis	1.06	0.64–1.73
Neonatal sepsis	0.86	0.64–1.16
Intraventricular hemorrhage	0.76	0.48–1.19

Abbreviations: CI, confidence interval; RR, relative risk.

Data from Flenady V, Hawley G, Stock OM, et al. Prophylactic antibiotics for inhibiting preterm labour with intact membranes. Cochrane Database Syst Rev 2013;(12):CD000246.

confidence interval [CI] 0.89–1.28).[12] However, subgroup analysis showed that cerebral palsy (CP) was significantly more frequent among infants of women allocated to macrolide and beta-lactam antibiotics combined compared with placebo (RR 2.83, 95% CI 1.02–7.0). Further, exposure to any macrolide antibiotics versus no macrolide antibiotics increased neonatal death (RR 1.52, 95% CI 1.05–2.19) and CP (RR 1.90, 95% CI 1.20–3.01). Exposure to any beta-lactam antibiotics versus no beta-lactam antibiotics resulted in more neonatal deaths (RR 1.51, 95% CI 1.06–2.15) and CP (RR 1.67, 95% CI 1.06–2.61).

Taken together, the evidence of a reduction in maternal infection associated with antibiotic prophylaxis in PTL comes at a cost of an increase in neonatal death and poorer long-term outcomes in children.

Special Consideration

In women who are known to be group-B streptococcus (GBS) colonized, prophylaxis with penicillin is recommended until imminent delivery is excluded; in women with unknown GBS status, rectovaginal cultures are recommended at diagnosis of PTL and GBS prophylaxis should be administered until culture results are available as well as to known carriers. The recommended antibiotic is penicillin (5 million units intravenously and then 2.5 million units every 4 hours or, if unavailable, ampicillin 2 g intravenously and then 1 g every 4 hours). In the presence of allergy to penicillin, the treatment should be based on sensitivity to erythromycin and clindamycin. Until sensitivity results, vancomycin should be used for prophylaxis.

CORTICOSTEROIDS

A single course of ACS is recommended for PTL before 34 weeks. Such treatment decreases the risk of neonatal death by 31% (95% CI 19%–42%), of respiratory distress syndrome by 34% (95% CI 27%–41%), of intraventricular hemorrhage by 46% (95% CI 31%–57%), of necrotizing enterocolitis by 54% (95% CI 26%–71%), and of neonatal infection in the first 48 hours by 44% (95% CI 15%–62%).[13,14] As for long-term outcomes, treatment was associated with a 51% reduction in developmental delay in childhood (95% CI 0%–76%) and a trend toward a lower risk of CP (RR 0.60, 95% CI 0.34–1.03).[13,14] ACS is safe and reduces the risk of adverse neonatal outcomes for all types of preterm birth; it is beneficial even in the presence of chorioamnionitis, where it has not been shown to increase potential harms, such as neonatal sepsis.[15]

Both betamethasone (2 doses of 12 mg given intramuscularly 24 hours apart) and dexamethasone (4 doses of 6 mg given intramuscularly 12 hours apart) have demonstrated similar efficacy.

Gestational Ages

The benefits of ACS demonstrated in the trials included in the systematic review were not consistent across all gestational ages because the sample sizes particularly at the 2 extremes of prematurity were underpowered to detect differences in the outcomes. The administration of ACS is recommended between 24 and 34 weeks' gestation. However, under particular circumstances, it may be beneficial even at 23 weeks.[16,17]

Repeated Courses

Benefits of ACS therapy have been established for infants born between 24 hours and 7 days after treatment. Two different approaches have been evaluated for patients undelivered after 7 days from the first course and who remain at increased risk for pre-term delivery: (1) a single rescue dose or course if the risk of preterm birth represents at more than 1 week from the first ACS course (A single course before 33 weeks when administered at least 2 weeks after the first course is associated with reduced respi-ratory and composite morbidity [RR 0.65, 95% CI 0.44–0.97])[18] and (2) multiple courses of ACS. The results of 10 RCTs on this topic, involving 4730 women and 5650 neonates, have been summarized recently in a Cochrane review.[19] Treatment of women who remained at risk of preterm birth 7 or more days after an initial course of ACS with repeat doses compared with no repeat treatment reduced the risk of in-fant respiratory distress syndrome (RR 0.83, 95% CI 0.75–0.91). In addition, serious infant morbidity included a composite of death, respiratory distress syndrome, severe intraventricular hemorrhage, periventricular leukomalacia, and necrotizing enteroco-litis was reduced by repeat doses (RR 0.84, 95% CI 0.75–0.94). Treatment with repeat doses was associated with a reduction in mean birth weight (mean difference −75.79 g, 95% CI −117.63 to 33.96). Four of the trials included reported data from an early childhood follow-up. No statistically significant differences were seen for chil-dren in the repeat corticosteroid group as compared to with controls. The authors in-vestigators concluded that short-term benefits support the use of repeat dose(s) of antenatal corticosteroids ACS for women who have received an initial course and remain at risk for preterm birth 7 or more days later. However, there is no proof of long-term benefit either. In addition, there are no data on overall health, neurodevelop-ment, and cardiovascular and metabolic function later in childhood or in adulthood af-ter exposure to repeat dose(s). Recently a gestational age–based decisional model observed that at more than 29 weeks, there is a suggestion of more risk than benefit for this policy.[20]

AMNIOCENTESIS

Since the original study by Miller and colleagues[21] in 1980, amniocentesis has been used in women with PTL to evaluate for the presence of microbial invasion of the am-niotic cavity. Several large cohort studies have shown that the prevalence of positive amniotic fluid cultures (including those for mycoplasma species) in patients with PTL averages 12.7%, and it is inversely related to the gestational age at sampling and directly related to the degree of cervical dilation.[22] The microorganisms usually follow an ascending route from the lower genital tract. While waiting for amniotic fluid culture results, several fast screening tests have been proposed for the detection of intra-amniotic infection: presence of microorganisms at a gram stain, white blood cell count of 50 cells/mm^3 or greater, and glucose level less than 14 mg/dL.[22] Proteomic profiling has also been proposed to predict intra-amniotic infection.[23,24] However, clinical use has been limited by lack of confirmation by enzyme-linked immunosorbent assay anal-ysis for altered expression patterns; moreover, results cannot be combined because of the heterogeneity in the type of sample and analytical platform.[25]

Because cultures may yield negative results despite the presence of intrauterine infection (eg, if the inoculum size is small, the bacterium is fastidious to grow, patients have been receiving antibiotics, or the infection is predominantly located within the chorion rather than intra-amniotic), several cytokines have been proposed as surro-gate markers of intra-amniotic infection. Such sterile intra-amniotic inflammation carries increased risks of spontaneous prematurity and shorter interval to delivery.[26] Moreover, adverse pregnancy and neonatal outcomes have been observed more frequently in the presence of intrauterine inflammation, independently from bacterio-logic culture results and gestational age.[22,27,28]

Among patients in PTL, biomarkers for increased risk of preterm delivery have been identified with proteomic profiling, transcriptomics, and metabolomics, both in amniotic fluid and maternal serum.[29,30] Characterization of the identified compounds has shown that different pathologic pathways are involved in PTL besides acute inflammation.[29]

Benefits

Amniocentesis can establish whether an intrauterine infection is present and, thus, assist the clinician in the counseling of patients, expediting delivery, initiation of guided antibiotic therapy, and alerting the neonatologist to the increased risk of an infected or compromised neonate. Such information may be particularly desired when PTL is associated with uterine tenderness, elevated maternal white blood cell count, or fetal tachycardia.

Risks

Although second trimester amniocentesis in women with PTL has not been shown to increase the risk of preterm delivery, information gained by the procedure may lead to a shortened interval to delivery without evidence of a benefit. Indeed there have been no case control, cohort, or RCT studies in which amniocentesis results have been used to guide the clinical management of patients with PTL. Of interest, among preterm infants, cord serum levels of interleukin-6, interleukin-8, interleukin-1 beta, tumor necrosis factor alpha, and C-reactive protein were not independently predictive of adverse newborn outcomes, CP, or neurodevelopmental delay at 2 years of age.[31,32]

TRANSFER TO APPROPRIATE FACILITY LEVEL

The only 2 interventions that have been able to reduce perinatal mortality in preterm birth are antenatal administration of corticosteroids and maternal transfer to facilities that provide the required level of specialized care. Neonatal outcomes of infants requiring neonatal intensive care unit management are better for those transferred in utero than those transferred as neonates, especially for preterm infants born at less than 30 weeks' gestation.[33–36] Out-born infants are at significantly higher risk of death (adjusted OR [aOR] 1.7), grade III or IV intraventricular hemorrhage (aOR 2.2), patent ductus arteriosus (aOR 1.6), respiratory distress syndrome (aOR 4.8), and nosocomial infection (aOR 2.5).[37–39]

Organization

In order to guarantee a reliable communication policy between referring hospitals, a network of assistance, based on a 24-hour availability transport system, should be established (**Table 4**). Each region should be responsible for developing transport protocols for specific clinical situations. The creation of a transfer network allows registering, by electronic databases, the requests for transport and how they are managed, for purposes of quality audit, education and research programs, and follow-up of clinical cases.[40]

All perinatal care providers must be familiar with the mechanisms for initiating transport and verifying the ability of the receiving institution to provide the necessary care. The reason for a maternal transport may be related to either the woman or the fetus or both.

Communication between the referring physician and the accepting physician before transport is essential to the provision effective care. Indeed one of the main causes of

Table 4
Principles for a good transfer network

Principles	Tools
Communications between professionals	Electronic database, informatics tools, maternal transfer form
24-h availability transport system	Link to territorial emergency facilities (ambulance or helicopter service)
Transport protocols	Clinical guidelines shared between different facilities
Good knowledge of transport system	Meeting and audit of cases in the network
Continuum of care	During transport an adequate level of assistance must be maintained; close monitoring of vital sign and clinical conditions
Back transport to referring hospital when problems are resolved	Good distribution of sanitary resources

substandard care in preterm delivery is lack of communication between professionals, resulting in poor care management and adverse clinical outcomes.[41]

Contraindications to maternal transport include the following:

- The woman's condition is insufficiently stable.
- The fetus' condition is unstable or may deteriorate rapidly.
- The birth is imminent.

During interhospital transfer, a continuum of care with adequate level of assistance must be maintained. The care of the woman during transport is the responsibility of the referring institution, and both mother and fetus need to be monitored. Assessments should include uterine activity, maternal vital signs, and fetal heart rate. A transfer network usually also provides a return transport, namely, when a woman or her neonate, after receiving intensive or specialized care at a referral center, is returned to the original referring hospital for continuing care after the problems that required the transfer have been resolved.

MAGNESIUM SULFATE

Prematurity is the leading risk factor for CP, which is the most common and costly form of chronic motor disability in childhood. It has been reported that more than 30% of cases of CP occur in infants delivered at less than 32 weeks or weighing less than 1500 g.[42] Possible human benefit from administration of magnesium sulfate was first shown in a case control study, which showed that children with CP were less likely to have been exposed to magnesium sulfate than control subjects (OR 0.14; 95% CI 0.05–0.51).[43] Subsequently, several RCTs have evaluated the efficacy of magnesium sulfate for prevention of CP. **Table 5** displays the characteristics of the studies in which magnesium sulfate was administered for neuroprotection of the fetus.[44–48]

A meta-analysis of the findings concluded that magnesium sulfate significantly reduces the risk of any CP (RR = 0.71, 95% CI 0.55–0.91), moderate or severe CP (RR = 0.64, 95% CI 0.44–0.92), as well as death or CP (RR = 0.85, 95% CI 0.74–0.98).[44] There was significant homogeneity among the studies. All studies included twins.

In addition to the dose of magnesium sulfate and the gestational age at inclusion, the RCTs differed for several inclusion criteria (such as clinical presentation: PTL, premature rupture of membranes, chorioamnionitis, preeclampsia, or severe fetal growth restriction)

Table 5
Characteristics of the RCTs on magnesium sulfate in preterm birth analyzed in reference to occurrence of perinatal death or CP

Study, Author, Year	Number of Subjects	Gestational Age	Regimen of MgSO$_4$: Load/Maintenance	RR of CP or Perinatal Death (95% CI)
Mittendorf et al,[45] 2002	59	<34 wk	4 g then 2–3 g/h	4.83 (0.60–38.90)
Crowther et al,[46] 2003	1255	<30 wk	4 g then 1 g/h	0.82 (0.66–1.02)
Marret et al,[47] 2006	688	<33 wk	4 g then none	0.80 (0.58–1.10)
Rouse et al,[48] 2008	2444	<32 wk	6 g then 2 g/h	0.90 (0.73–1.10)
Overall	—	—	—	0.85 (0.74–0.98)

Abbreviation: MgSO$_4$, magnesium sulfate.
Data from Refs.[45–48]

and timing of magnesium administration before birth. (In the largest trial of Rouse and colleagues,[48] women received magnesium as late as 20 minutes before delivery.)

It has been calculated that with the implementation of such prophylaxis in women at risk for delivery at less than 32 weeks, only 63 women would need to be treated to prevent one case of neonatal CP; the number would be higher if more inclusive criteria were used (eg, gestational age <34 weeks), whereas it would be lower if a more strict gestational age cutoff was used (eg, <30 weeks).[49] Magnesium sulfate administration did not significantly affect the risk of adverse maternal outcome (in terms of death, cardiac arrest or respiratory arrest, pulmonary edema, or severe postpartum hemorrhage). Similar conclusions were reached by 2 other meta-analyses on the subject.[50,51] Despite such evident benefits, a 2013 study showed that only 40% of candidate patients receive magnesium sulfate prophylaxis.[52]

The optimal treatment protocol (doses and duration) needed for maximal neuroprotection remains unknown. For practical purposes, each institution should develop a specific magnesium sulfate protocol, specifying inclusion criteria, treatment regimens, concurrent tocolysis, and monitoring.[8] **Box 1** displays the protocol used in the largest of the randomized trials.[48] In the absence of evidence for an optimal dose of magnesium sulfate, and the borderline increased risk of perinatal death associated with magnesium sulfate when used for tocolysis (RR 4.56, 95% CI 1.00–20.9),[5] other societies (Society of Obstetricians and Gynecologists of Canada [SOCG] and National Health and Medical Research Council of Australia [NHMRC])[49,53] suggest adopting the minimum dosage used in the published trials and when delivery seems imminent at less than 30 weeks.[53] Although the maternal serum concentration of magnesium is affected by maternal weight and the presence of multiple gestations and cord blood levels are inversely related to birth weight centile, it is unclear whether a correlation exists between the maternal serum level and a neuroprotective effect. Because it is unclear whether the duration of infusion and neonatal serum magnesium levels are associated with the risk of death,[54,55] it may be equally prudent to administer magnesium sulfate for the shortest duration.

MODE OF DELIVERY

When assessing the evidence from the literature for the optimal mode of delivery in prematurity, in terms of reduction of neonatal mortality and severe morbidity, several variables need to be taken into account, such as fetal presentation, indication for preterm birth (eg, PTL, severe fetal growth restriction, or preeclampsia), the initially intended route of delivery, and the fetal status on admission.

Box 1
Protocol for magnesium sulfate in neuroprophylaxis used in the RCT of Rouse and colleagues

Inclusion criteria

- Gestational age 24.0 to 31.6 weeks
- High risk for PTD within 2 hours caused by any indication (eg, PTL ≥4 cm dilation)

Exclusion criteria

- Active labor at greater than 8 cm dilation
- Major fetal anomalies
- Maternal contraindications to magnesium sulfate (pulmonary hypertension, myasthenia gravis, class II–IV cardiac disease, severe acute pulmonary disease, and renal insufficiency)

Management

- Discontinue any tocolysis.
- Use magnesium 6-g load over 20 to 30 minutes, followed by 2 g/h.
- Maximum duration of treatment is 12 hours.
- Discontinue magnesium if delivery is no longer considered imminent.
- Restart magnesium if delivery is deemed imminent again (reload if magnesium is discontinued >6 hours prior).
- Serum magnesium levels are not required.

Data from Rouse DJ, Hirtz DG, Thom E, et al. A randomized controlled trial of magnesium sulfate for the prevention of cerebral palsy. N Engl J Med 2008;359:895–905.

Fetal Growth Restriction

The issue has not been adequately studied, and the results are often contradictory. In a population of small-for-gestational-age (SGA) neonates born at 26 to 31 weeks, those delivered by cesarean section had increased survival rates; the benefit disappeared for SGA neonates born at greater than 33 weeks.[56] The survival advantage for SGA neonates at gestational ages of 26 to 31 weeks persisted after adjustment for sociodemographic and medical factors.

More recently, in 2885 cephalic SGA live-born neonates delivered between 25 and 34 weeks of gestation, cesarean delivery was not associated with improved neonatal outcomes in terms of intraventricular hemorrhage, subdural hemorrhage, seizures, or sepsis and was associated with an increased risk of respiratory distress syndrome after adjusting for confounders.[57]

It should be noted that studies originating from the pediatric literature use SGA as surrogate for fetal growth restriction. The features of fetal heart rate monitoring differ in the preterm fetus from the term fetus, making interpretation difficult during labor. Physiologic reserves available to combat hypoxia are less in a preterm fetus than those available to a term fetus, and even more so for a growth restricted fetus, so that a preterm fetus may suffer a hypoxic insult sooner.

It is commonly accepted that cesarean section offers survival advantage to a fetus so severely growth restricted as to require elective preterm delivery (particularly at <34 weeks) regardless of fetal presentation.[58] Vaginal delivery should be considered for the growth-restricted fetus when the woman is in labor. Induction of labor may also be possible under continuous fetal heart rate monitoring, in favorable obstetric situations and in the absence of severe fetal hemodynamic disturbances.[59]

Breech Presentation

From randomized studies there is insufficient evidence to recommend one mode of delivery over the other; however, the small number of women recruited limits the statistical power even of meta-analysis. A Cochrane systematic review of 4 RCTs (involving 116 women) in singleton pregnancies and refractory PTL at less than 37 weeks compared immediate caesarean versus planned vaginal birth. All trials were stopped early because of difficulties with recruitment. Women with breech presentation were more likely to experience major postpartum complications in the planned cesarean delivery group (RR 7.21, 95% CI 1.37–38.08). There was a trend for lower perinatal mortality with cesarean delivery (RR 0.29, 95% CI 0.07–1.14) across all gestational ages (between 26 and 32 weeks: RR 0.50 [0.02, 10.34], 28–36 weeks: RR 0.22 [0.03, 1.73]).[60]

Evidence from cohort studies consistently suggests that cesarean delivery offers a survival advantage in the presence of nonvertex presentation. A recent systematic review and meta-analysis of nonrandomized studies assessed the association between mode of delivery and neonatal mortality in women with preterm breech presentation between 25 and 36 weeks and included 7 studies and 3557 women. The weighted risk of neonatal mortality was 3.8% in the cesarean delivery group and 11.5% in the vaginal delivery group (pooled RR 0.63, 95% CI 0.48–0.81), suggesting that cesarean delivery significantly reduces neonatal mortality as compared with vaginal delivery.[61]

The largest and most recent data are derived from the National Institute of Child Health and Human Development (NICHD)-sponsored Consortium on Safe Labor, in which 2906 singleton pregnancies eligible for a vaginal delivery between 24 and 32 weeks were analyzed. Neonatal mortality in attempted vaginal delivery was compared with planned cesarean delivery stratified by presentation. For breech presentation, neonatal mortality was increased at 24 0/7 to 27 6/7 weeks' gestation (25.2% vs 13.2%, $P<.003$) and at 28 0/7 to 31 6/7 weeks (6.0% vs 1.5%, $P = .016$). Even at the lowest gestational ages (24.0–24.6 weeks), among breech presentations, planned cesarean delivery was associated with a lower incidence of neonatal death and asphyxia after controlling for other factors.[62]

At periviable gestational ages (<24 weeks), neonatal survival and neurodevelopmental disabilities among survivors vary greatly according to local protocols of perinatal care in terms of tocolysis, antenatal steroids, neonatal resuscitation, and intensive care support, among others.[62] The individual effect of mode of delivery in such cases is difficult to assess, and management should incorporate input from the family.[63]

Cephalic Presentation

In the largest cohort study to date (the NICHD-sponsored Consortium on Safe Labor) on 20,231 singleton, live-born, cephalic neonates delivered between 24 and 34 weeks of gestation (excluding congenital anomalies, operative vaginal deliveries, birth weight <500 g, and fetal growth restriction), associations between method of delivery and neonatal morbidities were estimated using logistic regression. After controlling for maternal age, ethnicity, education, primary payer, prepregnancy weight, gestational age, diabetes, and hypertension, cesarean delivery compared with vaginal delivery was associated with increased odds of respiratory distress (aOR 1.74, 95% CI 1.61–1.89) and 5-minute Apgar score less than 7 (aOR 2.04, 95% CI 1.77–2.35).[64]

In the NICHD-sponsored Consortium on Safe Labor mentioned earlier for vertex presentation, 79% attempted vaginal delivery and 84% were successful.[62] There was no difference in neonatal mortality, suggesting that attempted vaginal delivery for vertex presentation has a high success rate and there is no difference in neonatal mortality (unlike breech presentation).

Operative Vaginal Delivery

It is relatively contraindicated in preterm fetuses at less than 34 weeks. Data on vacuum extraction from Swedish national registers revealed that vacuum was used in 5.7% of the preterm deliveries and that intracranial hemorrhage (1.51%), extracranial hemorrhage (0.64%), and brachial plexus injury (0.13%) were higher compared with other modes of delivery.[65]

DELAYED CLAMPING OF UMBILICAL CORD
Timing of Cord Clamping

It is estimated that 25% to 60% of the total blood volume of the fetal-placental circulation is stored in the placenta. Early clamping of the cord (within the first 5–10 seconds of birth) results in a decrease to the neonate of 15 to 40 mL/kg of bodyweight.[66] Three quarters of the transfusion occurs in the first minute after birth.

Early cord clamping (clamping within the first 60 seconds from birth) was originally thought to be important in the active management of the third stage of labor; but because of the lack of evidence for it, the recommendation has been withdrawn in some guidelines.[67] Indeed, because delaying the clamping until the umbilical circulation has ceased approximates the natural physiology, early cord clamping should be considered the intervention and need for it should be demonstrated.

Delayed cord clamping leads to an expansion in intravascular volume that facilitates the cardiopulmonary transition, and it reduces iron and hematopoietic stem cells loss. Delayed cord clamping may not be desired in neonates at risk for polycythemia and neonatal jaundice, such as severe preterm fetal growth restriction, maternal alloimmunization, and macrosomia caused by maternal diabetes.

RCTs in both term and preterm infants have consistently demonstrated that delayed clamping is associated with significant benefits (**Table 6**).[68–70] In preterm infants, delayed cord clamping reduces the need for inotropic medications and increases systemic blood pressure. Delayed cord clamping also seems to be protective of motor disability in male very-low-birth-weight infants.[71] The optimal interval between cord clamping and whether such an interval is gestational age related are unknown. Additional data will probably come from the ongoing Australian Placental Transfusion Study, evaluating delayed cord clamping in neonates less than 30 weeks.

Table 6
Effects of delayed umbilical cord clamping from meta-analysis of RCTs

	RR (95% CI)
Preterm	
Need for blood transfusion	0.61 (0.46–0.81)
IVH (all grades)	0.59 (0.41–0.85)
NEC	0.62 (0.43–0.90)
Mortality (<32 wk)	0.42 (0.19–0.95)
Term	
Jaundice requiring phototherapy	1.59 (1.03–2.46)
Iron deficiency at 3–6 mo	0.56 (0.40–0.79)
Anemia	0.53 (0.40–0.70)

Abbreviations: IVH, intraventricular hemorrhage; NEC, necrotizing enterocolitis.
Data from Refs.[68–70]

Currently the World Health Organization (WHO) recommends delaying cord clamping for 1 to 3 minutes after birth with the infant held at or below the level of the placenta.[72] The American College of Obstetricians and Gynecologists' recommendations support delaying clamping in preterm neonates for 30 to 60 seconds after delivery.[73] Contraindications to delayed cord clamping are infants requiring immediate evaluation and resuscitation for nonreassuring status, in the presence of placental abnormalities (such as at cesarean sections done for placenta previa, vasa previa, or placental abruption), thick meconium-stained amniotic fluid, the presence of severe congenital anomalies, multiple pregnancy, severe fetal growth restriction with absent or reversed-end-diastolic flow in the umbilical artery at prenatal Doppler ultrasound, alloimmunization, and unstable maternal status.

Concerns

Implementation of delayed cord clamping has been sporadic, with most UK obstetricians clamping the cord within 20 seconds of birth both at term and preterm.

Several concerns have been raised, including

- Risk for hypothermia: Such risk can be avoided by putting the neonate immediately skin to skin on the maternal abdomen during delayed cord clamping and covering him with a warm blanket. Raising the neonate above the vaginal level is, however, contrary to the WHO's recommendations, as it could lead to baby-to-placenta transfusion. A recent trial has provided some reassurance, showing that in term neonates after vaginal delivery, gravity does not have an effect on the volume of placental transfusion.[66] Whether this also applies to preterm infants or those delivered by cesarean section is unknown.
- Delayed neonatal resuscitation: It is commonly perceived that early cord clamping is needed in infants who require immediate neonatal resuscitation, particularly those born extremely preterm or by cesarean section. A new strategy proposed is to milk the umbilical cord (3 times over a duration of <30 seconds); such a strategy achieves significant improvement in hemodynamic stability through 24 hours of age, higher hematocrit, lower need for transfusion, and overall improved outcome compared with a historic untreated cohort.[74] Alternatively, resuscitation of the compromised newborn can be initiated at the side of the mother with the umbilical cord intact.
- Cord blood gas analysis: The timing of cord clamping could affect the interpretation of cord blood gases; only a few small studies have addressed the issue, and the results are partly contradictory. Recently Di Tommaso and colleagues[75] reported that, in term neonates, blood gas analysis may be performed in the unclamped cord after birth without reducing the accuracy of the analysis.
- Uterotonic administration: There are no studies evaluating the transfusion of oxytocic drugs through the placenta and no reported evidence of any harmful effects on the baby.[76] Uterotonic agents following birth and before cord clamping increase the rate of placental transfusion and enhance the effect of delayed clamping.

In summary, the practice of delayed cord clamping can be easily adopted for most preterm and term vaginal deliveries.

SUMMARY

The aforementioned obstetric practices in women with PTL have the potential to contribute substantially to decreasing neonatal morbidities. The evidence in support of most practices is quite strong. Each institution should prepare specific protocols of care and conduct periodic audits to verify their consistent implementation.

REFERENCES

1. Iams JD, Berghella V. Care for women with prior preterm birth. Am J Obstet Gynecol 2010;203:89–100.
2. Neilson JP, West HM, Dowswell T. Betamimetics for inhibiting preterm labour. Cochrane Database Syst Rev 2014;(2):CD004352.
3. Flenady V, Wojcieszek AM, Papatsonis DN, et al. Calcium channel blockers for inhibiting preterm labour and birth. Cochrane Database Syst Rev 2014;(6):CD002255.
4. King JF, Flenady V, Cole S, et al. Cyclo-oxygenase (COX) inhibitors for treating preterm labour. Cochrane Database Syst Rev 2005;(2):CD001992.
5. Crowther CA, Brown J, McKinlay CJ, et al. Magnesium sulphate for preventing preterm birth in threatened preterm labour. Cochrane Database Syst Rev 2014;(8):CD001060.
6. Flenady V, Reinebrant HE, Liley HG, et al. Oxytocin receptor antagonists for inhibiting preterm labour. Cochrane Database Syst Rev 2014;(6):CD004452.
7. Duckitt K, Thornton S, O'Donovan OP, et al. Nitric oxide donors for treating preterm labour. Cochrane Database Syst Rev 2014;(5):CD002860.
8. American College of Obstetricians and Gynecologists. Magnesium sulfate use in obstetrics. Committee opinion No. 573. Obstet Gynecol 2013;122:727–8.
9. Haas DM, Caldwell DM, Kirkpatrick P, et al. Tocolytic therapy for preterm delivery: systematic review and network meta-analysis. BMJ 2012;345:e6226.
10. Nassar AH, Abu-Musa AA, Awwad J, et al. Two dose regimens of nifedipine for management of preterm labor: a randomized controlled trial. Am J Perinatol 2009;26:575–81.
11. Flenady V, Hawley G, Stock OM, et al. Prophylactic antibiotics for inhibiting preterm labour with intact membranes. Cochrane Database Syst Rev 2013;(12):CD000246.
12. Kenyon S, Pike K, Jones DR, et al. Childhood outcomes after prescription of antibiotics to pregnant women with spontaneous preterm labour: 7-year follow-up of the ORACLE II trial. Lancet 2008;372:1319–27.
13. Crowley P. Prophylactic corticosteroids for preterm birth. Cochrane Database Syst Rev 2000;(2):CD000065.
14. Roberts D, Dalziel S. Antenatal corticosteroids for accelerating fetal lung maturation for women at risk of preterm birth. Cochrane Database Syst Rev 2006;(3):CD004454.
15. Been J, Degraeuwe P, Kramer B, et al. Antenatal steroids and neonatal outcome after chorioamnionitis: a meta-analysis. BJOG 2011;118:113–22.
16. Hayes EJ, Paul DA, Stahl GE, et al. Effect of antenatal corticosteroids on survival for neonates born at 23 weeks of gestation. Obstet Gynecol 2008;111:921–6.
17. RCOG. Antenatal corticosteroids to reduce neonatal morbidity (Green-top 7). 2010; Available at: https://www.rcog.org.uk/globalassets/documents/guidelines/gtg_7.pdf. Accessed February 10, 2015.
18. Garite TJ, Kurtzman J, Maurel K, et al. Impact of a 'rescue course' of antenatal corticosteroids: a multicenter randomized, placebo-controlled trial. Am J Obstet Gynecol 2009;200:248.e1–9.
19. McKinlay CJ, Crowther CA, Middleton P, et al. Repeat antenatal glucocorticoids for women at risk of preterm birth: a Cochrane Systematic Review. Am J Obstet Gynecol 2012;206:187–94.

20. Zephyrin LC, Hong KN, Wapner RJ, et al. Gestational age-specific risks vs benefits of multicourse antenatal corticosteroids for preterm labor. Am J Obstet Gynecol 2013;209:330.e1–7.
21. Miller J, Pupkin M, Hill G. Bacterial colonization of amniotic fluid from intact fetal membranes. Am J Obstet Gynecol 1980;136:796–804.
22. Gomez R, Romero R, Mazor M, et al. The role of infection in preterm labor and delivery. In: Elder MG, Lamont RF, Romero R, editors. Preterm labor. New York: Churchill Livinstone; 1997. p. 85–125.
23. Cobo T, Palacio M, Navarro-Sastre A, et al. Predictive value of combined amniotic fluid proteomic biomarkers and interleukin6 in preterm labor with intact membranes. Am J Obstet Gynecol 2009;200:499.e1–6.
24. Buhimschi CS, Buhimschi IA, Abdel-Razeq S, et al. Proteomic profiling of intra-amniotic inflammation: relationship with funisitis and early-onset sepsis in the premature neonate. Pediatr Res 2007;61:318–24.
25. Kacerovsky M, Lenco J, Musilova I, et al. Proteomic biomarkers for spontaneous preterm birth: a systematic review of the literature. Reprod Sci 2014;21:283–95.
26. Romero R, Miranda J, Chaiworapongsa T, et al. Sterile intra-amniotic inflammation in asymptomatic patients with a sonographic short cervix: prevalence and clinical significance. J Matern Fetal Neonatal Med 2014. [Epub ahead of print].
27. Lee SE, Romero R, Jung H, et al. The intensity of the fetal inflammatory response in intra-amniotic inflammation with and without microbial invasion of the amniotic cavity. Am J Obstet Gynecol 2007;197:294.e1–6.
28. Lee J, Oh KJ, Yang HJ, et al. The importance of intra-amniotic inflammation in the subsequent development of atypical chronic lung disease. J Matern Fetal Neonatal Med 2009;22:917–23.
29. Pereira L, Reddy AP, Alexander AL, et al. Insights into the multifactorial nature of preterm birth: proteomic profiling of the maternal serum glycoproteome and maternal serum peptidome among women in preterm labor. Am J Obstet Gynecol 2010;202:555.e1–10.
30. Romero R, Mazaki-Tovi S, Vaisbuch E, et al. Metabolomics in premature labor: a novel approach to identify patients at risk for preterm delivery. J Matern Fetal Neonatal Med 2010;23:1344–59.
31. Varner MW, Marshall NE, Rouse DJ, et al. The association of cord serum cytokines with neurodevelopmental outcomes. Am J Perinatol 2015;30:115–22.
32. Sorokin Y, Romero R, Mele L, et al. Umbilical cord serum interleukin-6, C-reactive protein, and myeloperoxidase concentrations at birth and association with neonatal morbidities and long-term neurodevelopmental outcomes. Am J Perinatol 2014;31:717–26.
33. Lee SK, McMillan DD, Ohlsson A, et al. The benefit of preterm birth at tertiary care centers is related to gestational age. Am J Obstet Gynecol 2003;188:617–22.
34. Shlossman PA, Manley JS, Sciscione AC, et al. An analysis of neonatal morbidity and mortality in maternal (in utero) and neonatal transports at 24–34 weeks' gestation. Am J Perinatol 1997;14:449–56.
35. Chung JH, Phibbs CS, Boscardin WJ, et al. Examining the effect of hospital-level factors on mortality of very low birth weight infants using multilevel modeling. J Perinatol 2011;31:770–5.
36. Doyle LW, Bowman E, Callanan C, et al. Changing outcome for infants of birthweight 500–999 g born outside level 3 centres in Victoria. Aust N Z J Obstet Gynaecol 1997;37:253–7.
37. Chien LY, Whyte R, Aziz K, et al. Improved outcome of preterm infants when delivered in tertiary care centers. Obstet Gynecol 2001;98:247–52.

38. Towers CV, Bonebrake R, Padilla G, et al. The effect of transport on the rate of severe intraventricular hemorrhage in very low birth weight infants. Obstet Gynecol 2000;95:291–5.

39. Lorch SA, Baiocchi M, Ahlberg CE, et al. The differential impact of delivery hospital on the outcomes of premature infants. Pediatrics 2012;130:270–8.

40. Health Canada. Family-centred maternity and newborn care: national guidelines. Ottawa (Canada): Minister of Public Works and Government Services; 2000.

41. Cantwell R, Clutton-Brock T, Cooper G, et al. Saving Mothers' Lives: reviewing maternal deaths to make motherhood safer: 2006-2008. The Eighth Report of the Confidential Enquiries into Maternal Deaths in the United Kingdom. BJOG 2011;118(Suppl 1):1–203.

42. Drummond PM, Colver AF. Analysis by gestational age of cerebral palsy in singleton births in north-east England 1970-94. Paediatr Perinat Epidemiol 2002;16:172–80.

43. Nelson KB, Grether JK. Can magnesium sulfate reduce the risk of cerebral palsy in very low birthweight infants? Pediatrics 1995;95:263–9.

44. Doyle LW, Crowther CA, Middleton P, et al. Antenatal magnesium sulfate and neurologic outcome in preterm infants: a systematic review. Obstet Gynecol 2009;113:1327–33.

45. Mittendorf R, Dambrosia J, Pryde PG, et al. Association between the use of antenatal magnesium sulfate in preterm labor and adverse health outcomes in infants. Am J Obstet Gynecol 2002;186:1111–8.

46. Crowther CA, Hiller JE, Doyle LW, et al. Effect of magnesium sulfate given for neuroprotection before preterm birth: a randomized controlled trial. JAMA 2003;290: 2669–76.

47. Marret S, Marpeau L, Zupan-Simunek V, et al. Magnesium sulfate given before very-preterm birth to protect infant brain: the randomized controlled PREMAG trial. BJOG 2007;114:310–8.

48. Rouse DJ, Hirtz DG, Thom E, et al. A randomized controlled trial of magnesium sulfate for the prevention of cerebral palsy. N Engl J Med 2008;359:895–905.

49. Magee L, Sawchuck D, Synnes A, et al. SOGC clinical practice guideline. Magnesium sulphate for fetal neuroprotection. J Obstet Gynaecol Can 2011;33:516–29.

50. Conde-Agudelo A, Romero R. Antenatal magnesium sulfate for the prevention of cerebral palsy in preterm infants less than 34 weeks' gestation: a systematic review and meta-analysis. Am J Obstet Gynecol 2009;200:595–609.

51. Costantine MM, Weiner SJ, Eunice Kennedy Shriver National Institute of Child Health and Human Development Maternal-Fetal Medicine Units Network. Effects of antenatal exposure to magnesium sulfate on neuroprotection and mortality in preterm infants: a meta-analysis. Obstet Gynecol 2009;114:354–64.

52. Gibbins KJ, Browning KR, Lopes W, et al. Evaluation of the clinical use of magnesium sulfate for cerebral palsy prevention. Obstet Gynecol 2013;121:235–40.

53. Australian Government National Health and Medical Research Council. Antenatal magnesium sulphate prior to preterm birth for neuroprotection of the fetus, infant and child. National clinical practice guidelines. Available at: http://www.nhmrc. gov.au/_files_nhmrc/publications/attachments/cp128_mag_sulphate_child.pdf.

54. McPherson JA, Rouse DJ, Grobman WA, et al. Association of duration of neuroprotective magnesium sulfate infusion with neonatal and maternal outcomes. Obstet Gynecol 2014;124:749–55.

55. Basu SK, Chickajajur V, Lopez V, et al. Immediate clinical outcomes in preterm neonates receiving antenatal magnesium for neuroprotection. J Perinat Med 2011;40:185–9.

56. Lee HC, Gould JB. Survival rates and mode of delivery for vertex preterm neonates according to small- or appropriate- for-gestational-age status. Pediatrics 2006;118:e1836–44.

57. Werner EF, Savitz DA, Janevic TM, et al. Mode of delivery and neonatal outcomes in preterm, small for gestational age newborns. Obstet Gynecol 2012; 120:560–4.

58. Mercer BM. Mode of delivery for periviable birth. Semin Perinatol 2013;37: 417–21.

59. Perrotin F, Simon EG, Potin J, et al. Delivery of the IUGR fetus. J Gynecol Obstet Biol Reprod (Paris) 2013;42:975–84.

60. Alfirevic Z, Milan SJ, Livio S. Caesarean section versus vaginal delivery for preterm birth in singletons. Cochrane Database Syst Rev 2013;(9):CD000078.

61. Bergenhenegouwen LA, Meertens LJ, Schaaf J, et al. Vaginal delivery versus caesarean section in preterm breech delivery: a systematic review. Eur J Obstet Gynecol Reprod Biol 2014;172:1–6.

62. Reddy UM, Zhang J, Sun L, et al. Neonatal mortality by attempted route of delivery in early preterm birth. Am J Obstet Gynecol 2012;207:117.e1–8.

63. Raju TN, Mercer BM, Burchfield DJ, et al. Periviable birth: executive summary of a joint workshop by the Eunice Kennedy Shriver National Institute of Child Health and Human Development, Society for Maternal-Fetal Medicine, American Academy of Pediatrics, and American College of Obstetricians and Gynecologists. Obstet Gynecol 2014;123:1083–96.

64. Werner EF, Han CS, Savitz DA, et al. Health outcomes for vaginal compared with cesarean delivery of appropriately grown preterm neonates. Obstet Gynecol 2013;121:1195–2000.

65. Aberg K, Norman M, Ekeus C. Preterm birth by vacuum extraction and neonatal outcome: a population-based cohort study. BMC Pregnancy Childbirth 2014; 22(14):42.

66. Vain NE, Satragno DS, Gorenstein AN, et al. Effect of gravity on volume of placental transfusion: a multicentre, randomized, non-inferiority trial. Lancet 2014;384:235–40.

67. Ceriani Cernadas JM, Carroli G, Pellegrini L, et al. The effect of timing of cord clamping on neonatal venous hematocrit values and clinical outcome at term: a randomized, controlled trial. Pediatrics 2006;117(4):e779–86.

68. Hutton EK, Hassan ES. Late vs early clamping of the umbilical cord in full-term neonates: systematic review and meta-analysis of controlled trials. JAMA 2007; 21(297):1241–52.

69. Rabe H, Diaz-Rossello JL, Duley L, et al. Effect of timing of umbilical cord clamping and other strategies to influence placental transfusion at preterm birth on maternal and infant outcomes. Cochrane Database Syst Rev 2012;(8):CD003248.

70. Backes CH, Rivera BK, Haque U, et al. Placental transfusion strategies in very preterm neonates: a systematic review and meta-analysis. Obstet Gynecol 2014;124:47–56.

71. Mercer JS, Vohr BR, Erickson-Owens DA, et al. Seven-month developmental outcomes of very low birth weight infants enrolled in a randomized controlled trial of delayed versus immediate cord clamping. J Perinatol 2010;30:11–6.

72. World Health Organization. Guidelines on basic newborn resuscitation. Geneva (Switzerland): World Health Organization; 2012.

73. American College of Obstetricians and Gynecologists. Timing of umbilical cord clamping after birth. Committee opinion no. 543. Obstet Gynecol 2012;120: 1522–6.

74. Patel S, Clark EA, Rodriguez CE, et al. Effect of umbilical cord milking on morbidity and survival in extremely low gestational age neonates. Am J Obstet Gynecol 2014;211:519.e1–7.

75. Di Tommaso M, Seravalli V, Martini I, et al. Blood gas values in clamped and unclamped umbilical cord at birth. Early Hum Dev 2014;90:523–5.

76. Soltani H, Hutchon DR, Poulose TA. Timing of prophylactic uterotonics for the third stage of labour after vaginal birth. Cochrane Database Syst Rev 2010;(8):CD006173.

A Uniform Management Approach to Optimize Outcome in Fetal Growth Restriction

Viola Seravalli, MD, Ahmet A. Baschat, MD*

KEYWORDS

- Fetal growth restriction • Fetal acidemia • Fetal Doppler • Umbilical artery
- Middle cerebral artery • Biophysical profile score • Neonatal outcome • Fetal testing

KEY POINTS

- A uniform approach to diagnosis and management of fetal growth restriction (FGR) produces better outcomes, prevents unanticipated stillbirth, and allows appropriate timing of delivery.
- An estimated fetal weight less than the tenth percentile in association with either an elevated umbilical artery Doppler index, a decreased middle cerebral artery Doppler index, or a decreased cerebroplacental ratio should be considered evidence of FGR. Early-onset and late-onset FGR represent two distinct clinical phenotypes of placental dysfunction.
- Integration of different testing modalities allows adjustment of monitoring intervals based on Doppler parameters and a more precise prediction of acid-base status based on biophysical variables.
- Antenatal surveillance of the growth-restricted fetus requires adjustment of monitoring intervals based on signs of disease acceleration, when delivery is not yet indicated.
- Thresholds for interventions are defined by the balance of fetal risks of continuation of pregnancy versus the neonatal risks that follow delivery and depend on gestational age.

INTRODUCTION

The main challenges in the management of pregnancies complicated by fetal growth restriction (FGR) are accurate identification of the small fetus at risk for adverse outcome, prevention of unanticipated stillbirth, and appropriate timing of delivery. A

Authors declare no relationship with a commercial company that has a direct financial interest in the subject matter or materials discussed in the article or with a company making a competing product.
Department of Gynecology and Obstetrics, The Johns Hopkins Center for Fetal Therapy, The Johns Hopkins Hospital, 600 North Wolfe Street, Nelson 228, Baltimore, MD 21287, USA
* Corresponding author.
E-mail addresses: aabaschat@hotmail.com; abascha1@jhmi.edu

Obstet Gynecol Clin N Am 42 (2015) 275–288
http://dx.doi.org/10.1016/j.ogc.2015.01.005
0889-8545/15/$ – see front matter © 2015 Elsevier Inc. All rights reserved.

uniform management approach to diagnosis and management of FGR consistently produces better outcome than is reported in observational studies that rely on a range of diagnostic, surveillance, and delivery criteria.[1–5] Once the diagnosis of FGR has been made, surveillance tests need to be applied at appropriate intervals until the relative risks of delivery outweigh the benefits of ongoing monitoring. These factors are determined by the clinical phenotype of FGR across gestational ages.

CLINICAL PHENOTYPE OF FETAL GROWTH RESTRICTION IN RELATION TO GESTATIONAL AGE

FGR evolves from a preclinical phase to clinically apparent growth delay and may eventually lead to fetal deterioration before the spontaneous onset of labor. Growth delay due to decreased nutrient delivery affects liver size and therefore the abdominal circumference (AC) first, and then growth of the head and entire body.[6] Abnormal placental perfusion in the maternal compartment results in increased blood flow resistance in the uterine artery flow-velocity waveform.[7] Abnormal perfusion of the fetal villous vascular tree is associated with decreased umbilical artery (UA) end-diastolic velocity proportional to the degree of flow impairment.[8] Abnormal oxygen diffusion across the villous membrane leading to lower fetal arterial PaO_2 is associated with a decrease in middle cerebral artery (MCA) blood flow resistance,[9] whereas decreased CO_2 clearance additionally increases the MCA peak systolic velocity (**Fig. 1**).[10] The relative predominance of these mechanisms determines the clinical picture of FGR.[11–16]

FGR that is established by the second trimester is associated with a greater degree of vascular abnormality in the maternal and fetal compartments of the placenta. In the mother, high-resistance uterine artery flow velocity waveforms and a 40% to 70% rate of associated pre-eclampsia are characteristic. In the fetal compartment, an elevation

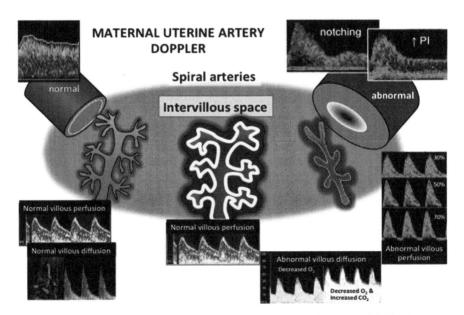

FETAL UMBILICAL AND MIDDLE CEREBRAL ARTERY DOPPLER

Fig. 1. Clinical correlates of maternal and fetal aspects of placental function.

of the UA pulsatility index (PI) is typical.[11,12] In FGR that is not established until 31 to 34 weeks (late-onset FGR), villous diffusion and perfusion defects coexist in various proportions,[17–21] leading to cerebral or UA Doppler abnormalities that may be present independent of each other (**Fig. 2**).[22–24] Because of this variable association between small fetal size and abnormal Doppler velocimetry, distinction between growth restriction and constitutional smallness can be challenging. Accordingly, management challenges in early-onset FGR revolve around prematurity and coexisting maternal hypertensive disease, whereas in late-onset disease, failure of diagnosis or surveillance leading to unanticipated stillbirth is the primary issue.[25,26]

DIAGNOSIS OF FETAL GROWTH RESTRICTION

The diagnosis of fetal growth delay can be based on fetal biometry alone or by also taking umbilical or cerebral artery Doppler indices into consideration. An AC less than the tenth percentile has the highest sensitivity for the diagnosis of FGR, whereas a sonographically estimated fetal weight (SEFW) less than the tenth percentile has greater specificity.[11] Most national societies agree on the tenth percentile for the SEFW as a diagnostic cutoff for small for gestational age (SGA). The disadvantage of this cutoff is the inclusion of a variable number of normal constitutionally small fetuses that do not require surveillance. Using an SEFW less than the third percentile or a decreased AC growth rate is more likely to identify "true FGR,"[27] but has the disadvantage that less severe forms of FGR at risk for deterioration are missed and therefore their risk for stillbirth remains. Combining an SEFW less than the tenth percentile with either an abnormal UA, MCA, or cerebroplacental ratio (CPR, defined as UA/MCA index), increases the identification of the small fetus at risk for adverse outcome. Although UA Doppler velocimetry is sufficient for the diagnosis of FGR before 32 weeks gestation, thereafter MCA Doppler is also required to represent the whole clinical spectrum found in early-onset and late-onset placental disease.[12,14,16,24] Because the CPR mathematically amplifies mild abnormalities in the umbilical and middle cerebral arteries, it is

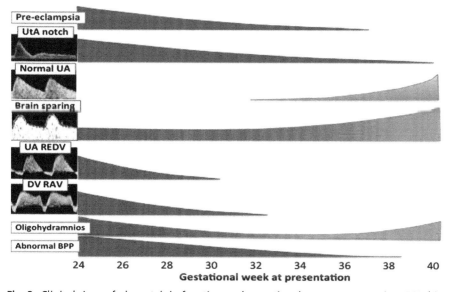

Fig. 2. Clinical signs of placental dysfunction and gestational age at presentation. BPP, biophysical profile; RAV, reversed a-wave velocity; UtA, uterine artery.

the most sensitive Doppler parameter, especially after 28 weeks of gestation, and its decrease should alert the clinician to the possibility of evolving brain sparing. Here, an SEFW less than the tenth percentile in association with either an elevated UA Doppler index, a decreased MCA Doppler index, or a decreased CPR should be considered evidence of FGR (**Table 1**).[11,12,14,16,24] The proportion of growth-restricted fetuses with normal UA blood-flow resistance but isolated MCA brain sparing is higher toward the late third trimester. Accordingly, MCA Doppler better identifies FGR after 34 weeks of gestation, when the predictive accuracy of CPR decreases.[12]

ASSESSMENT OF THE DEGREE OF FETAL DETERIORATION

Fetal surveillance tests are applied to pregnancies with suspected FGR to estimate the risk for hypoxemia, prelabor acidemia or stillbirth, as well as the rate of clinical deterioration. The required accuracy of this assessment is highest at early gestational ages, when prematurity-related risks are high and each additional day gained in utero can significantly increase chance of neonatal survival. An accurate estimation of pH is important to predict fetal compromise that precedes stillbirth and therefore critical to time delivery.

The association between the abnormalities in Doppler parameters and the deterioration of fetal acid-base status has been demonstrated in several studies,[28–31] predominantly in the preterm fetus. Abnormal umbilical flow patterns indicate an increased risk of hypoxemia and acidemia proportional to the severity of Doppler abnormality. Although Doppler findings in each of the examined vascular beds correlate with fetal acid-base status, there is a wide variation in fetal pH with abnormal results. Among Doppler parameters, the elevation of the precordial venous Doppler indices provides the best prediction of acidemia in fetuses with FGR.[31,32] Therefore, fetal Doppler assessment that is based on the UA indices alone is no longer appropriate in early-onset FGR, and the incorporation of venous Doppler is necessary to assess the rate and degree of fetal compromise. In preterm growth-restricted fetuses, MCA Doppler study has limited accuracy to predict acidemia and adverse outcome and should not be used to time delivery. Beyond 34 weeks, the UA waveform may be normal, and therefore, the best predictor of fetal adaptation to hypoxemia is considered the MCA PI. However, studies on fetal brain circulation in late-onset FGR[33,34] primarily evaluated the relationship of MCA Doppler with intrapartum fetal distress or neonatal acidosis rather than prelabor acid-base status. Accordingly, conclusions relating MCA Doppler to fetal pH are generally extrapolated.

Table 1 Implications of diagnostic cutoffs for management of fetal growth restriction		
Diagnostic Cutoff	**Advantage**	**Disadvantage**
AC <10th percentile	Highest sensitivity for FGR	Lowest specificity for FGR
SEFW <10th percentile	Acceptable sensitivity for FGR	Unnecessary monitoring of normal fetuses
SEFW <3rd percentile	Greater specificity for FGR	Less severe FGR is missed
SEFW <10th percentile & abnormal UA Doppler	Greatest specificity for FGR at risk for adverse outcome	Misses term FGR with normal UA Doppler
SEFW <10th percentile with abnormal UA or MCA	Greatest specificity for FGR at risk for adverse outcome across all gestational ages	Requires interpretation of umbilical and cerebral Doppler studies

The 5-component biophysical profile scoring (BPS) shows a reliable and reproducible relationship with the fetal pH, irrespective of gestational age.[35,36] An abnormal BPS of 4 or less is associated with a mean pH of less than 7.20 and a score of less than 2 has a sensitivity of 100% for acidemia.[36] When the relationship between the various testing modalities and fetal acid-base status is compared, biophysical parameters show a closer relationship with the pH, whereas there is a wide variation in fetal pH with abnormal Doppler results. On the other hand, the BPS alone has limited utility in the prediction of longitudinal deterioration,[37,38] which is better assessed with multi-vessel Doppler studies.

Fetal heart rate is one of the 5 components of the BPS. A nonreactive cardiotoco-gram (CTG) has been correlated with fetal hypoxemia and acidemia,[39,40] but it is associated with a wide range of pH values,[39] and as for the other components of the BPS, it does not anticipate the rate of deterioration. Computerized heart rate monitoring (cCTG) has been introduced to improve the interpretation of fetal heart rate traces, by determining quantitative parameters, such as the short-term variation, that cannot be visually assessed. In fetuses with intrauterine growth restriction, a short-term variation less than 3.5 ms appears the best predictor of an UA pH of less than 7.20.[41] However, cCTG as a stand-alone test in FGR offers limited accuracy, and it performs best when combined with venous Doppler or as a substitute for the traditional NST in the BPS.[42]

SELECTION OF MONITORING INTERVALS

The goal of fetal surveillance is to prevent stillbirth and irreversible fetal deterioration; this requires adjustment of monitoring intervals based on signs of disease accelera-tion, when delivery is not yet indicated.

With standardization of antenatal surveillance, a reduction in antenatal mortality might be achieved without worsening neonatal outcome.[3] The optimal surveillance pattern and timing of delivery remain the objects of much debate and research. There is no general consensus between national guidelines on the appropriate frequency of testing, and they are based on expert opinion of key authors because there is no high-quality evidence to guide practice.

In the authors' opinion, the best approach consists of a longitudinal surveillance starting at 24 to 26 weeks with integrated fetal testing, including multivessel Doppler examination, fetal heart rate analysis, and assessment of fetal activity through BPS, because the combination of tests improves the prediction of acidemia and stillbirth compared with single tests.[37,42–44]

Monitoring interval choice depends on gestational age at onset and signs of dete-rioration at Doppler study. When new features indicating disease acceleration or fetal deterioration develop, monitoring frequency needs to be increased until the delivery threshold is reached. Because early-onset and late-onset FGR represent 2 distinct clinical phenotypes of placental dysfunction, they show different signs of disease pro-gression. In early-onset FGR, fetal deterioration typically evolves from abnormal UA Doppler studies, to brain-sparing, abnormal venous Doppler parameters, abnormal computerized CTG, and finally, an abnormal 5-component BPS.[38,45–52] The rate of progression is determined by the interval between diagnosis to loss of UA end-diastolic velocity[49–51,53] and typically takes 4 to 6 weeks.[51] Once forward velocities in the ductus venosus (DV) become absent or reversed, fetal survival of longer than 1 week is unlikely.[54] Late-onset FGRs are characterized by a slower progression (up to 9 weeks), with predominant cerebral or UA Doppler abnormalities. There are no evident Doppler changes in the precordial veins and brain sparing may be the only observed Doppler sign of hypoxemia (see **Fig. 2**).[16,55] Importantly, however, terminal deterioration resulting in stillbirth occurs more rapidly and unanticipated in term FGR.[56] Therefore, a closer surveillance is required after 34 weeks, and new onset of Doppler abnormalities at this age should raise consideration for delivery.

The observed progression of Doppler abnormalities should determine the interval of monitoring as follows, until the threshold for delivery is reached.

Early-onset fetal growth restriction
- Elevated UA Doppler PI ($\geq$2 SDs above the mean for gestational age), no other abnormality: every 2 weeks Doppler, weekly BPS
- Low MCA PI or CPR: weekly Doppler + BPS
- UA absent end-diastolic velocity (AEDV): consider admission, 2 times per week Doppler + BPS
- UA reversed end-diastolic velocity (REDV), increased DV Doppler indices, and/or oligohydramnios (maximum vertical pocket of fluid <2 cm): admission, 3 times per week Doppler + BPS, daily CTG
- Absent/reversed DV a-wave: admission, daily Doppler + BPS, prepare for delivery

Late-onset fetal growth restriction (>34 weeks)
- Elevated UA Doppler PI ($\geq$2 SDs above the mean for gestational age), no other abnormality: weekly Doppler + BPP
- Low MCA PI or CPR: 2 to 3 times per week Doppler + BPS

PLANNING DELIVERY: GESTATIONAL AGE AS A DETERMINANT OF INTERVENTION THRESHOLDS

In pregnancies complicated by FGR, the thresholds for interventions are defined by the balance of fetal risks of continuation of pregnancy versus the neonatal risks that follow delivery. The principle neonatal risks are neonatal mortality, major neonatal morbidity, which is associated with long-term impacts on health, and adverse neonatal development. These risks change in specific gestation age epoch (**Fig. 3**, **Table 2**), and the outcome is comparable to that of appropriate for gestational age infants born at a 2-week shorter gestational age.[57] Accordingly, the threshold for delivery needs to be higher at earlier gestational age.

The neurodevelopmental outcome of growth-restricted babies has received growing attention in recent years, given the impact on quality of life.[4,58,59] In early-onset FGR, gestational age has been found to be one of the major determinants of neurodevelopment. However, it remains to be determined if interventions other than modulating disease course might improve neurodevelopment.

Taking in account the data on neonatal survival derived from 2 large observational studies (see **Fig. 3**),[3,5] the following delivery indications per gestational epoch are suggested.

24 to 26 Weeks Gestation

The survival rate of FGR neonates averages less than 50%.[5] In surviving babies, the risks for major neonatal complications are as high as 80%. With these neonatal morbidities, especially higher grades of intraventricular hemorrhage, the motor neurodevelopmental adverse outcomes are equally high. These risks gradually decrease and there is an improvement in survival by an average of 2% per gestational day that is gained in utero. The survival rates exceed 50% once the estimate of fetal weight exceeds 500 g or 26 weeks are reached. Because of these significant neonatal morbidities, delivery for fetal deterioration may not be considered in certain health care

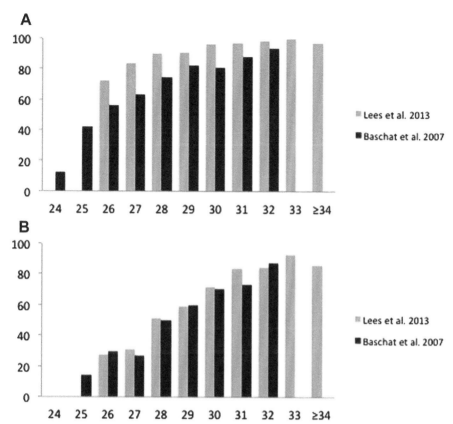

Fig. 3. Data on neonatal survival (*A*) and intact survival (*B*). (*Data from* Lees C, Marlow N, Arabin B, et al. Perinatal morbidity and mortality in early-onset fetal growth restriction: cohort outcomes of the trial of randomized umbilical and fetal flow in Europe (TRUFFLE). Ultrasound Obstet Gynecol 2013;42(4):400–8; and Baschat AA, Cosmi E, Bilardo CM, et al. Predictors of neonatal outcome in early-onset placental dysfunction. Obstet Gynecol 2007;109(2 Pt 1):253–61.)

settings. Maternal indications such as severe pre-eclampsia are the primary indications for delivery.

26 to 28 Weeks Gestation

Neonatal survival exceeds 50%. However, intact survival at 26 to 27 weeks remains around 30% (see **Fig. 3**).[3,5] Because neonatal morbidity rates are high, additional fetal deterioration before delivery does not appear to produce a statistical impact on survival. Although maternal disease remains an absolute delivery indication, fetal status may not qualify until acidemia is certain. Although an abnormal 5-component BPS (<6/10) is an indication to delivery from 26 weeks of gestation, because of its strong association with fetal acidemia, the evidence of venous Doppler abnormalities is not considered an indication to intervention until 28 weeks. The observed median time interval between the detection of abnormal venous Doppler indices and the deterioration of the BPS is 1 week,[52] which could potentially increase neonatal survival by 14% (see **Table 2**). Individualization of care in these pregnancies needs to be discussed with the patient, including the option of nonintervention.

Table 2
Management goals at different gestational ages

	24–26 wk	26–28 wk	28–30 wk	30–32 wk	32–34 wk	34–38 wk	>38 wk
Absolute delivery indications			Maternal indications, abnormal BPS				
Goal	Delay to reach viability	Delay to gain neonatal survival	Delay to improve neonatal morbidity		Delay for administration of steroids	Delay to decrease NICU admission rate	Delay not justified
Evidence	Birth-weight <500 g & gestational age <26 wk at delivery associated with >50% mortality	Each day in utero increases neonatal survival by median of 2% Fetal deterioration has no statistical impact on neonatal outcome	Each day in utero increases neonatal survival by median of 1% Reversed DV a-wave before delivery is associated with lower neonatal survival		SGA fetuses receiving prenatal steroids have lower rate of RDS, BPD, IVH, and mortality	SGA neonates delivered before 38 wk have a higher rate of NICU admission	Risks of surveillance failure, risks for progressive decline in growth, low neonatal morbidities favor delivery at 38 wk
Delivery threshold	Maternal conditions	Abnormal BPS (<6)	Reversed DV a-wave		UA REDV	UA AEDV	

Abbreviations: BPD, bronchopulmonary dysplasia; IVH, Intraventricular hemorrhage; NICU, neonatal intensive care unit; RDS, respiratory distress syndrome; SGA, small for gestational age.

28 to 32 Weeks Gestation

Neonatal survival exceeds 70% at 28 weeks and increases to more than 90% at 32 weeks (see **Fig. 3**). Survival gain per day in utero now averages 1% and neonatal mortality and morbidity progressively decrease. Fetal deterioration of venous Doppler parameters may be tolerated as long as DV a-wave velocities are antegrade. Reversal of the DV a-wave before delivery has an independent additional impact on neonatal morbidities, and persistence of this abnormality beyond 1 week carries significant risk for stillbirth. For this reason, the presence of a DV reversed a-wave is generally considered an indication to intervention from 28 weeks. However, delivery before 30 weeks gestation still carries a significantly higher risk for adverse neurodevelopment at age 2 because of neonatal complications and their impact on motor development.[4]

32 to 34 Weeks Gestation

Thirty-two to 34 weeks gestation is a time in fetal development whereby the cerebral circulation gains an additional structural layer, and, accordingly, there is a significant reduction in the rates of intraventricular hemorrhage. This reduction has measurable impact on motor development at age 3. Now, up until 34 weeks gestational age especially, the administration of antenatal steroids has an added benefit in reducing respiratory neonatal morbidity as well as intraventricular hemorrhage rates, and babies who have received steroids have improved survival. Moreover, recent evidence suggests that neurodevelopment is also improved by the administration of steroids[60]; this is most likely due to the beneficial impact on the respiratory performance and the decrease of ventilation related intraventricular bleeding.

Evidence of reversed UA end-diastolic velocity is generally considered a delivery indication from 32 weeks onward, whereas an AEDV is an indication from 34 weeks onward.

34 to 38 Weeks Gestation

At this gestational age, the gain in survival as well as neonatal morbidity is minimal; however, up to 38 weeks gestation, the rate of neonatal admissions to the intensive care nursery is still significantly greater for FGR infants, and the overall neonatal adverse outcome scores are higher. Accordingly, delivery thresholds should be based on clear maternal or fetal indications. The absence of UA end-diastolic velocity at Doppler study is considered an indication to delivery from 34 weeks onward. In late-onset FGR, the MCA Doppler is considered the best predictor of fetal adaptation to hypoxemia, and some national guidelines recommend the use of this parameter to time delivery in fetuses with normal UA Doppler.[61,62]

After 38 Weeks Gestation

Neonatal adverse events in SGA infants are negligible and, accordingly, ongoing pregnancy must be weighed carefully against the risks of unanticipated stillbirth if the patient remains undelivered. Risks of surveillance failure, risks for progressive decline in head growth, and low neonatal risks favor delivery. The Disproportionate Intrauterine Growth Intervention Study at Term (DIGITAT)[2] showed that among women with suspected intrauterine growth restriction at 36 to 41 weeks, a policy of labor induction affects neither the rate of adverse neonatal outcomes nor the rates of instrumental vaginal delivery or caesarean section, indicating that both approaches are acceptable. The consensus view from the DIGITAT is that the optimum time for induction in SGA with normal Doppler study is at around 38 weeks, because it is associated with the lowest neonatal morbidity[63] and seems to minimize the risk of stillbirth.[64]

Between 24 and 34 weeks, antenatal corticosteroids should be administered over a period of 48 hours for fetal lung maturity if delivery is being considered. At this age, delivery should be planned at a center with a neonatal intensive care unit. The route of delivery depends on the severity of fetal compromise, along with maternal condition and other obstetric factors. If prelabor acidemia is suspected, cesarean section is recommended. In FGR cases with abnormal UA Doppler, induction of labor can be offered, but rates of emergency caesarean section are increased. The use of prostaglandin for cervical preparation is usually discouraged. Because of the increased risk of intrapartum asphyxia in growth-restricted fetuses, continuous fetal heart rate monitoring is recommended from the onset of uterine contractions.

SUMMARY

Detection of FGR must be accompanied by uniform approaches to management to improve perinatal outcomes. The understanding of the clinical phenotype of early-onset and late-onset FGR is actively evolving. A decreased estimated fetal weight coupled with abnormal umbilical, MCA, or CPR studies provides the best identification of fetuses requiring surveillance. Doppler abnormalities precede biophysical deterioration and therefore allow adjustment of monitoring frequency. Concurrent deterioration of Doppler and biophysical variables best predict prelabor acidemia and therefore allow timing of delivery. The threshold for delivery is determined by the neonatal risks at each gestational epoch and decreases with advancing gestational age.

REFERENCES

1. Divon MY, Girz BA, Lieblich R, et al. Clinical management of the fetus with markedly diminished umbilical artery end-diastolic flow. Am J Obstet Gynecol 1989; 161(6 Pt 1):1523–7.
2. Boers KE, Vijgen SM, Bijlenga D, et al. Induction versus expectant monitoring for intrauterine growth restriction at term: randomised equivalence trial (DIGITAT). BMJ 2010;341:c7087.
3. Lees C, Marlow N, Arabin B, et al. Perinatal morbidity and mortality in early-onset fetal growth restriction: cohort outcomes of the trial of randomized umbilical and fetal flow in Europe (TRUFFLE). Ultrasound Obstet Gynecol 2013;42(4):400–8.
4. Thornton JG, Hornbuckle J, Vail A, et al. Infant wellbeing at 2 years of age in the Growth Restriction Intervention Trial (GRIT): multicentred randomised controlled trial. Lancet 2004;364(9433):513–20.
5. Baschat AA, Cosmi E, Bilardo CM, et al. Predictors of neonatal outcome in early-onset placental dysfunction. Obstet Gynecol 2007;109(2 Pt 1):253–61.
6. Baschat AA. Fetal responses to placental insufficiency: an update. BJOG 2004; 111(10):1031–41.
7. Meekins JW, Pijnenborg R, Hanssens M, et al. A study of placental bed spiral arteries and trophoblast invasion in normal and severe pre-eclamptic pregnancies. Br J Obstet Gynaecol 1994;101(8):669–74.
8. Morrow RJ, Adamson SL, Bull SB, et al. Effect of placental embolization on the umbilical arterial velocity waveform in fetal sheep. Am J Obstet Gynecol 1989; 161(4):1055–60.
9. Arbeille P, Maulik D, Fignon A, et al. Assessment of the fetal PO2 changes by cerebral and umbilical Doppler on lamb fetuses during acute hypoxia. Ultrasound Med Biol 1995;21(7):861–70.

10. Picklesimer AH, Oepkes D, Moise KJ, et al. Determinants of the middle cerebral artery peak systolic velocity in the human fetus. Am J Obstet Gynecol 2007; 197(5):526.e1–4.

11. Baschat AA, Weiner CP. Umbilical artery doppler screening for detection of the small fetus in need of antepartum surveillance. Am J Obstet Gynecol 2000; 182(1 Pt 1):154–8.

12. Bahado-Singh RO, Kovanci E, Jeffres A, et al. The Doppler cerebroplacental ratio and perinatal outcome in intrauterine growth restriction. Am J Obstet Gynecol 1999;180(3 Pt 1):750–6.

13. Seravalli V, Block-Abraham DM, Turan OM, et al. Second-trimester prediction of delivery of a small-for-gestational-age neonate: integrating sequential Doppler information, fetal biometry, and maternal characteristics. Prenat Diagn 2014;34(11): 1037–43.

14. Unterscheider J, Daly S, Geary MP, et al. Optimizing the definition of intrauterine growth restriction: the multicenter prospective PORTO Study. Am J Obstet Gynecol 2013;208(4):290.e1–6.

15. Parra-Saavedra M, Crovetto F, Triunfo S, et al. Association of Doppler parameters with placental signs of underperfusion in late-onset small-for-gestational-age pregnancies. Ultrasound Obstet Gynecol 2014;44(3):330–7.

16. Oros D, Figueras F, Cruz-Martinez R, et al. Longitudinal changes in uterine, umbilical and fetal cerebral Doppler indices in late-onset small-for-gestational age fetuses. Ultrasound Obstet Gynecol 2011;37(2):191–5.

17. Kovo M, Schreiber L, Ben-Haroush A, et al. The placental component in early-onset and late-onset preeclampsia in relation to fetal growth restriction. Prenat Diagn 2012;32(7):632–7.

18. Ogge G, Chaiworapongsa T, Romero R, et al. Placental lesions associated with maternal underperfusion are more frequent in early-onset than in late-onset pre-eclampsia. J Perinat Med 2011;39(6):641–52.

19. Egbor M, Ansari T, Morris N, et al. Morphometric placental villous and vascular abnormalities in early- and late-onset pre-eclampsia with and without fetal growth restriction. BJOG 2006;113(5):580–9.

20. Matsuo K, Malinow AM, Harman CR, et al. Decreased placental oxygenation capacity in pre-eclampsia: clinical application of a novel index of placental function preformed at the time of delivery. J Perinat Med 2009;37(6):657–61.

21. Parra-Saavedra M, Simeone S, Triunfo S, et al. Correlation between histological signs of placental underperfusion and perinatal morbidity in late-onset small for gestational age fetuses. Ultrasound Obstet Gynecol 2015;45(2):149–55.

22. Savchev S, Figueras F, Sanz-Cortes M, et al. Evaluation of an optimal gestational age cut-off for the definition of early- and late-onset fetal growth restriction. Fetal Diagn Ther 2014;36(2):99–105.

23. Unterscheider J, Daly S, Geary MP, et al. Predictable progressive Doppler deterioration in IUGR: does it really exist? Am J Obstet Gynecol 2013;209(6): 539.e1–7.

24. Hershkovitz R, Kingdom JC, Geary M, et al. Fetal cerebral blood flow redistribution in late gestation: identification of compromise in small fetuses with normal umbilical artery Doppler. Ultrasound Obstet Gynecol 2000;15(3):209–12.

25. Frøen JF, Gardosi JO, Thurmann A, et al. Restricted fetal growth in sudden intra-uterine unexplained death. Acta Obstet Gynecol Scand 2004;83(9):801–7.

26. Winje BA, Roald B, Kristensen NP, et al. Placental pathology in pregnancies with maternally perceived decreased fetal movement–a population-based nested case-cohort study. PLoS One 2012;7(6):e39259.

27. Divon MY, Chamberlain PF, Sipos L, et al. Identification of the small for gestational age fetus with the use of gestational age-independent indices of fetal growth. Am J Obstet Gynecol 1986;155(6):1197–201.

28. Bilardo CM, Nicolaides KH, Campbell S. Doppler measurements of fetal and uteroplacental circulations: relationship with umbilical venous blood gases measured at cordocentesis. Am J Obstet Gynecol 1990;162(1):115–20.

29. Akalin-Sel T, Nicolaides KH, Peacock J, et al. Doppler dynamics and their complex interrelation with fetal oxygen pressure, carbon dioxide pressure, and pH in growth-retarded fetuses. Obstet Gynecol 1994;84(3):439–44.

30. Hecher K, Snijders R, Campbell S, et al. Fetal venous, intracardiac, and arterial blood flow measurements in intrauterine growth retardation: relationship with fetal blood gases. Am J Obstet Gynecol 1995;173(1):10–5.

31. Rizzo G, Capponi A, Arduini D, et al. The value of fetal arterial, cardiac and venous flows in predicting pH and blood gases measured in umbilical blood at cordocentesis in growth retarded fetuses. Br J Obstet Gynaecol 1995;102(12):963–9.

32. Baschat AA, Güclü S, Kush ML, et al. Venous Doppler in the prediction of acid-base status of growth-restricted fetuses with elevated placental blood flow resistance. Am J Obstet Gynecol 2004;191(1):277–84.

33. Cruz-Martínez R, Figueras F, Hernandez-Andrade E, et al. Fetal brain Doppler to predict cesarean delivery for nonreassuring fetal status in term small-for-gestational-age fetuses. Obstet Gynecol 2011;117(3):618–26.

34. Severi FM, Bocchi C, Visentin A, et al. Uterine and fetal cerebral Doppler predict the outcome of third-trimester small-for-gestational age fetuses with normal umbilical artery Doppler. Ultrasound Obstet Gynecol 2002;19(3):225–8.

35. Ribbert LS, Snijders RJ, Nicolaides KH, et al. Relationship of fetal biophysical profile and blood gas values at cordocentesis in severely growth-retarded fetuses. Am J Obstet Gynecol 1990;163(2):569–71.

36. Manning FA, Snijders R, Harman CR, et al. Fetal biophysical profile score. VI. Correlation with antepartum umbilical venous fetal pH. Am J Obstet Gynecol 1993;169(4):755–63.

37. Baschat AA. Integrated fetal testing in growth restriction: combining multivessel Doppler and biophysical parameters. Ultrasound Obstet Gynecol 2003;21(1):1–8.

38. Baschat AA, Gembruch U, Harman CR. The sequence of changes in Doppler and biophysical parameters as severe fetal growth restriction worsens. Ultrasound Obstet Gynecol 2001;18(6):571–7.

39. Ribbert LS, Snijders RJ, Nicolaides KH, et al. Relation of fetal blood gases and data from computer-assisted analysis of fetal heart rate patterns in small for gestation fetuses. Br J Obstet Gynaecol 1991;98(8):820–3.

40. Vintzileos AM, Fleming AD, Scorza WE, et al. Relationship between fetal biophysical activities and umbilical cord blood gas values. Am J Obstet Gynecol 1991;165(3):707–13.

41. Guzman E, Vintzileos A, Martins M, et al. The efficacy of individual computer heart rate indices in detecting acidemia at birth in growth-restricted fetuses. Obstet Gynecol 1996;87(6):969–74.

42. Turan S, Turan OM, Berg C, et al. Computerized fetal heart rate analysis, Doppler ultrasound and biophysical profile score in the prediction of acid-base status of growth-restricted fetuses. Ultrasound Obstet Gynecol 2007;30(5):750–6.

43. Odibo AO, Goetzinger KR, Cahill AG, et al. Combined sonographic testing index and prediction of adverse outcome in preterm fetal growth restriction. Am J Perinatol 2014;31(2):139–44.

44. Turan S, Miller J, Baschat AA. Integrated testing and management in fetal growth restriction. Semin Perinatol 2008;32(3):194–200.
45. Arduini D, Rizzo G, Romanini C. Changes of pulsatility index from fetal vessels preceding the onset of late decelerations in growth-retarded fetuses. Obstet Gynecol 1992;79(4):605–10.
46. Harrington K, Thompson MO, Carpenter RG, et al. Doppler fetal circulation in pregnancies complicated by pre-eclampsia or delivery of a small for gestational age baby: 2. Longitudinal analysis. Br J Obstet Gynaecol 1999;106(5):453–66.
47. Hecher K, Bilardo CM, Stigter RH, et al. Monitoring of fetuses with intrauterine growth restriction: a longitudinal study. Ultrasound Obstet Gynecol 2001;18(6):564–70.
48. Senat MV, Schwärzler P, Alcais A, et al. Longitudinal changes in the ductus venosus, cerebral transverse sinus and cardiotocogram in fetal growth restriction. Ultrasound Obstet Gynecol 2000;16(1):19–24.
49. Visser GH, Bekedam DJ, Ribbert LS. Changes in antepartum heart rate patterns with progressive deterioration of the fetal condition. Int J Biomed Comput 1990;25(4):239–46.
50. Ferrazzi E, Bozzo M, Rigano S, et al. Temporal sequence of abnormal Doppler changes in the peripheral and central circulatory systems of the severely growth-restricted fetus. Ultrasound Obstet Gynecol 2002;19(2):140–6.
51. Turan OM, Turan S, Gungor S, et al. Progression of Doppler abnormalities in intrauterine growth restriction. Ultrasound Obstet Gynecol 2008;32(2):160–7.
52. Cosmi E, Ambrosini G, D'Antona D, et al. Doppler, cardiotocography, and biophysical profile changes in growth-restricted fetuses. Obstet Gynecol 2005;106(6):1240–5.
53. Baschat AA, Kush M, Berg C, et al. Hematologic profile of neonates with growth restriction is associated with rate and degree of prenatal Doppler deterioration. Ultrasound Obstet Gynecol 2013;41(1):66–72.
54. Turan OM, Turan S, Berg C, et al. Duration of persistent abnormal ductus venosus flow and its impact on perinatal outcome in fetal growth restriction. Ultrasound Obstet Gynecol 2011;38(3):295–302.
55. Hernandez-Andrade E, Stampalija T, Figueras F. Cerebral blood flow studies in the diagnosis and management of intrauterine growth restriction. Curr Opin Obstet Gynecol 2013;25(2):138–44.
56. Crimmins S, Desai A, Block-Abraham D, et al. A comparison of Doppler and biophysical findings between liveborn and stillborn growth-restricted fetuses. Am J Obstet Gynecol 2014;211(6):669.e1–10.
57. Visser GH, Bilardo CM, Lees C. Fetal growth restriction at the limits of viability. Fetal Diagn Ther 2014;36(2):162–5.
58. Baschat AA. Neurodevelopment following fetal growth restriction and its relationship with antepartum parameters of placental dysfunction. Ultrasound Obstet Gynecol 2011;37(5):501–14.
59. Arcangeli T, Thilaganathan B, Hooper R, et al. Neurodevelopmental delay in small babies at term: a systematic review. Ultrasound Obstet Gynecol 2012;40(3):267–75.
60. Sotiriadis A, Tsiami A, Papatheodorou S, et al. Neurodevelopmental outcome after a single course of antenatal steroids in preterm infants: a systematic review and meta-analysis. Obs Gynecol, in press.
61. Royal College of Obstetricians and Gynaecologists (RCOG). The investigation and management of the small-for-gestational-age fetus. Green-top Guideline No. 31. 2nd edition. 2013. Available at: https://www.rcog.org.uk/en/guidelines-research-services/guidelines/gtg31/.

62. New Zealand Maternal Fetal Medicine Network. Guideline for the management of suspected small for gestational age singleton pregnancies after 34 weeks gestation. 2013. Available at: http://www.asum.com.au/newsite/Files/Documents/Resources/NZMFM%20SGA%20Guideline_September%202013.pdf.

63. Boers KE, van Wyk L, van der Post JA, et al. Neonatal morbidity after induction vs expectant monitoring in intrauterine growth restriction at term: a subanalysis of the DIGITAT RCT. Am J Obstet Gynecol 2012;206(4):344.e1–7.

64. Trudell AS, Cahill AG, Tuuli MG, et al. Risk of stillbirth after 37 weeks in pregnancies complicated by small-for-gestational-age fetuses. Am J Obstet Gynecol 2013;208(5):376.e1–7.

Maternal Early Warning Systems

Alexander M. Friedman, MD

KEYWORDS

- Maternal early warning system • Modified early obstetric warning system
- Modified early warning criteria • Maternal morbidity • Maternal mortality

KEY POINTS

- Maternal mortality case reviews find that severe vital sign abnormalities often precede clinical recognition of critical illness.
- Early warning systems have been used in other specialties to identify patients at high risk for clinical decompensation.
- Specific early warning criteria have been developed for obstetric patients.
- Maternal early warning systems are being advocated by obstetric leadership.
- Although early warning systems are a promising strategy for improving maternal outcomes, research evidence is limited.

INTRODUCTION

The burden posed by severe morbidity and mortality during pregnancy and childbirth in the developed world has long been overlooked, and prevention has been neglected despite its vital importance in improving outcomes. As a result, recent data indicate that maternal death and severe morbidity—key indicators of population health—not only remain common[1] but are actually increasing in the United States.[2,3] Dramatic advances in neonatal and fetal care over the past 3 decades have not been matched by improved maternal care, with the Centers for Disease Control and Prevention estimating that 52,000 women suffer major morbidity annually.[2] National organizations, including the American Congress of Obstetricians and Gynecologists, American Board of Obstetrics and Gynecology, the Society for Maternal-Fetal Medicine, the Joint Commission, Amnesty International, and the Eunice Shriver Kennedy National Institute of Child Health and Human development have all recently issued recommendations to the obstetric community to increase awareness of maternal mortality and promote improved care of the mother. The failure to prioritize maternal care—a

Financial Disclosure: The author does not report any potential conflicts of interest.
Division of Maternal-Fetal Medicine, Department of Obstetrics and Gynecology, College of Physicians and Surgeons, Columbia University, 622 East 168th Street, New York, NY 10032, USA
E-mail address: amf2104@columbia.edu

Obstet Gynecol Clin N Am 42 (2015) 289–298
http://dx.doi.org/10.1016/j.ogc.2015.01.006   obgyn.theclinics.com

question of "Where is the 'M' in maternal-fetal medicine?"[4]—has led to educational, clinical, and research initiatives to improving maternal outcomes.[5] However, efforts to decrease maternal death and severe morbidity have been limited, and the only validated strategy that has emerged to systematically improve maternal outcomes is routine use of postcesarean thromboembolism prophylaxis.[6,7]

Many cases of major maternal morbidity and mortality may be preventable,[7–9] and obstetric early warning systems that alert care providers of abnormal physiologic parameters that may precede critical illness have been advocated,[7] as they may represent a means of improving clinical outcomes. Other specialties have used early warning systems to predict clinical deterioration with varying success.[10] In its 2007 triennial report on maternal death, the United Kingdom's Confidential Enquiry into Maternal Death recommended adoption of the modified early obstetric warning system (MEOWS)[11] which utilizes a combination of physiologic and neurologic parameters to identify obstetric inpatients who require urgent or emergent evaluation by a care provider. The parameters in MEOWS seek to identify patients with hypertensive disorders, hemorrhage, thromboembolism, sepsis, and cardiovascular and cerebrovascular complications, conditions that account for more than 50% of all maternal deaths and disproportionate major morbidity.[1,7,12] Given the need to implement strategies that will systematically improve maternal outcomes and the emerging interest and research literature on maternal early warning systems, this review covers the following topics:

1. The clinical rationale for early warning systems including the research literature on early alerts in other specialties
2. Clinical parameters and recommended care in maternal early warning systems
3. Research evidence supporting maternal early warning systems
4. Future directions in optimizing and validating maternal early warning systems

EARLY WARNING SYSTEMS IN OTHER SPECIALTIES

Early warning systems have been used in several specialties, primarily with the goal of identifying patients who may become critically ill and improving outcomes with early intervention. These systems are classified as either triggering systems, in which a patient is at risk based on one positive parameter, or scoring systems, in which different parameters contribute to a single numerical value and score cutoff levels predict risk.[13,14] The Pediatric Early Warning Score created by Duncan and colleagues[15] to predict actual or impending cardiopulmonary arrest in hospitalized children is shown in **Table 1**. In their cohort of more than 32,000 patients, a cutoff score of 5 was 78% sensitive and 95% specific in predicting actual or impending cardiopulmonary arrest with an area under the receiver operating characteristic (AUROC) curve of 0.90, yielding 68 true-positive and 1763 false-positive cases. Findings from their analysis show an important consideration in early warning systems: in a population with low risk for critical illness, even alert systems with test characteristics that perform relatively well may result in large numbers of false-positive cases.

Early warning systems and scores have been studied in several clinical settings including pediatrics,[14,16] general medical and surgical admission populations,[17–19] and medical[20] and surgical[21] specialties. The quality of data supporting the use of individual systems is generally poor.[22] The number of alert systems has proliferated, and studies generally lack appropriate methodology and adequate statistical powering given the relative infrequency of critical illness that may occur even in a large population. A systematic review of pediatric early warning systems found that the validity, reliability, and utility of pediatric alert criteria were weak.[13] A systematic review of early warning

Table 1
The Pediatric Early Warning Score system

Score	2	1	0	1	2
Age-specific items					
<3 mo					
HR	<90	90–109	110–150	151–180	>180
RR	<20	20–29	30–60	61–80	>80
SBP	<50	50–59	60–80	81–100	>100
3–12 mo					
HR	<80	80–99	100–150	151–170	>170
RR	<20	20–24	25–50	51–70	>70
SBP	<70	70–79	80–100	99–120	>120
1–4 y					
HR	<70	70–89	90–120	121–150	>150
RR	<15	15–19	20–40	41–60	>60
SBP	<75	75–89	90–110	111–125	>125
4–12 y					
HR	<60	60–69	70–110	111–130	>130
RR	<12	12–19	20–30	31–40	>40
SBP	<80	80–90	90–120	120–130	>130
>12 y					
HR	<50	50–59	60–100	101–120	>120
RR	<8	8–12	12–16	15–24	>24
SBP	<86	85–101	100–130	131–150	>150
General items					
Pulses	Absent	Doppler	Present	Bounding	
O2 saturation (%)	<85	85–95	>95		
Capillary refill	CRT >3	2–3	CRT <2		
LOC	<7	7–11	12–15		
Oxygen therapy	>50% or >4 L/min	Any <50% or <4 L/min	None		
Bolus fluid		Any	None		
Temperature	<35	35–<36	36	>38.5–<40	>40

The score is calculated by adding the demographic and medication subscores. Patients received 1 point for each of the following: abnormal airway (not tracheostomy), home oxygen, any previous admission to an ICU, central venous line in situ, transplant recipient, severe cerebral palsy, gastrostomy tube, and greater than 3 medical specialties involved in care. The medication subscore is from the number of medication administered in 24 hours. $\leq 3 = 0$, $4–6 = 1$, $7–9 = 2$, $9–12 = 3$, $12–15 = 4$, $\geq 16 = 5$.

Abbreviations: HR, heart rate (beats per minute); LOC, level of consciousness measured with the Glasgow Coma Scale; RR, respiratory rate (breaths per minute); SBP, systolic blood pressure (mm Hg).

From Duncan H, Hutchison J, Parshuram CS. The pediatric early warning system score: a severity of illness score to predict urgent medical need in hospitalized children. J Crit Care 2006;21:275; with permission.

systems for adults admitted to medical or surgical wards found that although predictive values for death (AUROC curve, 0.88–0.93) and cardiac arrest within 48 hours (AUROC curve, 0.74–0.86) were fairly high, the overall impact on health outcomes and resource utilization was unclear.[17] A Cochrane review of early warning systems and critical care outreach noted poor methodologic quality of most studies reviewed and a found a lack of evidence regarding the benefit of critical care outreach in studies included in the analysis.[10] For example, the medical emergency response improvement team (MERIT) study randomly selected 23 hospitals to a medical emergency team system with call parameters to see if unplanned intensive care unit (ICU) admissions, cardiac arrests, and deaths could be prevented, and found that although emergency team calling was greatly increased, there was no improvement in outcomes.[23]

Varying criteria across scoring systems and a lack of consistency in detecting deterioration of patients' conditions have been identified as major concerns[24] and led the Royal College of Physicians to design a national standard for nonpregnant adults for the United Kingdom called the National Early Warning Score (NEWS).[25] NEWS was designed to address specific concerns identified with the proliferation of different systems including: (1) varying parameters and weighting leading to unfamiliarity across hospitals or in different clinical settings within hospitals, (2) poor validation of early warning systems in detecting a broad range of acute severe illness across different clinical settings, (3) lack of clear definitions for an appropriate clinical response in the setting of a positive alert, and (4) an absence of uniform criteria to base postgraduate and undergraduate training. The NEWS parameters and scoring system are shown in **Table 2**. Based on the severity of abnormalities present, evaluation of the patient by a nurse, provider, or critical care specialist is recommended.

Although research literature on NEWS suggests it performs favorably compared with other alert systems,[26,27] its authors note that although a nationally standardized alert system may standardize care, simplify clinical management and communication, and be important for research validation, cut-points and scoring algorithms may be revised in the future.[25] Optimizing alert system performance is an important goal. A warning system that results in a large number of false-positive results relative to true cases detected early may potentially worsen clinical care, function as a nuisance alarm, and contribute to alarm fatigue. Alarm fatigue—wherein clinical providers becoming

Table 2
NEWS

Physiologic Parameters	3	2	1	0	1	2	3
Respiration rate	≤8		9–11	12–20		21–24	≥25
Oxygen saturation	≤91	92–93	94–95	≥96			
Any supplemental oxygen		Yes		No			
Temperature	≤35.0		35.1–36.0	36.1–38.0	38.1–39.0	≥39.1	
Systolic blood pressure	≤90	91–100	101–110	111–219			≥220
Heart rate	≤40		41–50	51–90	91–110	111–130	≥131
Level of consciousness				A			V, P, or U

Respiration rate (breaths per minute); Oxygen saturation (%); Temperature (degrees Celsius); Systolic blood pressure (mm Hg); Heart rate (beats per minute). Level of consciousness is based on the Alert Voice Pain Unresponsive scale, which assesses 4 possible outcomes to measure and record a patient's level of consciousness. A low score (NEWS of 1–4) should prompt an assessment by a registered nurse. A medium score (NEWS of 5–6 or any single parameter of 3) should prompt an urgent review by a clinician such as a ward-based physician or acute-team nurse. A high score (NEWS of 7 or more) should prompt emergency assessment by a critical care team with likely transfer of patient to higher acuity setting.

From National Early Warning Score (NEWS). Standardising the assessment of acute-illness severity in the NHS. London: Royal College of Physicians; 2012. Available at: https://www.rcplondon.ac.uk/sites/default/files/documents/national-early-warning-score-standardising-assessment-acute-illness-severity-nhs.pdf. Accessed December 1, 2014; with permission.

overwhelmed and desensitized to alerts of little to no clinical usefulness (nuisance · alarms) that can occur several hundred per day per patient depending on the hospital unit—is a recognized source of medical errors.[28,29] To establish the validity of an early warning system in any population (particularly in an obstetric population in which the rate of major morbidity and critical illness is low), a careful assessment of test characteristics is necessary.

MATERNAL EARLY WARNING SYSTEMS

Early warning systems to detect critical illness in obstetric patients have been specifically designed for this population because of (1) the physiologic changes that occur during pregnancy and (2) the small number of conditions responsible for most maternal severe morbidity and mortality. Recommendations for use of the NEWS include the restriction that it is not applicable to pregnant patients.[25] Adoption of maternal alert systems was strongly advocated in the 2007 *Saving Mothers' Lives* report from the Confidential Enquiries into Maternal and Child Health (CEMACH) in the United Kingdom. The report made hospital-based adoption of MEOWS a "top ten" recommendation, an urgent priority "which every commissioner, provider, policy maker and other stakeholder involved in providing maternity services should plan to introduce, and audit, as soon as possible."[30] The CEMACH report includes case reviews of maternal deaths and found that "in many cases in this Report, the early warning signs of impending maternal collapse went unrecognized."[30]

A MEOWS scoring system is shown in **Table 3**. In this system, 2 moderately abnormal parameters (yellow alerts) or 1 severely abnormal parameter (red alert) triggers a clinical response to urgently assess the patient's status and make a follow-up surveillance plan. The parameters are designed to detect patients suffering from conditions that may lead to severe maternal morbidity and mortality. In the United States, the conditions responsible for most adverse maternal outcomes include hemorrhage, venous thromboembolism, hypertensive diseases of pregnancy, sepsis, and cardiovascular causes as demonstrated in **Table 4**, which presents data on deaths from the Centers for Disease

Table 3
A modified early obstetric warning system

Physiologic Parameters	Yellow Alert	Red Alert
Respiration rate	21–30	<10 or >30
Oxygen saturation		<95
Temperature	35–36	<35 or >38
Systolic blood pressure	150–160 or 90–100	<90 or >160
Diastolic blood pressure	90–100	>100
Heart rate	100–120 or 40–50	>120 or <40
Pain score	2–3	
Neurologic response	Voice	Unresponsive, pain

Respiration rate (breaths per minute); Oxygen saturation (%); Temperature (degrees Celsius); Systolic blood pressure (mm Hg); Heart rate (beats per minute). Level of consciousness is based on the Alert Voice Pain Unresponsive scale, which assesses 4 possible outcomes to measure and record a patient's level of consciousness. Pain scores are as follows: (0 = no pain, 1 = slight pain on movement, 2 = intermittent pain at rest/moderate pain on movement). A single red score or 2 yellow scores triggers an evaluation.
From Singh S, McGlennan A, England A, et al. A validation study of the CEMACH recommended modified early obstetric warning system (MEOWS). Anaesthesia 2012;67:12–8; with permission.

Table 4
Causes of pregnancy-related death resulting in live births in the United States, 1998–2005

Condition	Deaths (%)
Pulmonary embolism	9.7
Hemorrhage	9.7
Amniotic fluid embolism	9.0
Hypertensive disorders	15.0
Infection	9.2
Anesthesia	1.2
Cardiomyopathy	13.3
Cerebrovascular accident	7.0
Cardiovascular conditions	12.5
Other/unknown	13.5

Data derived from the Centers for Disease Control and Prevention's Pregnancy Mortality Surveillance System. Maternal deaths (n = 2856) in this table resulted in a live birth. Maternal deaths associated with a stillbirth (n = 243) or with an undelivered pregnancy (n = 589) were not included.
From Berg CJ, Callaghan WM, Syverson C, et al. Pregnancy-related mortality in the United States, 1998 to 2005. Obstet Gynecol 2010;116:1302–9; with permission.

Control and Prevention's Pregnancy Mortality Surveillance System.[2,12,31] Data from state mortality reviews suggest that deaths from all of these causes may be reduced by improved care. For example, a California review found that 70% of hemorrhage deaths, 60% of preeclampsia/eclampsia deaths, and 63% of sepsis/infection deaths may have been preventable.[22] The MEOWS alert parameters may lead to detection of the following unrecognized conditions: hemorrhage (as demonstrated by hypotension and tachycardia), sepsis (fever, hypotension, tachycardia, hypoxia), venous thromboembolism (tachycardia, tachypnea, hypoxia), preeclampsia (hypertension, hypoxia), and cardiovascular complications (tachycardia, bradycardia, hypoxia, hypotension). The subsequent 2011 *Saving Mothers' Lives* report found that for many patients critically ill secondary to diagnoses such as sepsis and hemorrhage, MEOWS alerts had the potential to improve outcomes by facilitating early recognition.[7]

In the United States, the National Partnership for Maternal Safety, a national leadership group,[32] proposed a simplified early warning system adapted from MEOWS, the Maternal Early Warning Criteria (MEWC).[33] While MEOWS represents a simple scoring system, MEWC represents a trigger system. If a patient has any single abnormal parameter (**Table 5**) a prompt bedside assessment by a provider is required. The simplified MEWC parameters were chosen to minimize the rate of false alarms, facilitate implementation, and retain sensitivity, given that case reviews of maternal deaths frequently show frank vital sign abnormalities preceding recognized critical illness. Given the range of possible clinical care settings, from small nonteaching community hospitals to large quaternary referral academic centers, determining the optimal personnel and protocol response for alerts is the responsibility of the individual center. Based on the care setting, an alert response may be led by obstetric providers, anesthesiologists, hospitals, intensivists, emergency physicians, or a rapid response team.[34] Likewise, because of the varying clinical settings, outcome variables and process measures for this system have not been defined. The American Congress of Obstetricians and Gynecologists District II's Safe Motherhood Initiative, a collaboration to improve maternal outcomes in New York, a state with one of the highest mortality rates in the country, has endorsed MEWC for use in all hospitals providing obstetric services.

Table 5 MEWC	
Systolic BP, mm Hg	<90 or >160
Diastolic BP, mm Hg	>100
Heart rate, beats per minute	<50 or >120
Respiratory rate, breaths per minute	<10 or >30
Oxygen saturation, % on room air	<95
Oliguria, milliliters per hour for ≥2 h	<35
Neurologic: Maternal agitation, confusion, or unresponsiveness; Patient with preeclampsia reporting a nonremitting headache or shortness of breath	

The presence of any of the abnormal parameters above necessitates the prompt evaluation of the patient by a provider.

From Mhyre JM, D'Oria R, Hameed AB, et al. The maternal early warning criteria: a proposal from the national partnership for maternal safety. Obstet Gynecol 2014;124:782–6; with permission.

RESEARCH EVIDENCE SUPPORTING MATERNAL EARLY WARNING SYSTEMS

Emerging research literature has sought to characterize the potential benefits of maternal early warning systems. Singh and colleagues[35] assessed MEOWS parameters in an obstetric population to determine test characteristics (see **Table 3**) for screening for severe maternal morbidity. Their definition of morbidity included obstetric hemorrhage, severe preeclampsia, infection, and thromboembolism among other diagnoses. Of 673 obstetric admissions, 86 women (13%) suffered morbidity, and 200 women (30%) had a positive MEOWS screen (either 1 red alert or 2 yellow alerts). Morbidity was driven by 3 conditions—hemorrhage, pre-eclampsia, and infection—which accounted for 94% of morbidity cases. MEOWS was 89% sensitive for predicting morbidity (95% confidence interval [CI], 81%–95%) and 79% specific (95% CI, 76–82) with a positive predictive value of 39% (95% CI, 96%–99%). Although this trial demonstrated that MEOWS was reasonably sensitive for detecting morbidity, it was not designed to determine MEOWS efficacy in (1) identifying otherwise undetected acute or impending critical illness, (2) optimizing process measures related to managing morbidity (eg, time to administration of antihypertensives), or (3) improving clinically meaningful outcomes.

An analysis by Carle and colleagues[36] used early warning parameters to predict death for patients with obstetric diagnoses admitted to ICUs. This analysis found that the study model and the early warning system presented in the 2003–2005 Report on Confidential Enquiries into Maternal Deaths were highly predictive of death for ICU patients with AUROC curves of 0.96 (95% CI, 0.92–0.99) and 0.94 (95% CI, 0.88–0.99), respectively. Although these data lend support to the general validity of maternal early warning parameters being highly sensitive for critical illness and risk of death, determining the clinical benefit of early detection and intervention was outside the scope of the analysis.

Austin and colleagues[37] performed a retrospective cohort analysis of severely ill obstetric patients admitted to high-acuity units at a single referral center. Of 64 patients that met study inclusion criteria, 5 (7.6%) may have had a condition detectable by an early warning system before clinical deterioration and admission to a high-acuity setting. Given the small number of patients and the single-center design, interpretation of validity and generalizability is limited. Although the lack of data on validated outcomes improvement may lead to the clinicians questioning the value of dedicating resources to maternal early warning systems,[38] leadership has shown enthusiasm with survey research showing high rates of hospital adoption of MEOWS within the United Kingdom.[39]

DISCUSSION

Maternal early warning systems represent a promising strategy for reducing severe maternal morbidity and mortality. For a maternal early warning system to contribute to improved health outcomes, it must (1) identify patients at risk for critical illness and who benefit from timely intervention and (2) not result in such a high number of false-positive alerts that patient care is otherwise compromised. The clinical rationale for maternal early warning systems is largely based on case reviews of maternal mortality that show delayed response to abnormal vital sign parameters and other findings suggestive of acute decompensation.[7,8,30] Given the rare occurrence of maternal death in the developed world, well-powered data to assess the benefits of trends and interventions in improving safety are often limited to national vital statistics.

Limited current research evidence supports that early warning parameters may be clinically useful in identifying patients that may become critically ill or at high risk for mortality. However, these data are primarily from single centers, and further data are needed to improve generalizability and validity. Currently, no data show what the optimal responses are in particular settings to improve maternal care once an alert has been initiated. Hospitals will likely require different response protocols based on physician staffing, teaching status, bed size, nursing expertise, consultant services, and critical care availability. Furthermore, the identification of an at-risk patient does not ensure that (1) the correct diagnostic workup and evaluation will be performed in setting of a positive screening result or (2) that with the correct diagnosis, subsequent interventions will be appropriate. Given that severe maternal morbidity and mortality are rare, clinical decision support tools may be a necessary component for providing optimal responses, particularly at smaller, nonteaching centers.

Maternal early warning systems are a promising surveillance strategy designed to address the finding of multiple mortality reviews that clinical responses to acute deterioration in obstetric patients are often delayed or inadequate. These systems are increasingly being embraced and implemented by obstetric safety leadership. Future work needs to focus on refining alert parameters, optimal response strategies across clinical settings, and creating provider support tools for managing high-risk patients.

REFERENCES

1. Khan KS, Wojdyla D, Say L, et al. WHO analysis of causes of maternal death: a systematic review. Lancet 2006;367:1066–74.
2. Callaghan WM, Creanga AA, Kuklina EV. Severe maternal morbidity among delivery and postpartum hospitalizations in the United States. Obstet Gynecol 2012; 120:1029–36.
3. Berg CJ, Callaghan WM, Syverson C, et al. Pregnancy-related mortality in the United States, 1998 to 2005. Obstet Gynecol 2010;116:1302–9.
4. D'Alton ME. Where is the "M" in maternal-fetal medicine? Obstet Gynecol 2010; 116:1401–4.
5. D'Alton ME, Bonanno CA, Berkowitz RL, et al. Putting the "M" back in maternal-fetal medicine. Am J Obstet Gynecol 2012;208:442–8.
6. Clark SL, Belfort MA, Dildy GA, et al. Maternal death in the 21st century: causes, prevention, and relationship to cesarean delivery. Am J Obstet Gynecol 2008; 199:36.e1–5 [discussion 91–2.e7–11].

7. Cantwell R, Clutton-Brock T, Cooper G, et al. Saving mothers' lives: reviewing maternal deaths to make motherhood safer: 2006-2008. The eighth report of the confidential enquiries into maternal deaths in the United Kingdom. BJOG 2011;118(Suppl 1):1–203.

8. The California Pregnancy-Associated Mortality Review. Report from 2002 and 2003 maternal death reviews. Sacramento (CA): California Department of Public Health, Maternal Child and Adolescent Health Division; 2011.

9. Clark SL. Strategies for reducing maternal mortality. Semin Perinatol 2012;36: 42–7.

10. McGaughey J, Alderdice F, Fowler R, et al. Outreach and early warning systems (EWS) for the prevention of intensive care admission and death of critically ill adult patients on general hospital wards. Cochrane Database Syst Rev 2007;(3):CD005529.

11. The Confidential Enquiry Into Maternal and Child Health (CEMACH). Saving mother's lives: reviewing maternal deaths to make motherhood safer - 2003-2005. London: CEMACH; 2007.

12. Callaghan WM. Overview of maternal mortality in the United States. Semin Perinatol 2012;36:2–6.

13. Chapman SM, Grocott MP, Franck LS. Systematic review of paediatric alert criteria for identifying hospitalised children at risk of critical deterioration. Intensive Care Med 2010;36:600–11.

14. Seiger N, Maconochie I, Oostenbrink R, et al. Validity of different pediatric early warning scores in the emergency department. Pediatrics 2013;132:e841–50.

15. Duncan H, Hutchison J, Parshuram CS. The pediatric early warning system score: a severity of illness score to predict urgent medical need in hospitalized children. J Crit Care 2006;21:271–8.

16. Gold DL, Mihalov LK, Cohen DM. Evaluating the pediatric early warning score (PEWS) system for admitted patients in the pediatric emergency department. Acad Emerg Med 2014;21:1249–56.

17. Smith ME, Chiovaro JC, O'Neil M, et al. Early warning system scores for clinical deterioration in hospitalized patients: a systematic review. Ann Am Thorac Soc 2014;11:1454–65.

18. Subbe CP, Davies RG, Williams E, et al. Effect of introducing the Modified Early Warning score on clinical outcomes, cardio-pulmonary arrests and intensive care utilisation in acute medical admissions. Anaesthesia 2003;58:797–802.

19. Groarke JD, Gallagher J, Stack J, et al. Use of an admission early warning score to predict patient morbidity and mortality and treatment success. Emerg Med J 2008;25:803–6.

20. Bokhari SW, Munir T, Memon S, et al. Impact of critical care reconfiguration and track-and-trigger outreach team intervention on outcomes of haematology patients requiring intensive care admission. Ann Hematol 2010;89:505–12.

21. Patel MS, Jones MA, Jiggins M, et al. Does the use of a "track and trigger" warning system reduce mortality in trauma patients? Injury 2011;42:1455–9.

22. Gao H, McDonnell A, Harrison DA, et al. Systematic review and evaluation of physiological track and trigger warning systems for identifying at-risk patients on the ward. Intensive Care Med 2007;33:667–79.

23. Hillman K, Chen J, Cretikos M, et al. Introduction of the medical emergency team (MET) system: a cluster-randomised controlled trial. Lancet 2005;365:2091–7.

24. Patterson C, Maclean F, Bell C, et al. Early warning systems in the UK: variation in content and implementation strategy has implications for a NHS early warning system. Clin Med 2011;11:424–7.

25. National Early Warning Score (NEWS). Standardising the assessment of acute-illness severity in the NHS. London: Royal College of Physicians; 2012. Accessed December 1, 2014.
26. Smith GB, Prytherch DR, Meredith P, et al. The ability of the National Early Warning Score (NEWS) to discriminate patients at risk of early cardiac arrest, unanticipated intensive care unit admission, and death. Resuscitation 2013;84:465–70.
27. Badriyah T, Briggs JS, Meredith P, et al. Decision-tree early warning score (DTEWS) validates the design of the National Early Warning Score (NEWS). Resuscitation 2014;85:418–23.
28. Patient Safety Advisory Group. Medical device alarm safety in hospitals. Sentinel Event Alert 2013;(50):1–3.
29. ECRI Institute releases top 10 health technology hazards report for 2014. Available at: https://http://www.ecri.org/Press/Pages/2014_Top_Ten_Hazards.aspx. Accessed December 1, 2014.
30. Lewis G, editor. Saving mothers' lives: reviewing maternal deaths to make motherhood safer (2003-2005), the seventh confidential enquiry into maternal deaths in the United Kingdom. London: Confidential Enquiry into Maternal and Child Health; 2007.
31. Berg CJ, Chang J, Callaghan WM, et al. Pregnancy-related mortality in the United States, 1991-1997. Obstet Gynecol 2003;101:289–96.
32. D'Alton ME, Main EK, Menard MK, et al. The national partnership for maternal safety. Obstet Gynecol 2014;123:973–7.
33. Mhyre JM, D'Oria R, Hameed AB, et al. The maternal early warning criteria: a proposal from the national partnership for maternal safety. Obstet Gynecol 2014;124: 782–6.
34. ACOG II Safe Motherhood Initiative. Maternal Early Warning Systems. 2014. Available at: http://www.acog.org/-/media/Districts/District-II/PDFs/SMI/v2/OR-MEWS.pdf. Accessed December 1, 2014.
35. Singh S, McGlennan A, England A, et al. A validation study of the CEMACH recommended modified early obstetric warning system (MEOWS). Anaesthesia 2012;67:12–8.
36. Carle C, Alexander P, Columb M, et al. Design and internal validation of an obstetric early warning score: secondary analysis of the intensive care national audit and research centre case mix programme database. Anaesthesia 2013;68: 354–67.
37. Austin DM, Sadler L, McLintock C, et al. Early detection of severe maternal morbidity: a retrospective assessment of the role of an early warning score system. Aust N Z J Obstet Gynaecol 2014;54:152–5.
38. Mackintosh N, Watson K, Rance S, et al. Value of a modified early obstetric warning system (MEOWS) in managing maternal complications in the peripartum period: an ethnographic study. BMJ Qual Saf 2014;23:26–34.
39. Isaacs RA, Wee MY, Bick DE, et al. A national survey of obstetric early warning systems in the United Kingdom: five years on. Anaesthesia 2014;69:687–92.

Preeclampsia

Short-term and Long-term Implications

Jaimey M. Pauli, MD*, John T. Repke, MD

KEYWORDS

- Preeclampsia • Hypertension • Pregnancy • Prenatal screening
- Cardiovascular risk

KEY POINTS

- Preeclampsia is a hypertensive disease specific to pregnancy with a high risk of maternal and fetal morbidity and mortality, as well as long-term cardiovascular risks to both the patient and her child.
- The cause of preeclampsia is not fully understood, but is most likely to be abnormal placentation and release of placental factors that contribute to systemic endothelial function.
- Risk factor and biochemical/biophysical screening tests are available to approximate the risk of developing preeclampsia. Low-dose aspirin may reduce the risk of preeclampsia in high-risk patients; however, the ultimate cure remains delivery of the fetus and placenta.
- Diagnosis of preeclampsia is defined by hypertension with either proteinuria or signs of severe multiorgan dysfunction.
- Management of preeclampsia depends on gestational age at diagnosis and the presence of severe symptoms, and involves continuous maternal and fetal evaluation for worsening of disease prompting delivery. Postpartum hypertension and preeclampsia require vigilance on the part of both the medical provider and the patient to reduce morbidity.

Preeclampsia affects approximately 4% of all pregnancies[1,2] and is a major cause of maternal, fetal, and neonatal morbidity and mortality worldwide. It is a unique disease in several ways: it is one of only a small number of pathologic conditions that are specific to pregnancy; it is, by definition, a precursor of a potentially severe disease (eclampsia) but is lethal in its own right; it has had the same essential treatment (delivery) for hundreds of years; and its fundamental cause and prevention continue to elude researchers. It has recently become topical, both in mainstream and medical communities, at least in part because of its increasing incidence (25% increase in

Disclosures: None.

Division of Maternal Fetal Medicine, Department of Obstetrics and Gynecology, Penn State Milton S. Hershey Medical Center, 500 University Drive, Hershey, PA 17033, USA

* Corresponding author. 500 University Drive, H103, Hershey, PA 17033.

E-mail address: jpauli@hmc.psu.edu

Obstet Gynecol Clin N Am 42 (2015) 299–313

http://dx.doi.org/10.1016/j.ogc.2015.01.007

the United States in the last 20 years[3,4]) and severity of disease as it relates to the obesity epidemic currently facing the world.

DEFINITION

Preeclampsia is a hypertensive disease that is exclusive to pregnancy. It was traditionally defined as the triad of hypertension, proteinuria, and edema occurring after 20 to 24 weeks' gestation.[5] This definition has changed and been refined over the years as its pathology has been unraveled. Increase in systolic blood pressure of 30 mm Hg or diastolic blood pressure of 15 mm Hg is no longer part of the definition because these criteria are not predictive of adverse outcomes. Edema has also been removed from the definition, because it is too common a clinical finding during pregnancy to be clinically relevant.

It is now defined as new-onset hypertension (systolic blood pressure ≥140 mm Hg or diastolic blood pressure ≥90 mm Hg) and new-onset proteinuria after 20 weeks' gestation in a previously normotensive patient.[4] The hypertension should be documented to be persistent over 2 determinations at least 4 hours apart, unless it is greater than or equal to 160 mm Hg systolic or greater than or equal to 110 mm Hg diastolic. This severe increase may be confirmed in a shorter interval for prompt therapy. Proteinuria is defined as 300 mg of protein in 24 hours or a urine protein/creatinine ratio of 0.3 mg/dL. Urine dipstick of +1 is only to be used if the other methods are not available.

In the absence of proteinuria, preeclampsia may also be defined as new-onset hypertension with other signs of multisystem involvement (thrombocytopenia, liver dysfunction, renal insufficiency, pulmonary edema, cerebral or visual disturbances) (**Table 1**).

Preeclampsia is further divided into 2 categories: with and without severe features (**Box 1**).

Preeclampsia is part of a collection of hypertensive disorders of pregnancy, including gestational hypertension, chronic hypertension, and chronic hypertension with superimposed preeclampsia. Eclampsia (seizure associated with preeclampsia) and the HELLP (hemolysis, elevated liver enzymes, low platelets) syndrome are

Table 1 Definitions of preeclampsia		
Hypertension	**Proteinuria**	**Multisystem Involvement**
≥140 mm Hg systolic or ≥90 mm Hg diastolic	≥300 mg in 24 h	Thrombocytopenia
Previously normotensive patient >20 wk gestation	Protein/creatinine ratio ≥0.3 mg/dL	Renal insufficiency
BP measured two times at least 4 hours apart[a]	Dipstick 1+ (only if other methods not available)	Liver dysfunction
		Pulmonary edema
		Cerebral or visual disturbances

Abbreviation: BP, blood pressure.

[a] Greater than or equal to 160 mm Hg or greater than or equal to 110 mm Hg diastolic may be confirmed within minutes to facilitate treatment.

Adapted from American College of Obstetricians and Gynecologists, Task Force on Hypertension in Pregnancy. Hypertension in pregnancy. Report of the American College of Obstetricians and Gynecologists' Task Force on Hypertension in Pregnancy. Obstet Gynecol 2013;122(5):1122–31.

> **Box 1**
> **Severe features of preeclampsia**
>
> Systolic blood pressure greater than or equal to 160 mm Hg or diastolic blood pressure greater than or equal to 110 mm Hg on 2 occasions at least 4 hours apart while the patient is on bed rest
>
> Thrombocytopenia (<100,000 platelets/μL)
>
> Impaired liver function (liver enzymes levels increased to twice normal) or persistent right upper quadrant/epigastric pain unresponsive to medication and not accounted for by a different diagnosis)
>
> Progressive renal insufficiency (serum creatinine >1.1 mg/dL or doubling of creatinine level without other renal disease)
>
> Pulmonary edema
>
> Cerebral or visual disturbances
>
> *Adapted from* American College of Obstetricians and Gynecologists, Task Force on Hypertension in Pregnancy. Hypertension in pregnancy. Report of the American college of obstetricians and gynecologists' task force on hypertension in pregnancy. Obstet Gynecol 2013;122(5): 1122–31.

considered related disorders that may occur without or before the onset of documented hypertension.

Early-onset preeclampsia is defined as development before 34 weeks' gestation, and it affects up to 1% of pregnancies.[6] Compared with late-onset disease, early-onset disease is associated with increased risk of complications, especially early fetal growth restriction, intensive care, preterm delivery, and a 20-fold increased risk of maternal mortality.[6–8]

EPIDEMIOLOGY

Two-thirds of preeclampsia cases occur in otherwise healthy, nulliparous women, so there is no single most important recognizable risk factor.[1] However, there is a classic list of conditions that predispose a patient to preeclampsia (**Table 2**).[9,10]

One-third of cases in the United States are associated with obesity.[1] Studies have shown a progressive increase in risk of preeclampsia as body mass index (BMI) increases. O'Brien and colleagues[11] reported a doubling of preeclampsia risk for every increase of 5 to 7 kg/m^2 in prepregnancy BMI. Racial differences in rates of preeclampsia may to be more related to coexisting medical conditions such as hypertension. Other risk factors include unexplained fetal growth restriction, prior fetal growth restriction, prior fetal demise, molar pregnancy, and paternal contribution (although the last factor is controversial).[9–12]

PATHOPHYSIOLOGY

History has afforded many theories as to the cause of preeclampsia.[5] In ancient times, an imbalance of fluids, or humors, was thought to be linked to disease. Women were said to be porous and therefore prone to having too much fluid. The so-called wandering womb was thought to uproot itself and therefore cause problems wherever it landed (ie, the liver, spleen, or lungs). Restoring balance with lactation, menstruation, or bloodletting was the treatment of choice.

Although not formally defined in ancient times, the writings of Hippocrates have the likely first reference to eclampsia as convulsions and headache associated with

Table 2
Risk factors for preeclampsia

	Relative Risk[9]	Risk[10]
Nulliparity	3	—
Prior preeclampsia	7	—
Advanced maternal age	2	10%–40% (age >40 y)
Chronic hypertension	—	15%–40%
Chronic renal disease	—	15%–40%
Diabetes	3.5	10%–35%
Obesity	—	10%–15%
Multiple gestation	3	—
Vascular/connective tissue disorder (eg, lupus)	—	10%–20%
Antiphospholipid antibody syndrome/thrombophilia	9	10%–40%
Family history of preeclampsia	2–4	10%–15%
Patient born SGA	—	1.5-fold
Prior adverse pregnancy outcomes	—	2-fold to 3-fold

Abbreviation: SGA, small for gestational age.
Data from Duckitt K, Harrington D. Risk factors for pre-eclampsia at antenatal booking: systematic review of controlled studies. BMJ 2005;330(7491):565; and Barton J, Sibai B. Prediction and prevention of recurrent preeclampsia. Obstet Gynecol 2008;112(2):359–72.

pregnancy. Epilepsy was divided into 4 causative categories in the 1500s, one of which was the uterus. Eclampsia was defined in the early 1600s. The Frenchman Francois Mauriceau more extensively studied this disease, noting the increased risk in primigravidas, and again attributing the disease to an imbalance of humors via abnormal lochial flow or fetal death. Theories of the 1800s included cerebral congestion and toxic elements (toxemia), leading to more bloodletting and purging. The late 1800s recognized the connection between hypertension, edema, headache, and proteinuria as premonitory signs of the convulsions (ie, preeclampsia).

The twentieth century brought both good (placental disorder via abnormal spiral artery development)[13] and bad (the Hydatoxi lualba worm)[14] theories. The theory of endothelial dysfunction at the level of the placenta leading to toxin release and subsequent maternal disease was also introduced (**Fig. 1**).

At present, the most accepted theory of the pathologic cause of preeclampsia is abnormal placental development as a result of abnormal spiral artery remodeling and defective trophoblast invasion/differentiation. This process subsequently leads to a hypoperfusion/hypoxemia/ischemia sequence that causes a release of cytokines such as soluble fms-like tyrosine kinase-1 (sFlt-1) and vascular endothelial growth factor (VEGF) that induce systemic endothelial dysfunction and the systemic effects of the disease. Another corollary theory is that other immunologic factors (human leukocyte antigen [HLA] class 1 antigens, natural killer cells, antibodies to angiotensin AT 1 receptor) may play a role, supported by higher risk of preeclampsia in nulliparous patients, those who change partner, or those who have long interpregnancy intervals.[15,16]

SCREENING

Ideally, there would be a simple, accurate, low-cost test to predict who will develop preeclampsia so that an effective intervention can be initiated to improve maternal

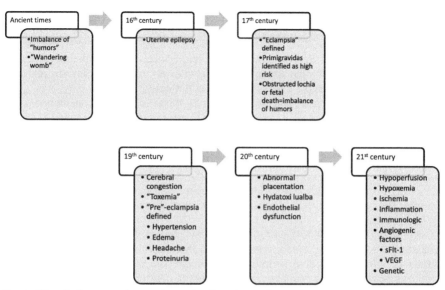

Fig. 1. Historical perspective on the pathophysiology of preeclampsia. VEGF, vascular endothelial growth factor.

and fetal/neonatal outcomes. Such a test has become something of a holy grail in obstetric research. However, all the screening tests in the world do not change the fact that the only proven intervention remains delivery. Proponents of the screening test suggest that improved antepartum surveillance, administration of antenatal steroids, and aspirin therapy are effective interventions that may alter outcomes, but knowing that a patient has an increased risk of preeclampsia in the first trimester may not fundamentally change management if the patient does develop preeclampsia.

Risk factor–based screening (see **Table 2**) is an appropriate evaluation tool when performing preconception counseling because identification of modifiable risk factors (eg, obesity) can lead to preconception intervention. Examples of this may be significant weight loss and optimization of diabetic control. This screening tool only carries a 29% to 37% detection rate, with a false-positive rate of 5% to 10%.[12,17] In addition, the risk is also related to the severity and duration of certain risk factors, such as hypertension.[10]

First trimester uterine artery Doppler velocimetry (flow wave velocity and notching) has been studied as a potential predictor of adverse perinatal outcomes, particularly preeclampsia. In a meta-analysis of more than 55,000 mostly low-risk women, abnormal flow wave velocity was specific (92%) but not sensitive (47%) for predicting early-onset preeclampsia.[6] Abnormal Doppler studies in these low-risk women increased the risk of early-onset preeclampsia from 0.4% to up to 6%. The investigators argued that initiation of low-dose aspirin therapy in this patient population has a number needed to treat of 173 to prevent 1 case of early-onset preeclampsia.[6] Another meta-analysis showed that increased pulsatility index with notching of the uterine artery Doppler in the second trimester best predicted overall preeclampsia in both low-risk and high-risk patients. Increased pulsatility index or bilateral notching best predicted the development of severe preeclampsia.[18]

Audibert and colleagues[19] studied combining maternal characteristics (gestational age, BMI, maternal age) with serum markers and uterine artery Doppler to develop a prediction model for preeclampsia in nulliparous women. In the first trimester, low levels of pregnancy-associated plasma protein A (PAPP-A), PIGF, and increased levels of inhibin A were all associated with increased risk of early and severe pre-eclampsia, with a sensitivity of 75% and false-positive rate of 10% when combined with clinical characteristics. This study did not find added benefit from first-trimester uterine artery Doppler studies. Other studies have failed to show a clinically relevant screening tool using multiple markers in the first trimester.[20]

Biochemical markers that have been studied for the prediction of preeclampsia are listed in **Box 2**. Although preeclampsia has been associated with decreased levels of angiogenic factors such as placental growth factor (PIGF) and increased levels of anti-angiogenic factors such as sFlt-1, their use as a screening tool to predict preeclampsia has not been proved.[15] Many other biomarkers secreted by the placenta, such as VEGF, PAPP-A, alpha fetoprotein, inhibin A, and A disintegrin and metalloprotease 12 (ADAM12) have been studied as predictors of preeclampsia in the first and second trimesters. The studies are mostly small and the clinical efficacy as a screening tool has not been established.[21]

Cell-free fetal DNA (cffDNA), a product of normal placental apoptosis, has also been evaluated as a screening tool for preeclampsia. Increased levels of cffDNA are noted in patients before the onset of symptoms of preeclampsia, purportedly from increased apoptosis related to placental hypoxia. To date, the clinical relevance of these levels as a predictive tool is promising but has not been adequately evaluated.[22]

DIAGNOSIS

Preeclampsia is diagnosed by new-onset hypertension ($\geq$140 mm Hg systolic or $\geq$90 mm Hg diastolic) with proteinuria after 20 weeks' gestation in a previously normotensive woman. Guidelines for accurate diagnosis include:

- Appropriate maternal positioning for blood pressure assessment (seated, resting for 5 minutes, legs not crossed, not talking)

Box 2
Potential biochemical/biophysical screening tools for preeclampsia

sFlt-1 ↑

PAPP-A ↓

Placental growth factor (PIGF)

VEGF ↑

Alpha fetoprotein (AFP) ↑

Inhibin A ↑

A disintegrin and metalloprotease 12 (ADAM12) ↑

Soluble endoglin ↑

Asymmetric dimethylarginine ↑

Serum placental protein 13 ↓

Cell-free fetal DNA (cffDNA) ↑

Uterine artery velocimetry (flow wave velocity, notching)

Data from Barton J, Sibai B. Prediction and prevention of recurrent preeclampsia. Obstet Gynecol 2008;112(2):359–72; and Goetzinger KR, Odibo AO. Screening for abnormal placentation and adverse pregnancy outcomes with maternal serum biomarkers in the second trimester. Prenat Diagn 2014;34:635–41.

- Persistence of the increased blood pressure (it is recommended that a single increased measurement be repeated to confirm that it is not isolated)

In 2013, the American College of Obstetricians and Gynecologists (ACOG) released new guidelines for hypertension in pregnancy[4] with the following updates in diagnostic criteria for preeclampsia:

- Mild preeclampsia is redefined as "preeclampsia without severe features."
- Severe preeclampsia is redefined as "preeclampsia with severe features."
- Proteinuria of greater than 5 g has been eliminated from the list of features defining severe disease.
  - This is because of lack of evidence that quantity of protein is associated with a significant change in outcomes.
- Fetal growth restriction has been removed from the list of features defining severe disease.
  - The guidelines state that management of fetal growth restriction is the same regardless of diagnosis of preeclampsia.
  - Again, in the absence of proteinuria, certain features still qualify a patient for the diagnosis of preeclampsia. These severe features are listed in **Box 1**.

Women with chronic hypertension have up to a 40% risk of developing superimposed preeclampsia.[4,23,24] This condition is generally defined as new-onset proteinuria, sudden escalation in blood pressure that was previously well controlled, or the appearance of severe symptoms (see **Box 1**).

MANAGEMENT

The ultimate management of preeclampsia (delivery) is primarily determined by 2 things: gestational age and the presence of severe features.[4] For patients who are term (≥37 weeks' gestation) at diagnosis, the recommendation is delivery. For patients with severe features, the recommendation is delivery if greater than or equal to 34 weeks' gestation. Expectant management is appropriate for certain patients if the patient is willing to undergo the risks of staying pregnant.

Expectant Management of Preeclampsia Without Severe Features

Expectant management of preeclampsia without severe features is summarized in **Fig. 2**. It involves close maternal and fetal monitoring with serum laboratory testing, fetal growth and well-being assessment, and surveillance for development of severe features. This management may occur as either an outpatient or inpatient depending on the patient's clinical status and reliability. Patients should be hospitalized and delivery considered if there is the development of any severe features, severe blood pressure increase, or abnormal fetal testing. Delivery should be effected if 37 weeks' gestation is attained, labor occurs, or there is persistent abnormal fetal testing or severe fetal growth restriction. Current evidence does not recommend strict bed rest, antihypertensive therapy for mild to moderate hypertension, or universal magnesium prophylaxis, because benefit has not been shown for these measures.

Expectant Management of Suspected Preeclampsia with Severe Features at less than 34 Weeks

Expectant management of suspected preeclampsia with severe features at less than 34 weeks is summarized in **Fig. 3**. Initial evaluation and stabilization should occur in the hospital. Continuous fetal monitoring, administration of antenatal steroids, and magnesium sulfate administration for seizure prophylaxis should occur during the

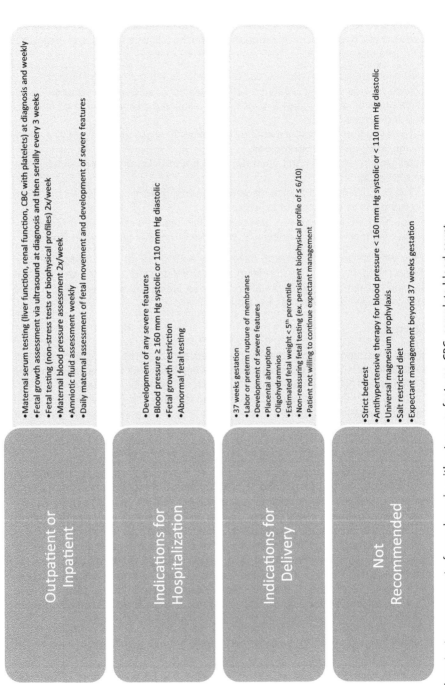

Outpatient or Inpatient
- Maternal serum testing (liver function, renal function, CBC with platelets) at diagnosis and weekly
- Fetal growth assessment via ultrasound at diagnosis and then serially every 3 weeks
- Fetal testing (non-stress tests or biophysical profiles) 2x/week
- Maternal blood pressure assessment 2x/week
- Amniotic fluid assessment weekly
- Daily maternal assessment of fetal movement and development of severe features

Indications for Hospitalization
- Development of any severe features
- Blood pressure ≥ 160 mm Hg systolic or 110 mm Hg diastolic
- Fetal growth restriction
- Abnormal fetal testing

Indications for Delivery
- 37 weeks gestation
- Labor or preterm rupture of membranes
- Development of severe features
- Placental abruption
- Oligohydramnios
- Estimated fetal weight < 5th percentile
- Non-reassuring fetal testing (ex. persistent biophysical profile of ≤ 6/10)
- Patient not willing to continue expectant management

Not Recommended
- Strict bedrest
- Antihypertensive therapy for blood pressure < 160 mm Hg systolic or < 110 mm Hg diastolic
- Universal magnesium prophylaxis
- Salt restricted diet
- Expectant management beyond 37 weeks gestation

Fig. 2. Expectant management of preeclampsia without severe features. CBC, complete blood count.

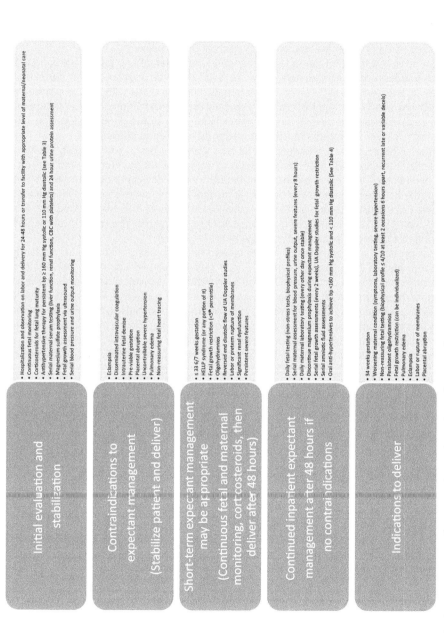

Initial evaluation and stabilization

- Hospitalization and observation on labor and delivery for 24-48 hours or transfer to facility with appropriate level of maternal/neonatal care
- Continuous fetal monitoring
- Corticosteroids for fetal lung maturity
- Antihypertensive therapy for persistent bp ≥160 mm Hg systolic or 110 mm Hg diastolic (see Table 3)
- Serial maternal serum testing (liver function, renal function, CBC with platelets) and 24 hour urine protein assessment
- Magnesium sulfate prophylaxis
- Fetal growth assessment via ultrasound
- Serial blood pressure and urine output monitoring

Contraindications to expectant management

(Stabilize patient and deliver)

- Eclampsia
- Disseminated intravascular coagulation
- Intrauterine fetal demise
- Pre-viable gestation
- Placental abruption
- Uncontrollable severe hypertension
- Pulmonary edema
- Non-reassuring fetal heart tracing

Short-term expectant management may be appropriate

(Continuous fetal and maternal monitoring, corticosteroids, then deliver after 48 hours)

- ≤ 33 6/7 weeks gestation
- HELLP syndrome (or any portion of it)
- Fetal growth restriction (<5th percentile)
- Oligohydramnios
- Reversed end diastolic flow of UA Doppler studies
- Labor or preterm rupture of membranes
- Significant renal dysfunction
- Persistent severe features

Continued inpatient expectant management after 48 hours if no contraindications

- Daily fetal testing (non-stress tests, biophysical profiles)
- Serial maternal assessment for blood pressure, urine output, severe features (every 8 hours)
- Daily maternal laboratory testing (every other day once stable)
- Discontinue magnesium prophylaxis during expectant management
- Serial fetal growth assessments (every 2 weeks), UA Doppler studies for fetal growth restriction
- Serial amniotic fluid assessments
- Oral anti-hypertensives to achieve bp <160 mm Hg systolic and < 110 mm Hg diastolic (See Table 4)

Indications to deliver

- 34 weeks gestation
- Worsening maternal condition (symptoms, laboratory testing, severe hypertension)
- Non-reassuring fetal testing (biophysical profile ≤ 4/10 at least 2 occasions 6 hours apart, recurrent late or variable decels)
- Persistent oligohydramnios
- Fetal growth restriction (can be individualized)
- Pulmonary edema
- Eclampsia
- Labor or rupture of membranes
- Placental abruption

Fig. 3. Expectant management of suspected preeclampsia with severe features (<34 weeks). UA, umbilical artery.

evaluation. Severe hypertension should be treated per protocol (**Tables 3** and **4**) and serial blood pressure, urine output, and serum laboratory assessment should occur. Patients who should not be expectantly managed include those with eclampsia, disseminated intravascular coagulation, intrauterine fetal demise, uncontrollable hypertension, placental abruption, and pulmonary edema. These patients should be stabilized and delivered. Fetal gestation age less than the institution-determined limit of viability (usually 23–24 weeks) is also an indication for delivery.

Short-term expectant management (continuous maternal and fetal monitoring with administration of antenatal steroids for 48 hours) may be appropriate for certain patients at less than 33 6/7 weeks. These patients include those with HELLP syndrome, abnormal umbilical artery Doppler studies, fetal growth restriction or oligohydramnios, and renal dysfunction. Worsening of maternal or fetal status during this period may warrant delivery regardless of the completion of the steroid course.

Continued expectant management at less than 34 weeks involves daily maternal assessment with laboratory testing, serial blood pressure monitoring, and vigilance for evolution of worsening severe features. Daily fetal assessment is also recommended with daily testing and serial growth, fluid, and Doppler assessment. Some patients may be managed with oral antihypertensives (see **Table 4**) to achieve blood pressure less than 160/110 mm Hg. Magnesium seizure prophylaxis should be discontinued during this period of expectant management.

For patients with preeclampsia with severe features being managed expectantly, delivery should occur by 34 weeks. Earlier delivery should occur for worsening of the maternal or fetal condition. Change in symptoms, laboratory testing, or ability to control hypertension in the patient should prompt delivery. Nonreassuring fetal testing, persistent oligohydramnios, and labor are fetal indications for delivery. Development of eclampsia, placental abruption, or pulmonary edema must be addressed immediately, the patient stabilized, and then the patient should be delivered. Management of fetal growth restriction in the context of severe preeclampsia is likely to require early delivery as well, but management may be individualized.

Intrapartum Management of Preeclampsia

Induction of labor for vaginal delivery is generally recommended for otherwise stable patients with a vertex fetus and no other obstetric contraindications. The likelihood of

Table 3
Acute antihypertensive therapy for severe hypertension

Drug	Dosage	Adverse Effects
Labetalol	10–20 mg IV initially, then 20–80 mg IV every 10–30 min up to a total of 300 mg 1–2 mg/min IV infusion	Bronchoconstriction Do not use in asthma or heart failure
Hydralazine	5 mg IV or IM, then 5–10 mg IV every 20–40 min, 0.5–10 mg/h IV infusion	Hypotension Headache Fetal distress
Nifedipine	10–20 mg orally Repeat in 30 min if needed, then 10–20 mg orally every 2–6 h	Reflex tachycardia Headache

Abbreviations: IM, intramuscular; IV, intravenous.

Data from American College of Obstetricians and Gynecologists, Task Force on Hypertension in Pregnancy. Hypertension in pregnancy. Report of the American College of Obstetricians and Gynecologists' Task Force on Hypertension in Pregnancy. Obstet Gynecol 2013;122(5):1122–31.

Table 4 Oral antihypertensive therapy	
Labetalol	200 to 2400 mg/d 2 or 3 divided doses
Nifedipine	10 to 20 mg every 6 hours 30 to 120 mg daily (slow release)
Methyldopa	0.5 to 3 g/d 2 or 3 divided doses
Thiazide diuretics	Dose depends on formulation Second-line agent

Data from American College of Obstetricians and Gynecologists, Task Force on Hypertension in Pregnancy. Hypertension in pregnancy. Report of the American College of Obstetricians and Gynecologists' Task Force on Hypertension in Pregnancy. Obstet Gynecol 2013;122(5):1122–31.

cesarean increases with decreasing gestational age (93%–97% for <28 weeks, 53%–65% for 28–32 weeks, and 31%–38% at 32–34 weeks' gestation)[25] and the patient's wishes as well as maternal and fetal condition must be taken into account.

Universal magnesium prophylaxis for all patients with preeclampsia with severe features is recommended during labor and for 24 hours postpartum. Any patient with eclampsia should receive an intravenous magnesium bolus of 4 to 6 g with 1 to 2 g/h maintenance for at least 24 hours. For patients with preeclampsia without severe features, universal magnesium prophylaxis is not recommended because of lack of evidence that it significantly prevents eclamptic seizures or development of severe preeclampsia. This evidence was based on small, poorly powered studies.[26,27] However, patients without severe features may progress in disease during labor and in the postpartum period, and should be carefully monitored with blood pressures, laboratory assessments, and clinical symptoms for development of severe features, and started on magnesium as indicated.

Postpartum Management

An area that has received increased attention recently is postpartum hypertension, the most common cause of which is gestational hypertension/preeclampsia or chronic hypertension.[4] This condition may be caused by persistence of the antenatal hypertensive disorder, or is also potentially a de novo postpartum condition, leading to the conclusion that delivery is not necessarily the immediate cure that it has previously been claimed to be. The potential complications of postpartum hypertension and preeclampsia are serious and can be life threatening, and include eclamptic seizure, stroke, congestive heart failure, renal failure, and permanent disability. The risk of this may persist for 4 weeks postpartum. Therefore, emphasis has shifted to continue close monitoring of patients with preeclampsia for a longer period of time, as well as patient and provider education regarding the signs and symptoms of postpartum hypertension/preeclampsia.

Current recommendations take into account that blood pressure that initially decreases after delivery may increase 3 to 6 days postpartum in patients with preeclampsia or other hypertensive disorders. The current hypertension guidelines suggest blood pressure monitoring for 72 hours postpartum and then again 7 to 10 days postpartum as well. Patients should be evaluated for other causes of hypertension (eg, thyroid disease, adrenal disease, cardiomyopathy, lupus, hemolytic uremic syndrome) Patients with persistent postpartum hypertension beyond 24 hours should have any medications that could be exacerbating blood pressure (eg, vasoconstrictive medications, nonsteroidal antiinflammatory drugs) discontinued. Patients who have signs or symptoms of preeclampsia or HELLP syndrome should be treated with magnesium prophylaxis for 24 hours. In addition, antihypertensives should be started for persistent blood pressures greater than or equal to 150 mm Hg systolic or greater than or equal to 100 mm Hg diastolic.[4,28] Examples of appropriate antihypertensive regimens are listed in **Table 4**.

Prevention of preeclampsia

Multiple studies have explored potential therapies for prevention of preeclampsia, including various antioxidant vitamins, calcium, and aspirin, as well as bed rest and activity restriction. No single therapy has proved to be overwhelmingly effective, but currently low-dose aspirin, as an antiplatelet and antiinflammatory agent, is the favorite. The proposed mechanism is the improvement in the disruption of the prostacyclin-thromboxane balance, reducing thromboxane-mediated vasoconstriction, as well an improvement in placental perfusion and reduction in ischemia-mediated endothelial damage.[29]

Several small studies showed reduced risk of preeclampsia and fetal growth restriction in high-risk patients (eg, prior preeclampsia, chronic hypertension, renal disease, diabetes) with low-dose aspirin (50–150 mg daily) given during pregnancy.[30,31] The large, randomized studies that followed did not show a significant benefit (although a trend was seen), but several meta-analyses pooling the available data do support the use of daily low-dose aspirin for prevention of preeclampsia and fetal growth restriction in high-risk women before 16 weeks. Risk reduction is reported as 10% to 20%.[10,29,32,33] The current recommendation from ACOG is to offer low-dose aspirin (60–80 mg daily starting in the late first trimester) to women with a prior birth at less than 34 weeks caused by preeclampsia or more than 1 prior pregnancy with preeclampsia, the justification of which is the low rate of adverse events from low-dose aspirin and low number needed to treat (depending on the study, as low as about 50) to prevent 1 case of preeclampsia.[4]

LONG-TERM RISKS

Cardiovascular disease is the number 1 cause of mortality in the United States.[34] Women with a history of preeclampsia have an increased risk of cardiovascular disease later in life, particularly if they have a history of early-onset, severe, or recurrent preeclampsia.[35] Gestational age at onset seems to be more significant than severity of disease, because patients in the early-onset group have the highest risk. Overall, preeclampsia leads to a 4-fold increase in risk for chronic hypertension and 2-fold increase in stroke (fatal and nonfatal), venous thromboembolism, and ischemic heart disease, as well as an increased risk of death.[35]

Women with prior preeclampsia have also been shown to have a higher number of white matter lesions years after the index pregnancy.[36] The association of these white matter lesions with posterior reversible encephalopathy syndrome or neurologic symptoms during the pregnancy was less clear. This group of women was also noted to have higher blood pressure years after the pregnancy compared with women with normotensive pregnancies, supporting prior data linking hypertension and white matter lesions in older populations. Visual disturbances affecting quality of life have been elucidated 10 years after pregnancy. An even longer-reaching risk is the finding that children of women with preeclampsia have higher blood pressure and an increased risk of stroke.[34]

Endothelial damage caused by preeclampsia may be the initial event that triggers the development of atherosclerosis later in life. In addition, patients with preeclampsia have higher levels of triglycerides and low-density lipoprotein cholesterol than normal pregnancies, as well as longer persistence of insulin resistance in the postpartum period.[34] These factors may also contribute to increased risk of cardiovascular disease and diabetes in later life. Other associations between future cardiovascular disease and preeclampsia include common genetic and pathologic influences such as obesity, metabolic syndrome, and renal disease that are known risk factors for preeclampsia.

RECURRENCE RISK

Recurrence rates of preeclampsia range widely, from 15% to 65%, likely because of the heterogeneity of the patient populations studied.[37–40] Women with severe preeclampsia in the second trimester are at increased risk of repeat preeclampsia, recurrence in the second trimester, chronic hypertension, and morbidity and mortality.[37] The recurrence risk in women with a history of early-onset preeclampsia has been shown to be related to chronic hypertension but not severity of the symptoms of the initial pregnancy.[38] Bramham and colleagues[39] identified risk factors for recurrent preeclampsia as black or Asian race, systolic blood pressure of greater than 130 mm Hg, current antihypertensive use, baseline proteinuria, and prior delivery at less than 34 weeks. Obese and overweight women are also at increased risk of recurrent preeclampsia.[40] Recurrence risk has also been shown to be inversely proportional to the gestational age at delivery of the index pregnancy.[40]

SUMMARY

Preeclampsia has threatened gravid patients and challenged the medical community since ancient times. Clinicians currently have a reasonable understanding of how to stratify patients based on risk of the disease or its recurrence as well as clear-cut guidelines for diagnosis. However, there are limited measures to offer in the way of prevention, and the fundamental cure beyond delivery continues to be elusive. Management of preeclampsia remains a challenge, because continuation of pregnancy for amelioration of prematurity of the fetus places the mother at ever increasing risk of potentially permanent or life-threatening complications. However, it is certain that constant vigilance is essential throughout antepartum, intrapartum, and postpartum care for signs and symptoms of development of the disease. Once the diagnosis has been made, it is the responsibility of the health care provider and the patient to continuously reevaluate the clinical status of both the patient and the fetus so that effective intervention can be made to bring about safe outcomes.

REFERENCES

1. Creasy RK. Creasy and Resnik's Maternal-Fetal Medicine: Principles and Practice: Expert Consult Premium Edition. 7th edition. Philadelphia: Elsevier Saunders; 2013.
2. Ananth CV, Keyes KM, Wapner RJ. Pre-eclampsia rates in the United States, 1980-2010: age-period-cohort analysis. BMJ 2013;347:f6564.
3. Wallis AB, Saftlas AF, Hsia J. Secular trends in the rates of preeclampsia, eclampsia, and gestational hypertension, United States, 1987-2004. Am J Hypertens 2008;21:521–6.
4. American College of Obstetricians and Gynecologists, Task Force on Hypertension in Pregnancy. Hypertension in pregnancy. Report of the American College of

Obstetricians and Gynecologists' Task Force on Hypertension in Pregnancy. Obstet Gynecol 2013;122(5):1122–31.

5. Bell MJ. A historical view of preeclampsia-eclampsia. J Obstet Gynecol Neonatal Nurs 2010;39:510–8.

6. Velauthar L, Plana MN, Kalidindi M, et al. First-trimester uterine artery Doppler and adverse pregnancy outcome: a meta-analysis involving 55 974 women. Ultrasound Obstet Gynecol 2014;43:500–7.

7. Crispi F, Llurba E, Domínguez C, et al. Predictive value of angiogenic factors and uterine artery Doppler for early- versus late-onset pre-eclampsia and intrauterine growth restriction. Ultrasound Obstet Gynecol 2008;31:303–9.

8. von Dadelszen P, Menzies JM, Payne B, et al. Predicting adverse outcomes in women with severe pre-eclampsia. Semin Perinatol 2009;33:152–7.

9. Duckitt K, Harrington D. Risk factors for pre-eclampsia at antenatal booking: systematic review of controlled studies. BMJ 2005;330(7491):565.

10. Barton J, Sibai B. Prediction and prevention of recurrent preeclampsia. Obstet Gynecol 2008;112(2):359–72.

11. O'Brien TE, Ray JG, Chan WS. Maternal body mass index and the risk of preeclampsia: a systematic overview. Epidemiology 2003;14(3):368.

12. Poon LC, Kametas NA, Chelemen T, et al. Maternal risk factors for hypertensive disorders in pregnancy: a multivariate approach. J Hum Hypertens 2010;24(2):104–10.

13. Meekins JW, Ijnenbor RP, Anssen MH, et al. A study of placental bed spiral arteries and trophoblast invasion in normal and severe pre-eclamptic pregnancies. BJOG 1994;101:669–74.

14. Ayala AR, Rodríguez de la Fuente F, Díaz Loya F, et al. Evidence that a toxemia-related organism (Hydatoxi lualba) is an artifact. Obstet Gynecol 1986;67(1):47–50.

15. Widmer M, Villar J, Benigni A, et al. Mapping the theories of preeclampsia and the role of angiogenic factors: a systemic review. Obstet Gynecol 2007;109:168–80.

16. McKeeman GC, Ardill JE, Caldwell CM, et al. Soluble vascular endothelial growth factor receptor-1 (sFlt-1) is increased throughout gestation in patients who have preeclampsia develop. Am J Obstet Gynecol 2004;191:1240–6.

17. North RA, McCowan LM, Dekker GA. Clinical risk prediction for pre-eclampsia in nulliparous women: development of model in international prospective cohort. BMJ 2011;342:d1875.

18. Cnossen JS, Morris RK, ter Riet G, et al. Use of uterine artery Doppler ultrasonography to predict pre-eclampsia and intrauterine growth restriction: a systematic review and bivariable meta-analysis. CMAJ 2008;178(6):701–11.

19. Audibert F, Boucoiran I, An N, et al. Screening for preeclampsia using first-trimester serum markers and uterine artery Doppler in nulliparous women. Am J Obstet Gynecol 2010;203:383.e1–8.

20. Myatt L, Clifton RG, Roberts JM, et al. First-trimester prediction of preeclampsia in nulliparous women at low risk. Obstet Gynecol 2012;119:1234–42.

21. Goetzinger KR, Odibo AO. Screening for abnormal placentation and adverse pregnancy outcomes with maternal serum biomarkers in the second trimester. Prenat Diagn 2014;34:635–41.

22. Martin A, Krishna I, Martina B, et al. Can the quantity of cell-free fetal DNA predict preeclampsia: a systematic review. Prenat Diagn 2014;34:685–91.

23. Sibai BM, Lindheimer M, Hauth J, et al. Risk factors for preeclampsia, abruption placentae, and adverse neonatal outcomes among women with chronic

hypertension. National Institute of Child Health and Human Development network of maternal-fetal medicine units. N Engl J Med 1998;339:667–71.

24. Ferrer RL, Sibai BM, Mulrow CD, et al. Management of mild chronic hypertension during pregnancy: a review. Obstet Gynecol 2000;96:849–60.

25. Sibai BM. Evaluation and management of severe preeclampsia before 34 weeks' gestation. Am J Obstet Gynecol 2011;205(3):191–8.

26. Sibai BM. Magnesium sulfate prophylaxis in preeclampsia: lessons learned from recent trials. Am J Obstet Gynecol 2004;190:1520–6.

27. Cahill AG, Macones GA, Odibo AO, et al. Magnesium for seizure prophylaxis in patients with mild preeclampsia. Obstet Gynecol 2007;110:601–7.

28. Sibai BM. Etiology and management of postpartum hypertension-preeclampsia. Am J Obstet Gynecol 2012;206(6):470–5.

29. Bujold E, Roberge S, Lacasse Y, et al. Prevention of preeclampsia and intrauterine growth restriction with aspirin started in early pregnancy: a meta-analysis. Am J Obstet Gynecol 2010;116(2):402–14.

30. Wallenburg HC, Dekker GA, Makovitz JW, et al. Low-dose aspirin prevents pregnancy induced hypertension and pre-eclampsia in angiotensin-sensitive primigravidae. Lancet 1986;1:1–3.

31. Schiff E, Peleg E, Goldenberg M, et al. The use of aspirin to prevent pregnancy-induced hypertension and lower the ratio of thromboxane A2 to prostacyclin in relatively high risk pregnancies. N Engl J Med 1989;321:351–6.

32. Trivedi NA. A meta-analysis of low-dose aspirin for prevention of preeclampsia. J Postgrad Med 2011;57:91–5.

33. Coomarasamy A, Honest H, Papaioannou S, et al. Aspirin for prevention of preeclampsia in women with historical risk factors: a systematic review. Obstet Gynecol 2003;1010(6):1319–32.

34. Ahmed R, Dunford J, Mehran R, et al. Pre-eclampsia and future cardiovascular risk among women: a review. J Am Coll Cardiol 2014;63:1815–22.

35. Bellamy L, Casas JP, Hingorani AD, et al. Pre-eclampsia and risk of cardiovascular disease and cancer in later life: systematic review and meta-analysis. BMJ 2007;335(7627):974.

36. Aukes A, De Groot J, Wiegman M, et al. Long-term cerebral imaging after pre-eclampsia. BJOG 2012;119:1117–22.

37. Sibai BM, Mercer B, Sarinoglu C. Severe preeclampsia in the second trimester: recurrence risk and long-term prognosis. Am J Obstet Gynecol 1991;165(5 Pt 1):1408.

38. van Rijn BB, Hoeks LB, Bots ML, et al. Outcomes of subsequent pregnancy after first pregnancy with early-onset preeclampsia. Am J Obstet Gynecol 2006; 195(3):723.

39. Bramham K, Briley AL, Seed P, et al. Adverse maternal and perinatal outcomes in women with previous preeclampsia: a prospective study. Am J Obstet Gynecol 2011;204(6):512.e1.

40. Mostello D, Kallogjeri D, Tungsiripat R, et al. Recurrence of preeclampsia: effects of gestational age at delivery of the first pregnancy, body mass index, paternity, and interval between births. Am J Obstet Gynecol 2008;199(1):55.e1.

Cardiac Disease in Pregnancy

Manisha Gandhi, MD[a], Stephanie R. Martin, DO[b],*

KEYWORDS

- Cardiac disease • Pregnancy • Valvular disease • Congenital heart disease

KEY POINTS

- Physiologic changes in pregnancy can place extra demands on cardiac function.
- Preconception counseling is key to improving pregnancy outcomes.
- The most commonly encountered cardiac events are pulmonary edema and dysrhythmias.
- A team approach to antepartum care is recommended and should include maternal-fetal medicine, cardiology, and anesthesia as indicated, particularly for patients with congenital cardiac disease.

INTRODUCTION

Cardiac disease complicates approximately 4% of all pregnancies in the United States; however, these patients are at a disproportionately increased risk for maternal deaths (10%–25%).[1,2] Congenital cardiac lesions are 3 times more common than acquired, adult-onset abnormalities in pregnant patients. Intensive care unit (ICU) admissions because of maternal cardiac disease comprise up to 15% of obstetric ICU admissions, but these patients account for up to 50% of all maternal deaths in the ICU.[3–9] The incidence of acute coronary events is also increasing in pregnancy because of older childbearing age along with a higher incidence of hypertension and obesity in women.[10]

Common complaints of normal pregnancy, such as dyspnea, fatigue, palpitations, orthopnea, and pedal edema, mimic symptoms of worsening cardiac disease and can create challenges for clinicians when evaluating pregnant patients with cardiac disease. Nevertheless, these patients are at risk of developing cardiac decompensation and adverse pregnancy outcomes based on the type of cardiac lesion. Pregnancy can have a negative influence on systolic and diastolic function in women with structural heart disease, which can persist 6 months after pregnancy.[11]

Disclosure: The authors have nothing to disclose.
[a] Division of Maternal-Fetal Medicine, Department of Obstetrics & Gynecology, Baylor College of Medicine, Texas Children's Pavilion for Women, 6651 Main Street Suite F1096, Houston, TX 77030, USA; [b] Maternal Fetal Medicine Services St Francis Medical Center/Centura Southstate, Southern Colorado Maternal Fetal Medicine, 6071 E Woodmen Road Suite 440, Colorado Springs, CO 80919, USA
* Corresponding author.
E-mail address: smartin@southerncoloradomfm.com

PHYSIOLOGIC CHANGES OF SINGLETON PREGNANCY

Comprehensive understanding of the normal physiologic adaptations to pregnancy is essential to the successful management of patients with cardiac disease. Conditions that may be asymptomatic while nonpregnant can deteriorate in the pregnant state. **Box 1** outlines key physiologic changes in a normal singleton gestation. Multiple gestations can be expected to have more dramatic physiologic changes.

COUNSELING THE PATIENT

Establishing baseline cardiac function is essential for pregnant cardiac patients. Functional status for patients with cardiac disease is commonly classified according to the New York Heart Association (NYHA) classification system, as outlined in **Box 2**. Patients in NYHA class I or II have less risk of complications compared with those in class III or IV.[12] **Box 3** classifies various cardiac abnormalities according to maternal death risk estimates; however, the patient's particular history is not included in these estimates.[13]

In a recent study of almost 600 pregnancies complicated by maternal cardiac disease, the investigators created a risk score to predict the likelihood of a maternal cardiovascular event in the presence of specific predictors for maternal complications[14]: **Box 4** outlines risk prediction according to the cardiac disease in pregnancy (CARPREG) risk score.

The most commonly encountered cardiac events are pulmonary edema and dysrhythmias. One large, multinational study of more than 1300 patients with cardiac disease showed that the most common obstetric complication is gestational hypertension or preeclampsia.[15] Maternal mortality is of highest risk for patients with coronary artery disease, pulmonary hypertension, endocarditis, cardiomyopathy, and dysrhythmias.[16,17]

Neonatal complications include small-for-gestational-age infants, delivery before 34 weeks' gestation, and neonatal death.[18] Fetal mortality approaches 2% in pregnancies with maternal heart disease.[15] Structural cardiac anomalies (excluding autosomal dominant disorders) occur in 2% to 18% of fetuses born to patients with a history of congenital cardiac disease. Therefore fetal echocardiogram is recommended for all pregnant patients with structural cardiac defects.

Even after delivery, these patients remain at high risk for complications in the postpartum period, with approximately 10% to 15% having at least 1 episode of heart failure during or after pregnancy.[15] In one study of 100 patients, postpartum complications were seen in about 4% of NYHA I/II patients and in 27% of NYHA III/IV patients.[19]

Preconception care
- Baseline evaluation of cardiac function.
- Counseling regarding pregnancy risk for mother and fetus.
- Consultation with cardiologist and maternal-fetal medicine specialist, if possible.
- Review of current medications to determine appropriateness of continuing during pregnancy.
- Routine preconception care as for all patients: assessment of immunization status, screening for genetic diseases as indicated, supplemental folic acid.

Antepartum care
- A team approach to antepartum care is recommended and should include maternal-fetal medicine, cardiology, and anesthesia as indicated, particularly for patients with congenital cardiac disease.
- Patients should be evaluated regularly for signs and symptoms of cardiac decompensation.
- Fetal echocardiogram between 20 and 24 weeks' gestation is indicated in the presence of congenital heart disease in mother.

Box 1
Expected physiologic changes occurring the antepartum, intrapartum, and postpartum periods

Antepartum

- Blood volume increases by 20% to 50%
- In nonpregnant women total blood volume is ~60 to 70 mL/kg
- Systemic vascular resistance decreases by 20%
  - Accounts for most of the reduction in blood pressure (BP).
  - Accommodates increase in circulating volume without increase in BP.
- BP (taken in sitting position)
  - BP greater than or equal to 140/90 mm Hg abnormal at any time in gestation.
  - BP decreases to lowest point at 28 wk.
  - After 28 wk, BP increases to nonpregnant level by term.
- Mean arterial pressure unchanged
- Heart rate increases by 10 to 15 beats per minute (bpm)
- Stroke volume increases by 30%
- Cardiac output (CO) increases by 30% to 50%
  - CO = heart rate × stroke volume. Most of the increase is from stroke volume.
  - Half of the expected increase occurs by 8 wk.
  - Peaks end of second trimester, sustained to term.
  - 6 L/min by term.
- Pulmonary capillary wedge pressure (preload to left heart) unchanged
- Central venous pressure (preload to right heart) unchanged
- Pulmonary vascular resistance decreases 30%
- Hypercoagulable state
  - Increased fibrinogen.
  - Platelets unchanged.
- Dilutional anemia despite 30% increase in red cell mass

Intrapartum

- During a contraction:
  - 300 to 500 mL of blood enters circulation.
  - Heart rate increases.
  - CO increases by 30%.
  - BP increases by 10 to 20 mm Hg.
- Supine position may decrease CO by 20%

Postpartum

- Postpartum diuresis between days 2 and 5
- CO increases by 50% in the immediate postpartum period
- Stroke volume increases 60% in the immediate postpartum period
- Reflex bradycardia occurs (15%)
- These changes persist for 2 wk after delivery

Box 2
NYHA functional classification system

Class I	No limitations of physical activity. Ordinary physical activity does not precipitate cardiovascular symptoms such as dyspnea, angina, fatigue, or palpitations
Class II	Slight limitation of physical activity. Ordinary physical activity precipitates cardiovascular symptoms. Patients are comfortable at rest
Class III	Less than ordinary physical activity precipitates symptoms that markedly limit activity. Patients are comfortable at rest
Class IV	Patients have discomfort with any physical activity. Symptoms are present at rest

Box 3
Maternal mortality associated with pregnancy

Group 1: Mortality less than 1%

  Atrial septal defect

  Ventricular septal defect

  Patent ductus arteriosus

  Mitral stenosis: NYHA classes I and II

  Pulmonic/tricuspid valve disease

  Corrected tetralogy of Fallot

  Bioprosthetic valve

Group 2: Mortality 5% to 15%

  2A

    Mitral stenosis: NYHA class III and IV

    Aortic stenosis

    Coarctation of aorta without valvular involvement

    Uncorrected tetralogy of Fallot

    Previous myocardial infarction

    Marfan syndrome with normal aorta

  2B

    Mitral stenosis with atrial fibrillation

    Artificial valve

Group 3: mortality 25% to 50%

  Pulmonary hypertension

    Primary

    Eisenmenger syndrome

  Coarctation of aorta with valvular involvement

  Marfan syndrome with aortic involvement

  Peripartum cardiomyopathy with persistent left ventricular dysfunction

Adapted from Clark SL, Phelan JP, Cotton DB, editors. Critical care obstetrics: structural cardiac disease in pregnancy. Oradell (NJ): Medical Economics Company; 1987.

Box 4
Risk prediction according to the CARPREG risk score

CARPREG risk score: predictors of maternal cardiovascular events
  NYHA functional class greater than II
  Cyanosis (room air saturation <90%)
  Prior cardiovascular event
  Systemic ventricular ejection fraction less than 40%
  Left heart obstruction
For each CARPREG predictor that is present, a point is assigned.

Risk estimation of maternal cardiovascular complications

No. of predictors	Risk of cardiac event in pregnancy (%)
0	5
1	27
>1	75

- Periodic ultrasonography to assess fetal growth.
- Antepartum fetal surveillance starting at 30 to 34 weeks if there are concerns for fetal growth restriction or maternal complications.

Labor and delivery care

- Attention to input and output. Maintain all intravenous (IV) fluids on a pump.
- Avoid supine positioning.
- Supplemental oxygen.
- Cesarean delivery is not routinely recommended in the setting of maternal cardiac disease.
- Endocarditis prophylaxis is no longer recommended for any genitourinary procedures, even in patients with the highest risk lesions.[20]

Table 1 outlines anesthetic considerations for specific cardiac lesions.

VALVULAR CARDIAC DISEASE

Valvular abnormalities may be congenital or acquired. However, most lesions are acquired secondary to rheumatic fever, which accounts for 90% of cardiac disorders in pregnancy worldwide. Heart failure is the most common complication and patients with valvular heart disease have a higher mortality than those with congenital heart disease.[12] The degree of risk for the development of complications (particularly dysrhythmias and pulmonary edema) depends on the specific valve lesion, number of valves involved, and the degree of valvular obstruction, particularly of the mitral and aortic valves. The mitral valve is most commonly affected, followed in order of decreasing frequency by the aortic, tricuspid, and pulmonic valves. Mitral stenosis carries the greatest potential for problems during pregnancy.

Potential complications include right heart failure if there is evidence of severe obstruction. No medical therapy or anticoagulation is typically recommended.

PULMONIC AND TRICUSPID LESIONS

Pulmonic stenosis/regurgitation and tricuspid stenosis/regurgitation are both typically well tolerated in pregnancy with minimal risk of right heart failure, and are rarely of any consequence in pregnancy.

Table 1
Anesthesia and cardiac lesions

Cardiac Lesion	Anesthesia
Pulmonic and tricuspid lesions	Epidural acceptable
Mitral stenosis	Epidural acceptable: may help in control of tachycardia in labor Avoid abrupt sympathetic blockade, which can decrease preload
Mitral insufficiency	Epidural acceptable
Aortic stenosis/IHSS	Epidural should be used with caution to avoid hypotension. Narcotic epidural may be acceptable
Aortic insufficiency	Epidural acceptable
Mechanical heart valves	Epidural acceptable but must be coordinated with last dose of anticoagulation to minimize the risk of epidural hematoma High-dose LMWH should be discontinued 24 h before epidural placement If the patient is on higher doses of UFH, document normal aPTT before placing epidural[22]
ASD, VSD, PDA	Epidural acceptable in absence of pulmonary hypertension or known Eisenmenger syndrome
Secondary pulmonary hypertension and Eisenmenger syndrome	Epidural is contraindicated. Narcotic-only epidural may be acceptable
Coarctation of the aorta	Epidural acceptable
Tetralogy of Fallot	Epidural acceptable if an intracardiac shunt is not present
Marfan syndrome	Epidural acceptable and may be recommended to minimize tachycardia caused by pain and avoid urge for Valsalva during delivery
Peripartum cardiomyopathy	Epidural acceptable and decreases preload and afterload. Also minimizes tachycardia from pain
Acute myocardial infarction	Epidural recommended to reduce afterload and to minimize pain and subsequent tachycardia

Abbreviations: aPTT, activated partial thromboplastin time; ASD, atrial septal defect; IHSS, idiopathic hypertrophic subaortic stenosis; LMWH, low-molecular-weight heparin; PDA, patent ductus arteriosus; UFH, unfractionated heparin; VSD, ventricular septal defect.

Recommended work-up and clinical findings
- Echocardiogram to evaluate severity of right outflow obstruction (>60 mm Hg consistent with severe obstruction)
Labor and delivery
- Reserve cesarean for usual obstetric indications, not shown to improve outcome

MITRAL STENOSIS

Mitral stenosis is the most common valvular lesion in pregnancy and typically a result of rheumatic heart disease. The stenosis of the mitral valve impedes flow of blood from the left atrium to the left ventricle, necessitating increased left atrial pressures to maintain adequate left ventricular filling through the restricted opening. Patients with moderate or severe stenosis are the most likely to develop cardiac complications. Patients may be asymptomatic until physiologic changes of pregnancy unmask the disease and symptomatic patients may undergo balloon valvulotomy during pregnancy.

Potential maternal complications include pulmonary edema, atrial fibrillation, and supraventricular tachycardia. Sixty percent develop the initial episode of pulmonary edema antepartum, at a mean gestational age of 30 weeks. Thromboembolism can develop as a result of left atrial dilatation and may present as a stroke. Things to avoid in patients with mitral stenosis include tachycardia, because increased heart rate decreases diastolic ventricular filling time. Fluid overload should be avoided because it may cause atrial fibrillation, pulmonary edema, and right ventricular failure. Decreases in systemic vascular resistance/hypotension and increases in pulmonary vascular resistance should also be avoided because they can lead to a decrease in cardiac output and hypoxia, respectively.

Medical therapy is typically recommended to prevent tachycardia and to maintain left ventricular filling (preload) to overcome obstruction. Pain management and β-blockers are recommended with a goal heart rate less than 100 beats per minute (bpm). Inadequate preload may not be able to overcome obstruction and can lead to inadequate left ventricular filling and reduction in cardiac output. Diuretics should be used to treat pulmonary edema as needed and digoxin to treat atrial fibrillation as needed. Anticoagulation should be considered if the left atrium is dilated or if there is chronic atrial fibrillation.

Recommended work-up and clinical findings
- Echocardiogram to establish severity of stenosis and size of left atrium.
- Symptoms unusual until valve area less than 2 cm^2.
- Moderate mitral stenosis: 1 to 1.5 cm^2 valve area.
- Severe mitral stenosis: less than 1 cm^2 valve area.
- Electrocardiogram (ECG) to exclude atrial fibrillation from enlarged left atrium. May show left atrial enlargement, right ventricular hypertrophy, and right atrial enlargement in cases of pulmonary hypertension.
- Auscultation: loud first heart sound, an opening snap, and rumbling diastolic murmur.

Labor and delivery
- Tocolytic agents that cause tachycardia are contraindicated for premature labor (eg, terbutaline).
- Hemodynamic monitoring for severe mitral stenosis.
- Consider assisted second stage of labor.
- Reserve cesarean for usual obstetric indications, not shown to improve outcome.

MITRAL INSUFFICIENCY

Mitral insufficiency is well tolerated in pregnancy and is commonly secondary to mitral valve prolapse. Long-standing regurgitation may lead to ventricular dysfunction or atrial enlargement.

Pulmonary edema or dysrhythmias are rare complications. For patients with mitral insufficiency, avoid arrhythmias, bradycardia, increase in systemic vascular resistance, and myocardial depressant drugs. Both bradycardia and increases in systemic vascular resistance can increase regurgitation.

Medical therapy is recommended in the presence of ventricular dysfunction or dysrhythmias, and anticoagulation can be considered if the left atrium is dilated or if there is chronic atrial fibrillation.

Recommended work-up and clinical findings
- ECG to assess severity of regurgitation and evaluate left atrial enlargement and ventricular function.

- ECG to exclude atrial fibrillation from enlarged left atrium. May show left atrial enlargement.

Labor and delivery

- Reserve cesarean section for usual obstetric indications, not shown to improve outcomes.

AORTIC STENOSIS/IDIOPATHIC HYPERTROPHIC SUBAORTIC STENOSIS

When isolated, aortic stenosis is most often caused by a congenital bicuspid aortic valve in women of childbearing age in developed countries. When multiple valves are involved, the lesion is typically rheumatic. Mild disease (valve area >1.5 cm^2; peak gradient <50 mm Hg) is typically tolerated well in pregnancy, whereas severe disease (valve area <1 cm^2; peak gradient >75 mm Hg or an ejection fraction <55%) is at significant risk and preconception correction is recommended. The stenotic valve leads to fixed cardiac output. The presence of symptoms worsens outcomes, and patients with uncorrected severe disease should limit activity. Complications may develop from underperfusion or excessive flow with underperfusion typically more life threatening than pulmonary edema from fluid overload. Therefore, diuretics should be used cautiously to avoid underperfusion.

Idiopathic hypertrophic subaortic stenosis is autosomal dominant in inheritance with similar risks and management to aortic stenosis. It is characterized by hypertrophy of the ventricular septum, which can obstruct left ventricular outflow.

Potential complications occur if the heart is unable to overcome obstruction and maintain adequate cardiac output. This condition can lead to angina caused by decreased coronary perfusion, syncope caused by poor cerebral perfusion, and sudden death caused by arrhythmias, and hypervolemia may lead to pulmonary edema. It is important to avoid hypotension in order to maintain coronary perfusion and to avoid decreased venous return via excessive blood loss, supine position, or Valsalva. Bradycardia should also be avoided because cardiac output is maintained by heart rate and stroke volume. If stroke volume is limited by obstruction, bradycardia can worsen cardiac output. In addition, hypervolemia should be avoided because it may lead to pulmonary edema.

Medical therapy is recommended in the presence of ventricular dysfunction or dysrhythmias. Anticoagulation is typically not needed.

Recommended work-up and clinical findings

- Echocardiogram to evaluate size of aortic valve opening, gradient of flow across the valve, and ejection fraction.
- ECG may show left ventricular hypertrophy and left atrial enlargement. Arrhythmias possible if there is significant left atrial enlargement.
- Harsh systolic ejection murmur.

Labor and delivery

- Reserve cesarean section for usual obstetric indications, not shown to improve outcomes.
- Avoid exertion. Consider shortened second stage of labor.
- Pulmonary edema may develop postpartum caused by the autotransfusion effect.

AORTIC INSUFFICIENCY

Aortic insufficiency is typically well tolerated in pregnancy although significant longstanding regurgitation may lead to left ventricular dysfunction. Complications are unlikely and are typically related to underlying left ventricular dysfunction. Similar to those with mitral insufficiency, avoid arrhythmias, bradycardia, increase in systemic vascular resistance, and myocardial depressant drugs.

Medical therapy is recommended in the presence of ventricular dysfunction or dysrhythmias. Anticoagulation is typically not needed.

Recommended work-up and clinical findings
- Echocardiogram to assess severity of regurgitation and evaluate left atrial enlargement and ventricular function.

Labor and delivery
- Reserve cesarean section for usual obstetric indications, not shown to improve outcomes.

MITRAL VALVE PROLAPSE

Mitral valve prolapse is one of the most common cardiac issues during pregnancy. Most women are asymptomatic but may have palpitations. Pregnancy is typically tolerated well and no changes in antenatal or intrapartum management are recommended.

MECHANICAL HEART VALVES

Patients may present with a history of mechanical valve replacement because of previous severe valvular disease. Prevention of valve thrombosis poses the primary management challenge in these pregnancies. Patients with mechanical valve prostheses require lifelong anticoagulation and warfarin is the typically recommended anticoagulant in the nonpregnant population. Nonmechanical tissue valves do not significantly increase risk for thromboembolism and do not require anticoagulation unless other risk factors (ie, atrial fibrillation) are present.

Patients with the highest risk for thrombosis[21]:

- Any mechanical mitral valve.
- A mechanical aortic valve with any of the following risk factors: atrial fibrillation, previous thromboembolism, ejection fraction less than 30%, a hypercoagulable state, older-generation thrombogenic valves, or multiple valves.
- The 10-year survival for patients with mechanical valves is 70%. Pregnancy does not seem to shorten expected survival.[22]

The maternal mortality risk is approximately 3% for those with mechanical heart valves in pregnancy.[23] In addition, valve failure may occur independently of pregnancy. Thrombosis of the valve is the primary concern. Too much and too little anticoagulation can pose risks for maternal and fetal complications. Rates of pregnancy loss are also increased, particularly with warfarin use. It is typically recommended to avoid warfarin beyond 6 weeks' gestation to avoid development of warfarin embryopathy. It is important to avoid insufficient anticoagulation, continuing anticoagulation intrapartum, waiting too long to resume anticoagulation postpartum (4–6 hours), and resuming warfarin alone postpartum. Unfractionated heparin (UFH) or low-molecular-weight heparin (LMWH) should be included until therapeutic anticoagulation levels are reached.

Medical therapy is recommended in the presence of ventricular dysfunction or dysrhythmias. Anticoagulation is necessary in the presence of mechanical valves and decisions are tailored to the patient's risk factors and preference as well as compliance.

Recommended work-up and clinical findings
- Echocardiogram to establish the location and type of valve and exclude thrombosis. Evaluation of left ventricular dysfunction is also important.

- ECG to establish baseline and exclude atrial fibrillation. Findings are variable, like aortic caged-ball or tilting disc valves (eg, Lillehei Kaster, Omniscience, Starr Edwards).
- Auscultation can reveal a variety of findings based on the type and location of the valve. Clicking of the valve may be audible.
  The 2012 Ninth American College for Chest Physicians (ACCP) guidelines for anticoagulation are summarized in **Box 5**.
- Daily low-dose aspirin may be added to patients at significant increased risk for thrombosis.
  Labor and delivery
- Reserve cesarean section for usual obstetric indications, not shown to improve outcomes. Operative delivery poses increased risk of bleeding related to need for anticoagulation.
- Consider switch to UFH at 36 weeks or before delivery. Discontinue UFH 4 to 6 hours before delivery and resume anticoagulation 4 to 6 hours postpartum.
- Start LMWH or UFH 4 to 6 hours postpartum. Start warfarin same day. Continue UFH or LMWH until warfarin therapeutic; 24 to 48 hours for a minimum of 72 hours.

CONGENITAL CARDIAC LESIONS

Most women with repaired congenital cardiac disease have uncomplicated pregnancies, although approximately a third display a decrease in functional class during pregnancy, with more than two-thirds of those patients subsequently improving postdelivery.[24,25] Approximately 1% have a late cardiac event, with dysrhythmias and heart failure being the most common cardiac events.[25]

Intracardiac communications in the form of atrial septal defects (ASDs) and ventricular septal defects (VSDs), as well as patent ductus arteriosus (PDA), allow shunting of blood across the defect. As a result, the heart must contend with larger volumes and additional demands. Over time this can lead to ventricular dysfunction, overdistension of the atria, cardiac failure or pulmonary overload, and pulmonary hypertension. Flow is typically in a left-to-right direction. As the pulmonary pressures increase, shunting can change direction and become right to left, as with Eisenmenger syndrome, which is addressed later. The shunt is described by the direction of flow as well as the proportion of pulmonary to systemic (right-to-left) flow.

Box 5
The 2012 ninth ACCP guidelines for anticoagulation

Option 1: high-dose LMWH therapy throughout gestation. Start enoxaparin 1 mg/kg every 12 hours. Goal anti-Xa level 4 hours postinjection is ~1 U/mL (0.7–1.2 U/mL).

Option 2: high-dose UFH throughout gestation. UFH subcutaneously every 12 hours. Goal anti-Xa level midinterval is 0.35 to 0.7 U/mL or goal midinterval activated partial thromboplastin time greater than or equal to 2 times control.

Option 3: either of the first two regimens through completed week 12, then change to warfarin until ~36 weeks or close to delivery. Goal INR ~3 (2.5–3.5). UFH or LMWH can then be resumed until delivery.

Adapted from Guyatt GH, Akl EA, Crowther M, et al. Executive summary: antithrombotic therapy and prevention of thrombosis, 9th edition: American College of Chest Physicians evidence-based clinical practice guidelines. Chest 2012;141(2 Suppl):7S–47S.

ATRIAL SEPTAL DEFECT, VENTRICULAR SEPTAL DEFECT, PATENT DUCTUS ARTERIOSUS

The ASD is the most common defect seen in pregnancy. Spontaneous closure is rare in adults and the ASD size and flow across the shunt can worsen in adults.[26] Pregnancy is generally well tolerated and does not change indications for closure. Patients with symptoms (paradoxic emboli, exercise intolerance, fatigue, heart failure, dysrhythmias) or pulmonary/systemic shunt flow ratio greater than 2:1 are candidates for closure of the defect.

Although VSDs are common in childhood, most close spontaneously or have been surgically repaired by adulthood. Smaller VSDs (<0.5 cm) restrict flow across the lesion and carry a lower risk for Eisenmenger syndrome if unrepaired into adulthood. Larger lesions (>1 cm) allow more equal flow between the left and right heart and are more likely associated with increased pulmonary pressures and Eisenmenger syndrome in adults. Because most large lesions have been repaired by adulthood, pregnancy is generally well tolerated.

Most cases of PDA are diagnosed and corrected in childhood and therefore this is typically an uncommon lesion in pregnancy. A small PDA is usually asymptomatic and tolerated well in pregnancy, whereas larger PDAs are associated with risks of ventricular overload and pulmonary hypertension similar to ASD and VSD.

Most complications of these cardiac lesions are associated with large defects. Patients with large defects and significant left-to-right shunts may develop atrial arrhythmias (atrial fibrillation) and congestive heart failure in pregnancy. Pulmonary hypertension may be present and may lead to Eisenmenger syndrome (discussed later). Emboli originating in the lower extremities and pelvis or from the defect, also known as paradoxic emboli, may travel across the defect to the brain, causing a stroke. Unrepaired patients have a 5% risk for venous thromboembolism (VTE).[27]

Hypertension, decrease in pulmonary vascular resistance, and supraventricular arrhythmias or tachycardia should be avoided in these lesions because an increase in systemic vascular resistance increases left-to-right shunting. If pulmonary hypertension is present, avoid increases in pulmonary vascular resistance (metabolic acidosis, excess catecholamines, hypoxemia, nitrous oxide, hypercarbia, pharmacologic vasoconstrictors, and lung hyperinflation) and hypotension. They may worsen right-to-left shunt and lead to Eisenmenger syndrome.

Medical therapy is recommended in the presence of ventricular dysfunction or dysrhythmias. Anticoagulation is typically not needed but the role of anticoagulation for patients with a history of paradoxic embolus and unrepaired defect is unclear. VTE prophylaxis is recommended for patients at prolonged bed rest or perioperatively.

Recommended work-up and clinical findings
- Echocardiogram to evaluate size of defect, severity of shunting, and measure pulmonary artery pressures. Pregnancy may falsely increase echocardiogram estimates of pulmonary artery pressures.[28]
- ECG:
  - ASD: partial right bundle branch block, right axis deviation, and sometimes right ventricular hypertrophy.
  - VSD/PDA: usually normal, may show left or right ventricular hypertrophy.
- Auscultation:
  - ASD: systolic ejection murmur at left sternal border and wide, fixed split second heart sound.
  - VSD: holosystolic thrill and murmur at left sternal border.
  - PDA: grade 3/6 continuous systolic and diastolic murmur in infraclavicular region (Gibson murmur).

Labor and delivery
- Reserve cesarean for usual obstetric indications, not shown to improve outcome.
- Consider air filters to all venous lines to decrease the risk for paradoxic embolism.[29]

CLASS 2 PULMONARY HYPERTENSION AND EISENMENGER SYNDROME

Secondary pulmonary hypertension results from excess flow into the pulmonary circulation from chronic left-to-right (systemic-to-pulmonary) shunting across an intracardiac communication (most commonly associated with ASD, VSD, and PDA). Pulmonary pressures may exceed systemic pressures and, when this happens, flow across the shunt reverses to right to left. The result is decreased pulmonary perfusion, hypoxemia, and worsening pulmonary hypertension as a result of hypoxemia. This reversal defines Eisenmenger syndrome. Maternal-fetal mortality is nearly 50% with Eisenmenger syndrome and occurs most often in the peripartum or recent postpartum period.[30] Therefore, pregnancy termination should be discussed with these patients.

These lesions are at higher risk because of decreased systemic vascular resistance of pregnancy leading to worsening of the right-to-left shunt, worsening hypoxemia, and death in 30% to 50% of patients. Death usually occurs in the first week postpartum. Most common causes of death are worsening and intractable hypoxemia, volume depletion, preeclampsia, and thromboembolism.

It is important to avoid hypotension. Decrease in the systemic vascular resistance causes massive right-to-left shunting, bypassing the pulmonary circulation and leading to severe hypoxemia and worsening pulmonary hypertension. Excessive blood loss and volume depletion should be avoided, because it can cause hypotension by decrease in venous return. Avoid increases in pulmonary vascular resistance (ie, hypoxemia, hypercarbia, metabolic acidosis, excess catecholamines) and avoid myocardial depressant drugs, iron deficiency, high altitude, and exercise.

Medical therapy via pulmonary artery vasodilators is recommended.[31] Pulmonary artery thrombosis is common in nonpregnant patients (21%–70%) and is more likely to occur in women.[32,33] Prophylactic anticoagulation should be considered in patients who continue the pregnancy.

Recommended work-up and clinical findings
- In patients with suspected secondary pulmonary hypertension, the following evaluation is recommended[31]:
- Pulse oximetry, including finger and toe oximetry, with and without administration of supplemental oxygen.
- ECG may show ventricular hypertrophy with associated ST-T wave changes or a right atrial abnormality.
- Chest radiograph abnormalities include dilatation of the central pulmonary arteries, abrupt termination of peripheral pulmonary artery branches (pruning), and right heart enlargement.
- Complete blood count and nuclear lung scintigraphy.
- Transthoracic and transesophageal echocardiography, cardiovascular MRI, or computed tomography.
- Cyanosis and clubbing as well as poor exercise tolerance are typical findings.
- Polycythemia is common.
Labor and delivery
- Outcomes seem to be similar with cesarean or vaginal delivery. Mortalities for any surgery in nonpregnant patients with Eisenmenger syndrome are high (19%).[34]

- Continuous pulse oximetry and supplemental oxygen to keep oxygen saturations at or more than 90%.
- Avoid air embolism: meticulous attention to IV infusions.

COARCTATION OF AORTA

Coarctation of the aorta is rarely seen in pregnancy, because most are corrected in childhood. The most common site for coarctation is distal to the left subclavian artery, so hypertension is measured equally in both arms. However, the femoral pulse is delayed compared with the brachial pulse, and the lower extremity pressures are low. Surgical repair is recommended for adults with a peak–to–peak gradient greater than 20 mm Hg (the difference between the peak pressure distal and proximal to the narrowing).[31] Postrepair, patients remain at risk for complications including recoarctation, aortic aneurysm and dissection, and hypertension. From 30% to 40% of patients also have a bicuspid aortic valve, and 10% of patients also have intracranial aneurysms (vs 2% in the general population). Therefore, all patients should have magnetic resonance angiography of the thoracic aorta and intracranial vessels performed at least once.[31]

Adults with uncorrected coarctation (native) are likely to have hypertension and coronary artery disease and are at risk for dissection and heart failure. This condition may be exacerbated by pregnancy. For patients with coarctation of the aorta, excessive blood loss, myocardial depressant drugs, bradycardia, and Valsalva efforts should be avoided.

Systemic hypertension should be treated as needed. Anticoagulation is typically not recommended.

Recommended work-up and clinical findings
- Echocardiogram to identify severity of the narrowing, evaluate left ventricular function, and exclude additional cardiac defects.
- ECG is usually normal, but may show left ventricular hypertrophy.
- Auscultation: may be normal. Various murmurs are possible based on presence of associated anomalies and size of collateral vessel development.
Labor and delivery
- Cesarean delivery rates are higher, primarily because of perceived risk of intracranial hemorrhage or aortic dissection.
- Vaginal delivery may be accomplished with attention to controlling pain and blood pressure fluctuations, maintaining adequate cardiac preload, and minimizing Valsalva efforts at delivery.

TETRALOGY OF FALLOT

Tetralogy of Fallot (TOF) includes a tetrad of findings of VSD, an overriding aorta, right ventricular outflow obstruction, and right ventricular hypertrophy. Most patients undergo intracardiac repair in the first year of life. The major long-term issues postrepair include right ventricular dysfunction and failure, tricuspid regurgitation, atrial and ventricular dysrhythmias, and sudden cardiac death.[31] Patients may also have persistent intracardiac shunting, pulmonary hypertension, aortic root dilatation, or aortic valve incompetence. The most common cause of death is sudden cardiac death and heart failure. Mortality is approximately 1% annually, 25 years postprocedure.

Spontaneous fetal loss rates are increased with TOF. Patients with surgically corrected TOF generally tolerate pregnancy well. However, patients with evidence of right ventricular dysfunction, severe pulmonary regurgitation, pulmonary hypertension, and hypoxemia are at increased risk for cardiac complications. These complications include dysrhythmias, cardiac failure, worsening cyanosis, pulmonary edema, and pulmonary embolus.[35] Patients with persistent intracardiac shunts are at additional risk (discussed elsewhere in this article).

Antidysrhythmic therapy should be administered as needed. Patients may already be on diuretic therapy, β-blockers, or antihypertensive medications and these should be reviewed and continued during pregnancy as needed. Anticoagulation is typically not indicated.

Recommended work-up and clinical findings
- Echocardiogram to establish cardiac anatomy, evaluate valvular and right ventricular function, assess pulmonary hypertension, and measure aortic root diameter.
- ECG is variable depending on the type of correction performed. It is important to establish the baseline and exclude atrial and ventricular dysrhythmias.

Labor and delivery
- Cesarean delivery is common and typically performed because of perceived cardiac risk. Data are lacking to shoe improved outcomes compared with vaginal delivery.

THE MARFAN SYNDROME

Marfan syndrome is an autosomal dominant condition and 80% of those affected have cardiac effects of the disease. Aneurysmal dilatation and dissection of the aorta account for most of the morbidity and mortality associated with the Marfan syndrome. From 60% to 80% of adults with the Marfan syndrome have aortic root dilatation with or without aortic regurgitation.

The risk of aortic rupture or dissection during pregnancy is ~10% if the aortic root diameter is greater than 4 cm.[36] Rupture and dissection can occur even with a normal aortic dimension (<1%). Secondary to this risk, all women with the Marfan syndrome should be counseled against pregnancy and termination discussed if the patient becomes pregnant.[37] An aortic root diameter greater than 4.5 cm is an indication for preconception repair if the patient desires pregnancy. The risk for dissection is decreased but not eliminated following surgical correction. In addition, pregnancy may hasten the rate of aortic root dilatation in patients with aortic roots greater than 4 cm.[38]

Aortic root dissection and rupture are the most significant risks of pregnancy in Marfan syndrome with dilated aortic root. Hypertension, tachycardia, and Valsalva should be avoided.

Labetalol or metoprolol is required for all patients to maintain the heart rate at less than 110 bpm after submaximal exercise and less than 90 bpm resting. Anticoagulation is typically not indicated.

Recommended work-up and clinical findings
- Echocardiogram to establish size of aortic root. This echocardiogram should be followed serially even if the baseline diameter is normal.
- The Marfan syndrome is associated with other clinical abnormalities, including joint hypermobility, ectopia lentis, pectus excavatum, arm span exceeding height, scoliosis, and arachnodactyly.

Labor and delivery
- Avoid tachycardia: consider continuous β-blocker.
- Assisted second stage to minimize Valsalva effort. Avoid pushing in labor.

- Cesarean may benefit patients with aortic root diameter greater than 4 cm, aortic root dissection, or heart failure.[39]

PERIPARTUM CARDIOMYOPATHY

Peripartum cardiomyopathy is typically defined as the development of cardiac failure in the last month of pregnancy or within 5 months postpartum without an identifiable cause for cardiac failure or recognizable heart disease before the last month of pregnancy. There is evidence of left ventricular systolic dysfunction with an ejection fraction less than 45%, shortening fraction less than 30%, and left ventricular end-diastolic dimension greater than 2.7 cm/m^2 body surface area.[40] Ninety percent of cases occur in first 2 months postpartum, with half of deaths occurring in the first 6 weeks postpartum.

There is a high rate of recurrence in subsequent pregnancies even with apparent recovery of cardiac function. A stress echocardiogram can be considered to evaluate cardiac function before subsequent pregnancies. Patients with incomplete recovery (ejection fraction <50%) have a high rate of decompensation and should be counseled against future pregnancies.

Patients with peripartum cardiomyopathy are at risk for worsening cardiac failure and pulmonary edema. Patients with an initial ejection fraction of less than 25% are at greatest risk for subsequent cardiac transplantation.[41] Failure to normalize cardiac function within 6 months postpartum carries a mortality of 85% by 5 years. Causes of death commonly include dysrhythmias, progressive cardiac failure, and thromboembolic phenomena. Atrial fibrillation is the most common dysrhythmia in patients with peripartum cardiomyopathy.[42] Hypertension, excessive fluid, and increasing cardiac demand should be avoided.

Goals of medical therapy include the following:

- Reduce preload: diuretic therapy (ie, furosemide 20–40 mg by mouth every day).
- Reduce afterload: vasodilator therapy (ie, hydralazine 25–100 mg by mouth every day, amlodipine 5–10 mg by mouth every day; postpartum use, enalapril 5 mg twice a day).
- Improve contractility: digoxin 0.25 to 0.5 mg by mouth every day.
- Reduce myocardial oxygen requirement: goal heart rate 80 to 100 bpm (metoprolol 25–100 mg by mouth every day, carvedilol 3.25 to 25 mg by mouth every day).
- Pentoxifylline 400 mg by mouth 3 times a day may reduce inflammation and reduce mortality risk.[43,44]

Anticoagulation should be considered in the presence of significant ventricular dilatation or atrial dysrhythmia. The risk for VTE associated with peripartum cardiomyopathy is highest during the first 4 weeks postpartum.[45]

Recommended work-up and clinical findings
- Echocardiogram: refer to key points. Establish baseline and repeat every trimester or with worsening symptoms.
- ECG is nonspecific, possibly atrial fibrillation.
- Chest radiograph shows cardiomegaly and pulmonary edema.
- Patients typically present with shortness of breath, orthopnea, fatigue, and leg edema.
- B-type natriuretic peptide level is markedly increased.
Labor and delivery

- Reserve cesarean for usual obstetric indications, not shown to improve outcome.
- Consider assisted second stage if there is significant cardiac dysfunction.

ACUTE MYOCARDIAL INFARCTION

Acute myocardial infarction (MI) is a rare event in women of childbearing age, but the risk increased by pregnancy. Major risk factors include an age greater than 30 years, hypertension, and diabetes. Eighty percent occur in the antepartum or postpartum period. Findings that are typically associated with acute MI include atherosclerosis (40%), coronary artery dissection (27%), coronary thrombus (21%), and normal coronary artery architecture (13%–29%).[46,47] Diagnosis is established with increased troponin levels (and/or increased CKMb [Creatinine kinase from myocardium] levels) plus abnormal ECG. Most are associated with ST segment elevation.

Potential complications include cardiac arrest and possibility of a perimortem cesarean section. Maternal mortality from in-hospital MI is about 5% to 7%.[48,49] Patients are at risk for cardiac failure or dysrhythmias.

Medical therapy typically includes the following:

- Management algorithm once acute MI suspected (goal is completion of MONA in <10 minutes):
    M: morphine sulfate 2 to 4 mg IV
    O: oxygen nasal cannula or mask
    N: nitroglycerin sublingual 0.5 mg every 5 minutes × 3
    A: aspirin 160 to 325 mg chewed
- Follow with 12-lead ECG (repeat in 5–10 minutes if MI is suspected and initial ECG normal). If ECG shows ST elevation or new left bundle branch block, treat as acute MI in consultation with cardiologists.
- β-Blockers, IV nitroglycerin.
- Anticoagulation with IV heparin, antiplatelet therapy (clopidogrel), and antithrombin therapy.
- Consider reperfusion therapy in consultation with cardiologists.
- If viable fetus, monitor fetal heart rate throughout therapy.

Recommended work-up and clinical findings
- Echocardiogram to exclude unrecognized structural cardiac abnormality, evaluate ventricular function.
- ECG to establish diagnosis: ST segment elevation or depression, Q wave abnormalities.
- Laboratory work-up should include troponin, complete blood count with platelet count, prothrombin time and International Normalized Ratio (INR), activated partial thromboplastin time, electrolytes, magnesium, blood urea nitrogen, creatinine, blood glucose, and serum lipid profile.
Labor and delivery
- Expert opinion recommends postponing delivery until 2 to 3 weeks postinfarct to minimize additional cardiac demands.[47]
- If vaginal delivery attempted, consider assisted second stage to minimize cardiac work.
- Delivery route should be individualized. Cesarean delivery may be associated with increased mortality risk.[50]
- Avoid hypertension or tachycardia.
- Avoid methergine and prostaglandins because they may cause coronary vasoconstriction.

REFERENCES

1. Berg CJ, Atrash HK, Koonin LM, et al. Pregnancy-related mortality in the United States, 1987–1990. Obstet Gynecol 1996;88(2):161–7.
2. Berg CJ, Chang J, Callaghan WM, et al. Pregnancy-related mortality in the United States, 1991–1997. Obstet Gynecol 2003;101(2):289–96.
3. El-Solh AA, Grant BJ. A comparison of severity of illness scoring systems for critically ill obstetric patients. Chest 1996;110(5):1299–304.
4. Loverro G, Pansini V, Greco P, et al. Indications and outcome for intensive care unit admission during puerperium. Arch Gynecol Obstet 2001;265(4):195–8.
5. Mabie WC, Sibai BM. Treatment in an obstetric intensive care unit. Am J Obstet Gynecol 1990;162(1):1–4.
6. Mahutte NG, Murphy-Kaulbeck L, Le Q, et al. Obstetric admissions to the intensive care unit. Obstet Gynecol 1999;94(2):263–6.
7. Naylor DF Jr, Olson MM. Critical care obstetrics and gynecology. Crit Care Clin 2003;19(1):127–49.
8. Tang LC, Kwok AC, Wong AY, et al. Critical care in obstetrical patients: an eight-year review. Chin Med J (Engl) 1997;110(12):936–41.
9. Zeeman GG, Wendel GD Jr, Cunningham FG. A blueprint for obstetric critical care. Am J Obstet Gynecol 2003;188(2):532–6.
10. Roos-Hasselink JW, Dukevot JJ, Thomas SA. Pregnancy in high risk cardiac conditions. Heart 2009;95:680–6.
11. Cornette J, Ruys TP, Rossi A, et al. Hemodynamic adaptation to pregnancy in women with structural heart disease. Int J Cardiol 2012;168(2):825–31.
12. Hsieh TT, Chen KC, Soong JH. Outcome of pregnancy in patients with organic heart disease in Taiwan. Asia Oceania J Obstet Gynaecol 1993;19(1):21–7.
13. Clark SL. Structural cardiac disease in pregnancy. In: Clark SL, Cotton DB, Phelan JP, editors. Critical care obstetrics. Oradell (NJ): Medical Economics Books; 1987. p. 92.
14. Siu SC, Sermer M, Colman JM, et al. Prospective multicenter study of pregnancy outcomes in women with heart disease. Circulation 2001;104(5):515–21.
15. Roos-Hesselink JW, Ruys TP, Stein JI, et al. Outcome of pregnancy in patients with structural or ischaemic heart disease: results of a registry of the European Society of Cardiology. Eur Heart J 2012;34(9):657–65.
16. Dye TD, Gordon H, Held B, et al. Retrospective maternal mortality case ascertainment in West Virginia, 1985 to 1989. Am J Obstet Gynecol 1992;167(1):72–6.
17. de Swiet M. Maternal mortality from heart disease in pregnancy. Br Heart J 1993;69(6):524.
18. Siu SC, Colman JM, Sorensen S, et al. Adverse neonatal and cardiac outcomes are more common in pregnant women with cardiac disease. Circulation 2002;105(18):2179–84.
19. Subbaiah M, Sharma V, Kumar S, et al. Heart disease in pregnancy: cardiac and obstetric outcomes. Arch Gynecol Obstet 2013;288(1):23–7.
20. Wilson W, Taubert KA, Gewitz M, et al. Prevention of infective endocarditis: guidelines from the American Heart Association: a guideline from the American Heart Association Rheumatic Fever, Endocarditis, and Kawasaki Disease Committee, Council on Cardiovascular Disease in the Young, and the Council on Clinical Cardiology, Council on Cardiovascular Surgery and Anesthesia, and the Quality of Care and Outcomes Research Interdisciplinary Working Group. Circulation 2007;116(15):1736–54.

21. Douketis JD, Berger PB, Dunn AS, et al. The perioperative management of antithrombotic therapy: American College of Chest Physicians evidence-based clinical practice guidelines (8th edition). Chest 2008;133(6 Suppl):299S–339S.

22. North RA, Sadler L, Stewart AW, et al. Long-term survival and valve-related complications in young women with cardiac valve replacements. Circulation 1999; 99(20):2669–76.

23. Chan WS, Anand S, Ginsberg JS. Anticoagulation of pregnant women with mechanical heart valves: a systematic review of the literature. Arch Intern Med 2000;160(2):191–6.

24. Wacker-Gußmann A, Threimer M, Yigitbasi M, et al. Women with congenital heart disease: long-term outcomes after pregnancy. Clin Res Cardiol 2012; 102(3):215–22.

25. Balint OH, Siu SC, Mason J, et al. Cardiac outcomes after pregnancy in women with congenital heart disease. Heart 2010;96:1656–61.

26. McMahon CJ, Feltes TF, Fraley JK, et al. Natural history of growth of secundum atrial septal defects and implications for transcatheter closure. Heart 2002; 87(3):256–9.

27. Webb G, Gatzoulis MA. Atrial septal defects in the adult: recent progress and overview. Circulation 2006;114(15):1645–53.

28. Penning S, Robinson KD, Major CA, et al. A comparison of echocardiography and pulmonary artery catheterization for evaluation of pulmonary artery pressures in pregnant patients with suspected pulmonary hypertension. Am J Obstet Gynecol 2001;184(7):1568–70.

29. Franklin WJ, Gandhi M. Congenital heart disease in pregnancy. Cardiol Clin 2012; 30:383–94.

30. Presbitero P, Somerville J, Stone S, et al. Pregnancy in cyanotic congenital heart disease. Circulation 1994;89(6):2673–6.

31. Warnes CA, Williams RG, Bashore TM, et al. ACC/AHA 2008 Guidelines for the Management of Adults with Congenital Heart Disease: a report of the American College of Cardiology/American Heart Association Task Force on Practice Guidelines (writing committee to develop guidelines on the management of adults with congenital heart disease). Circulation 2008;118(23):e714–833.

32. Silversides CK, Granton JT, Konen E, et al. Pulmonary thrombosis in adults with Eisenmenger syndrome. J Am Coll Cardiol 2003;42(11):1982–7.

33. Perloff JK, Hart EM, Greaves SM, et al. Proximal pulmonary arterial and intrapulmonary radiologic features of Eisenmenger syndrome and primary pulmonary hypertension. Am J Cardiol 2003;92(2):182–7.

34. Vongpatanasin W, Brickner ME, Hillis LD, et al. The Eisenmenger syndrome in adults. Ann Intern Med 1998;128(9):745–55.

35. Veldtman GR, Connolly HM, Grogan M, et al. Outcomes of pregnancy in women with tetralogy of Fallot. J Am Coll Cardiol 2004;44(1):174–80.

36. Task Force on the Management of Cardiovascular Diseases During Pregnancy of the European Society of Cardiology. Expert consensus document on management of cardiovascular diseases during pregnancy. Eur Heart J 2003;24(8): 761–81.

37. Bonow RO, Carabello BA, Chatterjee K, et al. ACC/AHA 2006 guidelines for the management of patients with valvular heart disease: a report of the American College of Cardiology/American Heart Association Task Force on Practice Guidelines (writing committee to revise the 1998 guidelines for the management of patients with valvular heart disease) developed in collaboration with the Society of Cardiovascular Anesthesiologists endorsed by the Society for Cardiovascular

Angiography and Interventions and the Society of Thoracic Surgeons. J Am Coll Cardiol 2006;48(3):e1–148.

38. Meijboom LJ, Vos FE, Timmermans J, et al. Pregnancy and aortic root growth in the Marfan syndrome: a prospective study. Eur Heart J 2005;26(9):914–20.

39. Vahanian A, Baumgartner H, Bax J, et al. Guidelines on the management of valvular heart disease: the task force on the management of valvular heart disease of the European Society of Cardiology. Eur Heart J 2007;28(2):230–68.

40. Pearson GD, Veille JC, Rahimtoola S, et al. Peripartum cardiomyopathy: National Heart, Lung, and Blood Institute and Office of Rare Diseases (National Institutes of Health) workshop recommendations and review. JAMA 2000;283(9):1183–8.

41. Habli M, O'Brien T, Nowack E, et al. Peripartum cardiomyopathy: prognostic factors for long-term maternal outcome. Am J Obstet Gynecol 2008;199(4):415.

42. Isezuo SA, Abubakar SA. Epidemiologic profile of peripartum cardiomyopathy in a tertiary care hospital. Ethn Dis 2007;17(2):228–33.

43. Sliwa K, Skudicky D, Candy G, et al. The addition of pentoxifylline to conventional therapy improves outcome in patients with peripartum cardiomyopathy. Eur J Heart Fail 2002;4(3):305–9.

44. Sliwa K, Fett J, Elkayam U. Peripartum cardiomyopathy. Lancet 2006;368(9536): 687–93.

45. Howlett JG, McKelvie RS, Costigan J, et al. The 2010 Canadian Cardiovascular Society guidelines for the diagnosis and management of heart failure update: heart failure in ethnic minority populations, heart failure and pregnancy, disease management, and quality improvement/assurance programs. Can J Cardiol 2010;26(4):185–202.

46. Roth A, Elkayam U. Acute myocardial infarction associated with pregnancy. J Am Coll Cardiol 2008;52(3):171–80.

47. Roth A, Elkayam U. Acute myocardial infarction associated with pregnancy. Ann Intern Med 1996;125(9):751–62.

48. Ladner HE, Danielsen B, Gilbert WM. Acute myocardial infarction in pregnancy and the puerperium: a population-based study. Obstet Gynecol 2005;105(3): 480–4.

49. James AH, Jamison MG, Biswas MS, et al. Acute myocardial infarction in pregnancy: a United States population-based study. Circulation 2006;113(12): 1564–71.

50. Badui E, Enciso R. Acute myocardial infarction during pregnancy and puerperium: a review. Angiology 1996;47(8):739–56.

Pregnancy Risks Associated with Obesity

John F. Mission, MD[a], Nicole E. Marshall, MD, MCR[b], Aaron B. Caughey, MD, PhD[b],*

KEYWORDS

- Obesity • Pregnancy • Prenatal care • Gestational diabetes • Macrosomia

KEY POINTS

- Obesity has been shown to be associated with increased rates of preeclampsia, gestational diabetes, fetal macrosomia, stillbirth, postterm pregnancy, and increased rates of cesarean delivery.
- Providing prenatal care to obese women is done by all types of prenatal providers and needs to take into consideration the increased risks of complications and challenges of providing such care.
- Because of the issues related to obesity in pregnancy, best practice would be for preconception care to lead to weight loss before pregnancy.

INTRODUCTION

Obesity has increased dramatically in the United States over the last several decades.[1] In 1990, states with the highest rates of obesity approached 15%. Today, approximately two-thirds of Americans are overweight or obese.[2] The obesity epidemic extends to the pregnant population, with 40% of women qualifying as either overweight or obese,[3] and 28% of pregnant women qualifying as obese. In 1999, 1 in every 10 pregnant women weighed more than 250 lb, whereas 1 in 20 pregnant women weighed more than 300 lbs.[4]

Obesity is defined as having a body mass index (BMI) of 30.0 kg/m^2 or greater, whereas overweight is defined as a having a BMI of 25.0 to 29.9 kg/m^2.[1] Obesity can further be subclassified into class I (BMI of 30.0–34.9 kg/m^2), class II (BMI of 35.0–39.9 kg/m^2), and class III (BMI of $\geq$40.0 kg/m^2).[5] Recently, these categories have been expanded to include an additional category of super obesity (BMI of $\geq$50.0 kg/m^2). Commonly, those with class II and class III obesity who are not in the super-obese range

Disclosures: The authors have no sources or funding or conflicts of interest to disclose.
[a] Maternal-Fetal Medicine, Department of Obstetrics, Gynecology & Reproductive Sciences, Magee-Womens Hospital of UPMC, 300 Halket Street, Pittsburgh, PA 15213, USA;
[b] Department of Obstetrics and Gynecology, Oregon Health & Science University, 3181 Southwest Sam Jackson Park Road, Portland, OR 97239, USA
* Corresponding author. Department of Obstetrics and Gynecology, Oregon Health & Science University, Mail Code L466, 3181 Southwest Sam Jackson Park Road, Portland, OR 97239.
E-mail address: caughey@ohsu.edu

Obstet Gynecol Clin N Am 42 (2015) 335–353
http://dx.doi.org/10.1016/j.ogc.2015.01.008
0889-8545/15/$ – see front matter © 2015 Elsevier Inc. All rights reserved.

obgyn.theclinics.com

are labeled as having severe obesity. In addition, if a BMI is 35.0 kg/m^2 or greater and there is a concomitant health condition such as diabetes, this is commonly deemed morbid obesity.

Obesity has been associated with many complications during pregnancy, including preeclampsia, gestational diabetes mellitus (GDM), fetal macrosomia, stillbirth, post-term pregnancy, and cesarean delivery. This article seeks to review the association of obesity with maternal and fetal adverse outcomes in both the antepartum and the intrapartum environments as well as provides recommendations for care of the obese gravida.

MATERNAL COMPLICATIONS OF OBESITY IN PREGNANCY
Hypertensive Disorders of Pregnancy

There is a longstanding, wide-ranging body of literature that supports a relationship between increasing maternal weight and the hypertensive disorders of pregnancy. Several observational studies demonstrate an association between obesity and gestational hypertension, with a reported 2.5-fold to a 3.2-fold increased risk.[6,7] A link has also been drawn between obesity and preeclampsia,[6–14] with several studies also demonstrating a linear relationship between BMI and preeclampsia risk.[11,15] One systematic review found the risk of preeclampsia to double with each increase of 5 to 7 kg/m^2 in BMI,[16] and one retrospective cohort study found that obese patients of Latina descent have an even greater increase in preeclampsia risk.[17] In another prospective cohort study, increases in BMI between the first and second pregnancies were found to also increase preeclampsia risk.[18] Weight has also been found to correlate with the incidence of both severe preeclampsia[7] and eclampsia.[10]

Diabetes

Many observational studies have examined the link between obesity and gestational diabetes risk, with most showing an association between obesity and an increased risk of GDM.[6–8,10,13,14] One observational study found a linear relationship between BMI and incidence of GDM, and a systematic review and meta-analysis found that the overall risk for GDM in obese patients was 3.76 times higher than in nonobese patients (OR 3.31–4.28), with the prevalence of GDM increasing by 0.82% for every increase of 1 kg/m^2 in BMI.[19] Obesity has been shown to be associated with higher rates of GDM in all racial/ethnic groups, with particularly high incidences in Latina and Asian women.[17]

Given that obesity predisposes to insulin resistance, many obese patients will have preexisting type 2 diabetes mellitus (T2DM) before pregnancy.[20,21] Several studies have described the detrimental effect of increasing maternal obesity on perinatal outcomes in women with diabetes. One study examining gestational diabetic women in Japan revealed increased rates of adverse outcomes with increasing BMI.[22] In the United States, another retrospective study demonstrated that increasing BMI among diabetic gravidas increased rates of preeclampsia, macrosomia, and cesarean section.[23]

The most recent recommendations from the American Diabetes Association are to screen patients with "severe" obesity for pregestational diabetes at the initial prenatal visit, with a screening test at 24 to 28 weeks for GDM if the initial screening test is normal.[24] These guidelines do not specify a BMI cutoff above which patients should receive screening, but using the definitions from above, that would be class II obesity and higher. Additional candidates for early screening according to these guidelines include women with glycosuria, a diagnosis of polycystic ovary syndrome, a strong family history of T2DM, or a prior history of GDM or delivery of a large-for-gestational-age (LGA) infant.[24] For gravidas with class I obesity, it is reasonable to perform early screening in women who also possess any of the additional risk factors listed above. In addition, because of increased prevalence and an obesity impact at lower BMI, it is also common to perform an early screen on all Latina, Asian, and Native American women with class I obesity and higher. Diagnostic criteria for T2DM include a hemoglobin A1c greater than 6.5%, a fasting glucose greater than 126 mg/dL, a 2-hour plasma glucose greater than 200 after a fasting 75 g glucose tolerance test, or a random plasma glucose greater than 200 in a patient with classic symptoms of hyperglycemia.[24,25] If a patient meets these criteria at the beginning of her pregnancy, current guidelines recommend diagnosing the patient with overt T2DM rather than GDM.[24] Patients who qualify for early screening but who present for care in the second trimester may not merit a diagnosis of T2DM with a positive test. Nonetheless, these patients should still be screened at their initial prenatal visit.[26]

Even in obese women without frankly diagnosed diabetes mellitus or GDM, a recent study demonstrated higher fasting and postprandial blood glucose levels.[27] Other studies have demonstrated an association between glucose levels not diagnostic of GDM and the risk of macrosomia, potentially providing a basis for the increased risk of macrosomia reported in obese patients.[28,29] Because the treatment of mild GDM is a carbohydrate-controlled diet and low-impact exercise, it is hard not to see an advantage of this intervention in all obese pregnant women.

Venous Thromboembolism

Venous thromboembolism (VTE) is a major cause of maternal mortality, and pregnancy is a well-established risk factor for VTE. Among all pregnant patients, the risk of VTE in pregnancy and the puerperium is increased 4-fold to 5-fold.[30] VTE has an overall incidence of 1.7 per 1000 deliveries and is responsible for 1.1 deaths per 100,000 deliveries.[31] Several observational studies have investigated the potential relationship between obesity and VTE risk, primarily indicating an increased risk of VTE in obese gravidas, with odds ratios (ORs) ranging from 1.7 to 5.3 greater than normal-weight patients.[32-34] Whether increasing degrees of obesity increase the risk of VTE is currently unknown.

FETAL AND NEONATAL COMPLICATIONS OF OBESITY IN PREGNANCY
Miscarriage and Stillbirth

Obesity has been associated with a modest increase in the risk of first-trimester miscarriage (OR 1.20; confidence interval [CI] 1.01–1.46)[35] and recurrent miscarriage.[35,36] A stronger link has been demonstrated between obesity and stillbirth,[13,14,37,38] with one meta-analysis showing just more than twice the risk of stillbirth compared with patients with normal BMI.[39] In addition, many studies cite an even higher risk among morbidly obese women,[14,40,41] and with increasing BMI,[42] suggesting that increasing BMI correlates with an increasing risk of stillbirth.[40] Another meta-analysis demonstrated that each 5-unit increase in BMI increased the risk ratio of stillbirth by 1.2.[13] This increased risk has been identified among diabetic women[44] as well as patients without diabetes and in fetuses without congenital anomalies.[45] Postulated theories to explain this association include hyperlipidemia leading to vascular inflammation and obesity-associated sleep apnea with subsequent desaturation events.[38] Increased perinatal mortality has been shown to extend to the neonatal period, with some studies demonstrating an increased risk of neonatal death.[37,45]

Fetal Anomalies

In addition to the link between obesity and stillbirth, many studies have shown an association between obesity and birth defects. Two meta-analyses on the topic have been recently published and document an increased risk of neural tube defects in offspring of the obese gravida, with pooled ORs of 1.70[46] and 1.87[47]; specific rates of spina bifida were noted to be even higher with an OR of 2.24.[47] In a more recent population-based study, increasing BMI was shown again to be associated with an increasing risk for neural tube defects.[48]

Other congenital abnormalities have been found to have a more moderate association with obesity, including cardiovascular defects,[47–50] orofacial clefts,[47,48,50,51] anorectal atresia, hydrocephaly, limb reduction defects,[47] diaphragmatic hernia, and omphalocele.[52] Interestingly, obesity has been associated with a decrease in gastroschisis.[47,50,52] Theories to explain these associations include the potential impact of nutritional deficiencies associated with obesity; similar metabolic as well as common fetal structural abnormalities are seen in diabetes, including insulin-resistance, hyperglycemia, and nutritional deficiencies. One study demonstrated lower rates of folate supplementation in women with a BMI greater than 35; dietary differences may also account for variation in folate levels.[53]

In addition to an increase in prevalence of fetal structural anomalies, obtaining adequate views of fetal anatomy by ultrasound has been shown to be more difficult in obese patients.[54] Inadequate views of fetal anatomy decrease the prenatal detection of anomalies, including potentially lethal malformations, thus limiting opportunities for patient counseling and appropriate perinatal care.

Fetal Macrosomia

Obesity is a well-established risk factor for fetal macrosomia, conferring between a 2-fold and 3-fold increased risk.[6,13,14,55–57] This relationship persists even after adjusting for gestational diabetes[58] and gestational weight gain and has also been described among obese adolescent gravidas.[59] Morbid obesity and increasing BMI have been shown to be associated with higher rates of macrosomia,[6,14,60] with other studies showing trends toward increasing LGA[8] and birth weight greater than 4000 g[11] with increasing BMI.

OBESITY AND DISORDERS OF GESTATIONAL AGE
Preterm Birth

Overall, the literature is conflicting regarding the association between preterm delivery and obesity. Although some studies support an increased risk,[13,61] others do not,[10,62] particularly when controlling for confounding comorbidities, such as hypertensive disorders, diabetes mellitus, and smoking.[63,64] Mild increases in preterm premature rupture of membranes among obese women leading to early delivery have been demonstrated as well.[65,66] Specifically, examining medically indicated preterm birth (PTB), several studies show higher rates among obese women,[65,67,68] with one meta-analysis showing an adjusted odds ratio (aOR) of 1.3 for induced PTB in overweight and obese women.[69] Some studies suggest that obese women are less likely to experience spontaneous PTB,[65,67] with a recent meta-analysis showing an OR of 0.83.[70] This decrease in spontaneous PTB was also observed among obese adolescents[71] and twin pregnancies, with an aOR of 0.86.[72] However, a more recent population-based cohort study of almost 1.6 million births demonstrated higher rates of spontaneous extremely PTB between 22 and 27 weeks' gestation among obese gravidas.[68] Overall, obesity seems to be associated with increased rates of very early spontaneous PTB as well as an increased risk of medically indicated preterm delivery due to comorbid illnesses.

Prolonged and Postterm Pregnancy

Obesity has been associated with prolonged and postterm pregnancy, with several large population-based studies demonstrating an increased risk of prolonged pregnancy beyond 41 weeks' gestation as well as postterm pregnancy at or beyond 42 weeks' gestation.[15,40,55,73–76] Two causes have been proposed for this association. One involves gestational dating; because obese women are more likely to be oligo-ovulatory, many may have actually ovulated several days or a week beyond the usual fourteenth day of the menstrual cycle. Thus, standard dating tools may lead to an overestimation of the gestational age in obese women, a problem that can be decreased with routine early dating ultrasounds in obese women.

The second proposed mechanism is that obese women have hormonal differences, in particular, elevated estrogen levels, which may interfere with the onset of spontaneous labor. For example, obesity has been shown to be associated with higher rates of induction of labor,[7,13,40,55,77] with one meta-analysis demonstrating labor induction rates that were 1.9 times higher in obese patients.[77] This finding is particularly impactful, because several studies have also shown higher rates of cesarean section following induction of labor in obese gravidas.[74,78]

INTRAPARTUM COMPLICATIONS OF OBESITY IN PREGNANCY
Dysfunctional Labor

Obesity has been shown to be associated with prolonged or dysfunctional labor. One study investigating prostaglandin inductions found increasing BMI to be associated with longer duration of labor, higher oxytocin requirements, and higher cesarean delivery rates.[79] The link between obesity and longer labor inductions was seen in another prospective study of induction of labor.[80] Other studies have demonstrated a link between obesity and a longer first stage of labor,[81–83] in both latent labor[84] and active labor.[85] For nulliparous gravidas who reach the second stage, increasing BMI was not found to be associated with a longer second stage of labor or increased cesarean risk,[86] with one study even demonstrating a shorter second stage of labor in obese women.[83] Whether these longer labors are due to differences in hormonal balance or variation in volume of distribution needs further elucidation.

Shoulder Dystocia

The literature is conflicting regarding the risk of shoulder dystocia among obese gravidas. Although 2 large retrospective cohort studies found that shoulder dystocia risk is increased among obese women,[55,87] an even larger population-based cohort study including more than 400,000 pregnant women found obesity to be associated with increased rates of macrosomia but not an increased incidence of shoulder dystocia.[14] The lack of association between obesity and shoulder dystocia is further supported by a large case-control study,[88] a large retrospective cohort study,[74] and a smaller study examining women without gestational diabetes.[56] One potential reason for these differing findings may be related to whether birthweight is controlled for in multivariable models. Because macrosomia is on the causal pathway from obesity to shoulder dystocia, some methodologists would recommend not controlling for birthweight. As birthweight is unknown before delivery, obese women are at increased risk of macrosomia compared with normal weight woman, and therefore, the risk of shoulder dystocia is likely elevated in obese gravidas.

Operative Vaginal Delivery

Few studies support a link between obesity and operative vaginal delivery. One small case-control study in India showed a statistically significant increase in instrumental deliveries among obese women,[89] whereas another population-based study only found an increased risk of operative vaginal delivery among morbidly obese gravidas.[6] A larger study did not find an association between BMI and operative vaginal delivery risk.[40] One reason for differing findings may be that the association is related to clinician bias, which may vary geographically and in different cultures.

Cesarean Delivery

Although the causal relationship between obesity and operative vaginal delivery remains unclear, an increased risk of cesarean delivery in obese patients has been repeatedly demonstrated,[6,55,90] especially in morbidly obese women.[8,15,55] There appears to be a dose-response effect, with multiple studies showing an increasing risk of cesarean delivery with increasing BMI.[40] One meta-analysis demonstrated obese gravidas had a cesarean risk that was 2.05 times higher than patients with normal weight (OR 1.86–2.27), whereas severe obese gravidas had a cesarean risk that was 2.89 times higher than normal weight patients (OR 2.28–3.79).[91] Another meta-analysis demonstrated the risk of cesarean section to be 2.26 times higher for women with a BMI of 30–35 (OR 2.04–2.51) and 3.38 times higher for women with a BMI greater than 35 (OR 2.49–4.57).[92] A more recent retrospective study examining women with "super obesity," defined as having a BMI greater than 50, found super-obese women to be at increased risk of having a cesarean section in comparison with obese women, with a rate of cesarean section of nearly 50%.[93] Examining the interaction of race and obesity, increased rates of cesarean section have been noted among obese African American women (OR = 1.50) and Asian women (OR = 1.73).[17]

Cesarean section in the first stage of labor has been shown to be higher in obese women, with a rate of 31% compared with 13% in normal weight women, whereas the rate of cesarean section in the second stage remains similar comparing obese, overweight, and normal weight women.[94] Obese women have also been shown to have an increased risk of emergent cesarean delivery.[7,13,40,55,92]

Cesarean Complications

Cesarean deliveries in obese gravidas can be more technically challenging, and increasing BMI has been associated with increasing operative times in one study.[95] Higher rates of postoperative wound complications have been described among obese women. The risk of infection has been reported to be 1.43 times higher after a cesarean delivery and more than doubled in obese diabetic women.[96] Several studies demonstrated increased rates of cesarean complication with increasing BMI.[97,98] In women with a BMI greater than 50, one study cited a 30% wound complication rate with 90% of complications involving wound disruptions, with higher risks seen in smokers and patients with subcutaneous drains in place.[99] Wound separations can be decreased by closing the subcutaneous fat with suture in patients with adipose depth greater than 2 cm.[100] In addition, a prospective, randomized controlled trial examining the use of drains in obese women after cesarean section did not demonstrate any improvement in complication rates using this technique.[101]

Some practitioners have suggested using vertical skin incisions or higher transverse incisions to improve wound complications, and one study examining morbidly obese women undergoing cesarean delivery found an increased use of vertical skin incisions in older, heavier patients.[102] Vertical skin incisions have been associated with higher rates of classic hysterotomy.[103] Although 2 studies found no difference in wound complications with supraumbilical vertical skin incisions,[103,104] a larger study found a lower rate of wound complications in patients with a vertical skin incision after adjusting for confounding factors.[105] Prospective studies are needed to elucidate the ideal skin incision for cesarean delivery in obese women.

Trial of Labor After Cesarean Section

Several studies have compared trial of labor after cesarean section (TOLAC) success rates in obese and normal weight women. One study found obese women to have lower TOLAC success rates in comparison with normal weight women (54.6% vs 70.5%).[106] Another case series described a 13% vaginal birth after cesarean section (VBAC) success rate in women weighing greater than 300 lb,[107] much lower than rates seen in patients weighing less than 200 or between 200 and 300 lb.[108] Another study found increasing BMI to be inversely associated with successful TOLAC.[109] In morbidly obese women attempting TOLAC, more complications have also been demonstrated in patients with failed TOLAC, including higher infectious morbidity,[107,110] composite morbidity, and neonatal injury.[109] Similar risks were reported in a study comparing obese women attempting VBAC and elective repeat cesarean delivery.[110] Given equivalent costs and an increased risk of complications with failed TOLAC in comparison with an elective repeat cesarean delivery, it may be reasonable for obese gravidas with low likelihood for TOLAC success to elect for a repeat cesarean delivery, particularly if they are interested in permanent sterilization with their delivery. This factor must be weighed against the risks for future pregnancy morbidity as well as the lower morbidity of a successful VBAC.

Postpartum Hemorrhage

Although 2 retrospective cohort studies found no increased risk in postpartum hemorrhage (PPH) in obese women,[14,74] most literature demonstrates a mild increase in the risk of PPH, including 4 retrospective cohort studies,[11,12,15,55,111] as well as a meta-analysis done in 2008 that showed an OR of 1.2 (95% CI 1.16–1.24).[77] Several studies have also demonstrated a higher risk for hemorrhage in morbidly obese women.[13] In addition, a recent population-based cohort study of 1.1 million women supported the increased risk of PPH and also demonstrated an increasing risk of atonic PPH with increasing BMI.[112] The increased volume of distribution for uterotonics in obese women and the difficulty in identification of the fundus and with performing bimanual massage likely contribute to this risk.

Anesthesia Complications

Analgesia is an important consideration for all laboring patients. Given the previously discussed associations of obesity with complications of labor and an increased risk of cesarean section, anesthesia becomes a particularly important issue for the obese gravida. Placing regional anesthesia has been shown to be more difficult in obese patients, often requiring multiple attempts at needle insertion and more frequently resulting in failure of regional anesthesia placement.[113] Intubation for general anesthesia can also be more difficult in obese patients.[113] Thus, the obese patient may benefit from placement of a functioning epidural catheter early in labor.[114] In addition to providing analgesia and alleviating elevated blood pressures during labor, a working epidural catheter can help to avoid the risks of general anesthesia for a patient who needs an emergency cesarean section. As operative times for cesarean deliveries in obese patients can be prolonged,[115,116] the use of combined spinal epidural anesthesia can offer flexibility in prolonging anesthesia as necessary for longer surgeries.[116] In any case, it is important to consult with anesthesia providers early in labor to discuss management options and ensure more time to place a functioning epidural,[21] or even to obtain antenatal anesthesia consultation for very challenging obese patients.[117]

WEIGHT MANAGEMENT AND PREGNANCY

Ideally, weight loss with the goal of a normal BMI should be attempted before conception, because the degree of weight loss required to yield improvements in hypertension, hyperlipidemia, and diabetes could potentially be harmful during pregnancy. The American College of Obstetricians and Gynecologists (ACOG) recommends weight loss through a healthy diet of caloric restriction in combination with aerobic exercise.[118] Weight change between the first and second pregnancies has been studied, with upward changes in BMI categories between pregnancies associated with increased risks of preeclampsia,[18] LGA birth,[119] and risk of cesarean delivery,[120] whereas decreasing BMI categories between pregnancies attenuates the risk of LGA birth[119] and cesarean delivery.[120]

Gestational weight gain in pregnancy has also been extensively studied, with the Institute of Medicine (IOM) releasing guidelines for weight gain during pregnancy according to prepregnancy BMI. For obese gravidas, the recommended weight gain is between 11 and 20 lb, with some recommending even less weight gain for women with higher classes of obesity.[121]

Many studies have examined the impact of weight gain greater and less than that recommended by the IOM. Excessive weight gain of 25 or more pounds in obese women increases the risk of cesarean delivery and preeclampsia.[122] An increase in LGA babies has also been seen in women who exceeded the recommended gestational weight gain guidelines (aOR 6.71, 95% CI 4.83–9.31).[123] Decreased complications overall have been demonstrated in obese gravidas with weight gain less than 10 lb.[124] Another study demonstrated decreased rates of preeclampsia, cesarean delivery, and LGA but increased small for gestational age among patients with class II and III obesity who gained less than 10 lbs.[125]

To achieve recommended gestational weight gain goals, referral to a nutritionist can be helpful for obese gravidas. In addition, many antenatal dietary interventions have been investigated to limit gestational weight gain.[126–129] A recent meta-analysis showed that antenatal dietary interventions can decrease total gestational weight gain by 6.5 kg without adverse impact on neonatal birth weight.[130] This evidence suggests that dietary restrictions in pregnancy may potentially improve maternal and neonatal outcomes and lower the likelihood of neonatal harm.

Gastric Bypass Surgery

Bariatric surgery refers to a heterogeneous group of procedures that include laparoscopic adjustable gastric banding, vertical-banded gastroplasty, Roux-en-Y gastric bypass, and biliopancreatic diversion/duodenal switch. Such procedures are appropriate for women with a BMI of 40 or greater or with BMI of 35 or greater with comorbidities such as diabetes, coronary artery disease, and severe sleep apnea.[131] Recent randomized controlled trials have also demonstrated that bariatric surgery may achieve better glycemic control than medical treatment alone.[132,133]

Many studies have demonstrated improved pregnancy outcomes with gastric bypass surgery before conception, particularly when comparing women with prior gastric bypass surgery to obese controls.[134] Among maternal outcomes examined when comparing obese controls and women after various types of bariatric surgery, decreases in the rates of preeclampsia,[135,136] chronic hypertensive disorders of pregnancy, and gestational diabetes[137] have been reported after bariatric surgery, whereas one smaller case-control study did not find a decrease in these outcomes.[138] Decreased rates of cesarean section have been demonstrated as well.[139] In examining perinatal outcomes, it was found that gastric bypass is associated with decreased rates of macrosomia,[138,140] although another study found no difference in macrosomia rates after gastric banding.[141]

Concerns exist in the literature for some worsened pregnancy outcomes in women with a prior history of bariatric surgery. Studies comparing outcomes of women who have had prior gastric bypass surgery to controls with normal BMI show increased rates of complications.[142–145] In particular, in one study examining 298 women with bariatric surgery to 158,912 controls in the general obstetric population, patients were more likely to have had a prior cesarean delivery, develop gestational diabetes, and give birth via cesarean delivery.[142] However, these studies may reflect intrinsically different pregnancy outcomes between patients with normal BMI and obese patients with a history of bariatric surgery. A more appropriate comparison group might include only obese gravidas who have not had surgery. Bariatric surgery has also been shown to be associated with increased rates of small for gestational age fetuses.[137] However, rates of preterm delivery[138,141] and intrauterine fetal demise were similar after bariatric surgery.[143]

The current recommendations according to ACOG are to avoid pregnancy for 12 to 18 months after bariatric surgery to avoid the risks to the fetus of rapid maternal weight loss,[131] although pregnancy outcomes may be similar among patients with a surgery-to-conception interval of less than 18 months and patients who wait longer than 18 months to conceive[146] or even patients who conceive at less than 12 months after surgery.[147] Common nutritional deficiencies after Roux-en-Y gastric bypass include protein, iron, vitamin B12, vitamin D, and calcium, and monitoring for these deficiencies should be considered.[131] In addition, absorptive surfaces along the gastrointestinal tract often change following bariatric surgery. Care should be taken when prescribing nonsteroidal anti-inflammatory drugs to avoid gastric ulceration in women with smaller gastric pouches.[148]

The presentation of operative complications resulting from bariatric surgery, such as anastomotic leaks, bowel obstructions, internal hernias, ventral hernias, band erosion, and band migration, can mimic the common nausea and vomiting of pregnancy. For patients who have nausea or vomiting due to adjustable gastric bands, these bands can be adjusted to improve emptying and alleviate symptoms.[149] All patients with a history of gastric bypass who present with nausea and vomiting should be evaluated carefully for these complications because maternal deaths have been reported resulting from postoperative complications of bariatric surgery during pregnancies following bariatric surgery.[150]

PREGNANCY MANAGEMENT

Although obesity is associated with a wide range of complications, these women are certainly not just under the purview of maternal-fetal medicine specialists. Because obesity is increasingly common, all clinicians who provide prenatal care will care for these patients. Given the wide range of issues that may impact pregnancy in obese women, the following issues should be addressed throughout gestation.

In the first trimester, there are several additional tests or considerations for the obese gravida. First, because of the increased risk of undiagnosed T2DM, class II obese and higher patients should be screened at their initial prenatal visit, with either hemoglobin A1C, fasting glucose, or a 2-hour glucose tolerance test. Given the increased risks of preeclampsia and other hypertensive disorders of pregnancy, providers should consider checking baseline preeclampsia laboratory tests, including a uric acid test and a liver function test, as well as a 24-hour urine protein collection to ensure normal values at baseline. In addition, a rigorous attempt to determine baseline blood pressure and to ensure proper cuff size should be made to screen for chronic hypertension. Because of the concern for oligo-ovulation in obese patients[151] and the increased risk of dizygotic twinning among obese patients,[152] an early first-trimester dating ultrasound in obese women is recommended to help determine timing of aneuploidy screening and third-trimester management.

Prenatal diagnosis also can be complicated in obese women. The new noninvasive prenatal testing using cell-free fetal DNA in the maternal circulation appears to be less effective in obese women with a lower rate having an adequate fetal fraction of the cell-free DNA and therefore not getting a result. For prenatal diagnosis, amniocentesis is always more challenging in obese women as is transabdominal chorionic villus sampling (CVS). Although CVS has not been specifically associated with increased rates of pregnancy loss among obese patients, interestingly, women with a BMI of 40 or greater have been shown to have a 2-fold increase in pregnancy loss rates after amniocentesis.[153]

Obese pregnant women should undergo nutrition counseling, preferably by a trained nutritionist. Pregnant women have been shown to change behavior to reduce adverse pregnancy outcomes after counseling,[154] so clinicians should focus on the potential benefits to pregnancy outcomes from appropriate diet, exercise, and gestational weight gain. As previously described, the IOM currently recommends 11 to 20 lb of weight gain in pregnancy in obese women, with perhaps even lower levels in higher levels of obesity.[121]

In the second trimester, obese women should have a fetal anatomy ultrasound, given their elevated risk of fetal anomalies. Such women should also be counseled that the images are more challenging because of their habitus, which may lead to a greater chance of anomalies not being able to be identified or additional ultrasounds required to complete screening. Throughout the second trimester, along with diabetes screening, a continued focus on diet, exercise, and gestational weight gain should persist to reinforce these goals.

In the third trimester, obese women should be monitored closely for development of preeclampsia and gestational hypertension. If fundal heights are challenging to follow, some clinicians will obtain a third-trimester growth ultrasound to screen for macrosomia or intrauterine growth restriction. Because these women are at increased risk for stillbirth, some individuals have proposed antenatal testing, but there is no specific evidence from clinical trials to support this practice.

Concerning labor and delivery, obese women should receive an early anesthesia consult to ensure adequate anesthesia in an emergent setting can be obtained. Obese women may have different labor curves than women of normal weight, and this should be considered when diagnosing failed induction, active phase arrest, and failure to descend. Particularly, for the latter diagnosis, care should be taken to identify the ischial spines as landmarks for the estimation of fetal station, because the fetuses of obese women may seem to be higher on vaginal examination than of nonobese women.

Throughout pregnancy and the postpartum period, obese patients are at increased risk for VTE. Thromboprophylaxis for 1 week postpartum can be considered in morbidly obese patients with additional risk factors for VTE, although these recommendations are based on expert opinion.[155] In the postpartum period, patients can benefit from continued focus on diet and exercise to support the idea that these lifestyle changes are not just for pregnancy, but rather should be a lifelong behavioral change. For obese patients with pregnancies complicated by GDM or either chronic or gestational hypertension, addressing these issues postpartum is important. Obese women should be specifically encouraged to breastfeed for maternal benefits, including decreased postpartum weight retention and lifelong reduction of T2DM[156] as well as decreasing their child's risk for obesity and metabolic syndrome. Postpartum contraception requires special attention in obese women, who have been reported to be less likely to use contraception.[157] As in women of normal weight, the intrauterine device is often the most consistent form of contraception, and obese women benefit in particular from the progestogenic impact on the uterine endometrium.

SUMMARY

Obesity is an increasingly common condition complicating pregnancy, and the consequences of obesity for the mother and neonate are numerous. Pregnancy represents a unique opportunity to counsel women appropriately to reduce these complications not only during their pregnancy but also in the future. Further research is needed to characterize optimal strategies to improve neonatal and maternal outcomes among obese women.

REFERENCES

1. Division of Nutrition PA, and Obesity, National Center for Chronic Disease Prevention and Health Promotion. Overweight and Obesity [Center for Disease Control Website]. 2012. Available at: http://www.cdc.gov/obesity. Accessed May 1, 2012.
2. Weight-control Information Network NIoDaDaKD. Overweight and Obesity Statistics, NIH Publication Number 04-4158. 2010. Available at: http://www.win.niddk.nih.gov/statistics/index.htm. overweight. Accessed May 1, 2012.
3. Kim SY, Dietz PM, England L, et al. Trends in pre-pregnancy obesity in nine states, 1993–2003. Obesity (Silver Spring) 2007;15(4):986–93.
4. Lu GC, Rouse DJ, DuBard M, et al. The effect of the increasing prevalence of maternal obesity on perinatal morbidity. Am J Obstet Gynecol 2001;185(4): 845–9.
5. Gunatilake RP, Perlow JH. Obesity and pregnancy: clinical management of the obese gravida. Am J Obstet Gynecol 2011;204(2):106–19.
6. Weiss JL, Malone FD, Emig D, et al. Obesity, obstetric complications and cesarean delivery rate–a population-based screening study. Am J Obstet Gynecol 2004;190(4):1091–7.
7. Athukorala C, Rumbold AR, Willson KJ, et al. The risk of adverse pregnancy outcomes in women who are overweight or obese. BMC Pregnancy Childbirth 2010;10:56.
8. Alanis MC, Goodnight WH, Hill EG, et al. Maternal super-obesity (body mass index > or = 50) and adverse pregnancy outcomes. Acta Obstet Gynecol Scand 2010;89(7):924–30.
9. Sibai BM, Gordon T, Thom E, et al. Risk factors for preeclampsia in healthy nulliparous women: a prospective multicenter study. The National Institute of Child Health and Human Development Network of Maternal-Fetal Medicine Units. Am J Obstet Gynecol 1995;172(2 Pt 1):642–8.
10. Baeten JM, Bukusi EA, Lambe M. Pregnancy complications and outcomes among overweight and obese nulliparous women. Am J Public Health 2001; 91(3):436–40.

11. Bhattacharya S, Campbell DM, Liston WA. Effect of body mass index on pregnancy outcomes in nulliparous women delivering singleton babies. BMC Public Health 2007;7:168.
12. Mbah AK, Kornosky JL, Kristensen S, et al. Super-obesity and risk for early and late pre-eclampsia. BJOG 2010;117(8):997–1004.
13. Sebire NJ, Jolly M, Harris JP, et al. Maternal obesity and pregnancy outcome: a study of 287,213 pregnancies in London. Int J Obes Relat Metab Disord 2001; 25(8):1175–82.
14. Ovesen P, Rasmussen S, Kesmodel U. Effect of prepregnancy maternal overweight and obesity on pregnancy outcome. Obstet Gynecol 2011;118(2 Pt 1):305–12.
15. Denison FC, Price J, Graham C, et al. Maternal obesity, length of gestation, risk of postdates pregnancy and spontaneous onset of labour at term. BJOG 2008; 115(6):720–5.
16. O'Brien TE, Ray JG, Chan WS. Maternal body mass index and the risk of preeclampsia: a systematic overview. Epidemiology 2003;14(3):368–74.
17. Ramos GA, Caughey AB. The interrelationship between ethnicity and obesity on obstetric outcomes. Am J Obstet Gynecol 2005;193(3 Pt 2):1089–93.
18. Getahun D, Ananth CV, Oyelese Y, et al. Primary preeclampsia in the second pregnancy: effects of changes in prepregnancy body mass index between pregnancies. Obstet Gynecol 2007;110(6):1319–25.
19. Torloni MR, Betran AP, Horta BL, et al. Prepregnancy BMI and the risk of gestational diabetes: a systematic review of the literature with meta-analysis. Obes Rev 2009;10(2):194–203.
20. American Diabetes Association. Gestational diabetes mellitus. Diabetes Care 2004;27(Suppl 1):S88–90.
21. American College of Obstetricians, Gynecologists. ACOG Committee Opinion number 315, September 2005. Obesity in pregnancy. Obstet Gynecol 2005; 106(3):671–5.
22. Sugiyama T, Nagao K, Metoki H, et al. Pregnancy outcomes of gestational diabetes mellitus according to pre-gestational BMI in a retrospective multi-institutional study in Japan. Endocr J 2014;61(4):373–80.
23. Marshall NE, Guild C, Cheng YW, et al. The effect of maternal body mass index on perinatal outcomes in women with diabetes. Am J Perinatol 2014;31(3): 249–56.
24. American Diabetes Association. Standards of medical care in diabetes–2010. Diabetes Care 2010;33(Suppl 1):S11–61.
25. American Diabetes Association. Diagnosis and classification of diabetes mellitus. Diabetes Care 2012;35(Suppl 1):S64–71.
26. Super DM, Edelberg SC, Philipson EH, et al. Diagnosis of gestational diabetes in early pregnancy. Diabetes Care 1991;14(4):288–94.
27. Harmon KA, Gerard L, Jensen DR, et al. Continuous glucose profiles in obese and normal-weight pregnant women on a controlled diet: metabolic determinants of fetal growth. Diabetes Care 2011;34(10):2198–204.
28. Metzger BE, Lowe LP, Dyer AR, et al. Hyperglycemia and adverse pregnancy outcomes. N Engl J Med 2008;358(19):1991–2002.
29. Ehrlich SF, Crites YM, Hedderson MM, et al. The risk of large for gestational age across increasing categories of pregnancy glycemia. Am J Obstet Gynecol 2011;204(3):240.e1–6.
30. Pomp ER, Lenselink AM, Rosendaal FR, et al. Pregnancy, the postpartum period and prothrombotic defects: risk of venous thrombosis in the MEGA study. J Thromb Haemost 2008;6(4):632–7.

31. James AH, Jamison MG, Brancazio LR, et al. Venous thromboembolism during pregnancy and the postpartum period: incidence, risk factors, and mortality. Am J Obstet Gynecol 2006;194(5):1311–5.

32. Simpson EL, Lawrenson RA, Nightingale AL, et al. Venous thromboembolism in pregnancy and the puerperium: incidence and additional risk factors from a London perinatal database. BJOG 2001;108(1):56–60.

33. Larsen TB, Sorensen HT, Gislum M, et al. Maternal smoking, obesity, and risk of venous thromboembolism during pregnancy and the puerperium: a population-based nested case-control study. Thromb Res 2007;120(4):505–9.

34. Knight M. Antenatal pulmonary embolism: risk factors, management and outcomes. BJOG 2008;115(4):453–61.

35. Lashen H, Fear K, Sturdee DW. Obesity is associated with increased risk of first trimester and recurrent miscarriage: matched case-control study. Hum Reprod 2004;19(7):1644–6.

36. Metwally M, Saravelos SH, Ledger WL, et al. Body mass index and risk of miscarriage in women with recurrent miscarriage. Fertil Steril 2010;94(1):290–5.

37. Kristensen J, Vestergaard M, Wisborg K, et al. Pre-pregnancy weight and the risk of stillbirth and neonatal death. BJOG 2005;112(4):403–8.

38. Fretts RC. Etiology and prevention of stillbirth. Am J Obstet Gynecol 2005; 193(6):1923–35.

39. Chu SY, Kim SY, Lau J, et al. Maternal obesity and risk of stillbirth: a meta-analysis. Am J Obstet Gynecol 2007;197(3):223–8.

40. Mantakas A, Farrell T. The influence of increasing BMI in nulliparous women on pregnancy outcome. Eur J Obstet Gynecol Reprod Biol 2010;153(1):43–6.

41. Cedergren MI. Maternal morbid obesity and the risk of adverse pregnancy outcome. Obstet Gynecol 2004;103(2):219–24.

42. Yao R, Ananth CV, Park BY, et al. Obesity and the risk of stillbirth: a population-based cohort study. Am J Obstet Gynecol 2014;210(5):457.e1–9.

43. Aune D, Saugstad OD, Henriksen T, et al. Maternal body mass index and the risk of fetal death, stillbirth, and infant death: a systematic review and meta-analysis. JAMA 2014;311(15):1536–46.

44. Roman AS, Rebarber A, Fox NS, et al. The effect of maternal obesity on pregnancy outcomes in women with gestational diabetes. J Matern Fetal Neonatal Med 2011;24(5):723–7.

45. Tennant PW, Rankin J, Bell R. Maternal body mass index and the risk of fetal and infant death: a cohort study from the North of England. Hum Reprod 2011;26(6):1501–11.

46. Rasmussen SA, Chu SY, Kim SY, et al. Maternal obesity and risk of neural tube defects: a metaanalysis. Am J Obstet Gynecol 2008;198(6):611–9.

47. Stothard KJ, Tennant PW, Bell R, et al. Maternal overweight and obesity and the risk of congenital anomalies: a systematic review and meta-analysis. JAMA 2009;301(6):636–50.

48. Blomberg MI, Kallen B. Maternal obesity and morbid obesity: the risk for birth defects in the offspring. Birth Defects Res A Clin Mol Teratol 2010;88(1):35–40.

49. Mills JL, Troendle J, Conley MR, et al. Maternal obesity and congenital heart defects: a population-based study. Am J Clin Nutr 2010;91(6):1543 9.

50. Block SR, Watkins SM, Salemi JL, et al. Maternal pre-pregnancy body mass index and risk of selected birth defects: evidence of a dose-response relationship. Paediatr Perinat Epidemiol 2013;27(6):521–31.

51. Stott-Miller M, Heike CL, Kratz M, et al. Increased risk of orofacial clefts associated with maternal obesity: case-control study and Monte Carlo-based bias analysis. Paediatr Perinat Epidemiol 2010;24(5):502–12.

52. Waller DK, Shaw GM, Rasmussen SA, et al. Prepregnancy obesity as a risk factor for structural birth defects. Arch Pediatr Adolesc Med 2007;161(8): 745–50.

53. Farah N, Kennedy C, Turner C, et al. Maternal obesity and pre-pregnancy folic acid supplementation. Obes Facts 2013;6(2):211–5.

54. Chung JH, Pelayo R, Hatfield TJ, et al. Limitations of the fetal anatomic survey via ultrasound in the obese obstetrical population. J Matern Fetal Neonatal Med 2012;25(10):1945–9.

55. Usha Kiran TS, Hemmadi S, Bethel J, et al. Outcome of pregnancy in a woman with an increased body mass index. BJOG 2005;112(6):768–72.

56. Jensen DM, Damm P, Sorensen B, et al. Pregnancy outcome and prepregnancy body mass index in 2459 glucose-tolerant Danish women. Am J Obstet Gynecol 2003;189(1):239–44.

57. Jolly MC, Sebire NJ, Harris JP, et al. Risk factors for macrosomia and its clinical consequences: a study of 350,311 pregnancies. Eur J Obstet Gynecol Reprod Biol 2003;111(1):9–14.

58. Ehrenberg HM, Mercer BM, Catalano PM. The influence of obesity and diabetes on the prevalence of macrosomia. Am J Obstet Gynecol 2004;191(3):964–8.

59. Sukalich S, Mingione MJ, Glantz JC. Obstetric outcomes in overweight and obese adolescents. Am J Obstet Gynecol 2006;195(3):851–5.

60. Khashan AS, Kenny LC. The effects of maternal body mass index on pregnancy outcome. Eur J Epidemiol 2009;24(11):697–705.

61. Kumari AS. Pregnancy outcome in women with morbid obesity. Int J Gynaecol Obstet 2001;73(2):101–7.

62. Bianco AT, Smilen SW, Davis Y, et al. Pregnancy outcome and weight gain recommendations for the morbidly obese woman. Obstet Gynecol 1998;91(1): 97–102.

63. Madan J, Chen M, Goodman E, et al. Maternal obesity, gestational hypertension, and preterm delivery. J Matern Fetal Neonatal Med 2010;23(1):82–8.

64. Aly H, Hammad T, Nada A, et al. Maternal obesity, associated complications and risk of prematurity. J Perinatol 2010;30(7):447–51.

65. Nohr EA, Bech BH, Vaeth M, et al. Obesity, gestational weight gain and preterm birth: a study within the Danish National Birth Cohort. Paediatr Perinat Epidemiol 2007;21(1):5–14.

66. Zhong Y, Cahill AG, Macones GA, et al. The association between prepregnancy maternal body mass index and preterm delivery. Am J Perinatol 2010;27(4): 293–8.

67. Hendler I, Goldenberg RL, Mercer BM, et al. The Preterm Prediction Study: association between maternal body mass index and spontaneous and indicated preterm birth. Am J Obstet Gynecol 2005;192(3):882–6.

68. Cnattingius S, Villamor E, Johansson S, et al. Maternal obesity and risk of preterm delivery. JAMA 2013;309(22):2362–70.

69. McDonald SD, Han Z, Mulla S, et al. Overweight and obesity in mothers and risk of preterm birth and low birth weight infants: systematic review and meta-analyses. BMJ 2010;341:c3428.

70. Torloni MR, Betran AP, Daher S, et al. Maternal BMI and preterm birth: a systematic review of the literature with meta-analysis. J Matern Fetal Neonatal Med 2009;22(11):957–70.

71. Salihu HM, Luke S, Alio AP, et al. The impact of obesity on spontaneous and medically indicated preterm birth among adolescent mothers. Arch Gynecol Obstet 2010;282(2):127–34.

72. Salihu HM, Lynch O, Alio AP, et al. Obesity subtypes and risk of spontaneous versus medically indicated preterm births in singletons and twins. Am J Epidemiol 2008;168(1):13–20.
73. Stotland NE, Washington AE, Caughey AB. Prepregnancy body mass index and the length of gestation at term. Am J Obstet Gynecol 2007;197(4):378.e1–5.
74. Arrowsmith S, Wray S, Quenby S. Maternal obesity and labour complications following induction of labour in prolonged pregnancy. BJOG 2011;118(5): 578–88.
75. Halloran DR, Cheng YW, Wall TC, et al. Effect of maternal weight on postterm delivery. J Perinatol 2012;32(2):85–90.
76. Caughey AB, Stotland NE, Washington AE, et al. Who is at risk for prolonged and postterm pregnancy? Am J Obstet Gynecol 2009;200(6):683.e1–5.
77. Heslehurst N, Simpson H, Ells LJ, et al. The impact of maternal BMI status on pregnancy outcomes with immediate short-term obstetric resource implications: a meta-analysis. Obes Rev 2008;9(6):635–83.
78. Roos N, Sahlin L, Ekman-Ordeberg G, et al. Maternal risk factors for postterm pregnancy and cesarean delivery following labor induction. Acta Obstet Gynecol Scand 2010;89(8):1003–10.
79. Pevzner L, Powers BL, Rayburn WF, et al. Effects of maternal obesity on duration and outcomes of prostaglandin cervical ripening and labor induction. Obstet Gynecol 2009;114(6):1315–21.
80. Nuthalapaty FS, Rouse DJ, Owen J. The association of maternal weight with cesarean risk, labor duration, and cervical dilation rate during labor induction. Obstet Gynecol 2004;103(3):452–6.
81. Hilliard AM, Chauhan SP, Zhao Y, et al. Effect of obesity on length of labor in nulliparous women. Am J Perinatol 2012;29(2):127–32.
82. Chin JR, Henry E, Holmgren CM, et al. Maternal obesity and contraction strength in the first stage of labor. Am J Obstet Gynecol 2012;207(2):129.e1–6.
83. Carlhall S, Kallen K, Blomberg M. Maternal body mass index and duration of labor. Eur J Obstet Gynecol Reprod Biol 2013;171(1):49–53.
84. Norman SM, Tuuli MG, Odibo AO, et al. The effects of obesity on the first stage of labor. Obstet Gynecol 2012;120(1):130–5.
85. Vahratian A, Zhang J, Troendle JF, et al. Maternal prepregnancy overweight and obesity and the pattern of labor progression in term nulliparous women. Obstet Gynecol 2004;104(5 Pt 1):943–51.
86. Robinson BK, Mapp DC, Bloom SL, et al. Increasing maternal body mass index and characteristics of the second stage of labor. Obstet Gynecol 2011;118(6): 1309–13.
87. Mazouni C, Porcu G, Cohen-Solal E, et al. Maternal and anthropomorphic risk factors for shoulder dystocia. Acta Obstet Gynecol Scand 2006;85(5):567–70.
88. Robinson H, Tkatch S, Mayes DC, et al. Is maternal obesity a predictor of shoulder dystocia? Obstet Gynecol 2003;101(1):24–7.
89. Mandal D, Manda S, Rakshi A, et al. Maternal obesity and pregnancy outcome: a prospective analysis. J Assoc Physicians India 2011;59:486–9.
90. Beyer DA, Amari F, Ludders DW, et al. Obesity decreases the chance to deliver spontaneously. Arch Gynecol Obstet 2011;283(5):981–8.
91. Chu SY, Kim SY, Schmid CH, et al. Maternal obesity and risk of cesarean delivery: a meta-analysis. Obes Rev 2007;8(5):385–94.
92. Poobalan AS, Aucott LS, Gurung T, et al. Obesity as an independent risk factor for elective and emergency caesarean delivery in nulliparous women–system-atic review and meta-analysis of cohort studies. Obes Rev 2009;10(1):28–35.

93. Marshall NE, Guild C, Cheng YW, et al. Maternal superobesity and perinatal outcomes. Am J Obstet Gynecol 2012;206(5):417.e1–6.
94. Fyfe EM, Anderson NH, North RA, et al. Risk of first-stage and second-stage cesarean delivery by maternal body mass index among nulliparous women in labor at term. Obstet Gynecol 2011;117(6):1315–22.
95. Conner SN, Tuuli MG, Longman RE, et al. Impact of obesity on incision-to-delivery interval and neonatal outcomes at cesarean delivery. Am J Obstet Gynecol 2013;209(4):386.e1–6.
96. Leth RA, Uldbjerg N, Norgaard M, et al. Obesity, diabetes, and the risk of infections diagnosed in hospital and post-discharge infections after cesarean section: a prospective cohort study. Acta Obstet Gynecol Scand 2011;90(5):501–9.
97. Stamilio DM, Scifres CM. Extreme obesity and postcesarean maternal complications. Obstet Gynecol 2014;124(2 Pt 1):227–32.
98. Conner SN, Verticchio JC, Tuuli MG, et al. Maternal obesity and risk of postcesarean wound complications. Am J Perinatol 2014;31(4):299–304.
99. Alanis MC, Villers MS, Law TL, et al. Complications of cesarean delivery in the massively obese parturient. Am J Obstet Gynecol 2010;203(3):271.e1–7.
100. Chelmow D, Rodriguez EJ, Sabatini MM. Suture closure of subcutaneous fat and wound disruption after cesarean delivery: a meta-analysis. Obstet Gynecol 2004;103(5 Pt 1):974–80.
101. Ramsey PS, White AM, Guinn DA, et al. Subcutaneous tissue reapproximation, alone or in combination with drain, in obese women undergoing cesarean delivery. Obstet Gynecol 2005;105(5 Pt 1):967–73.
102. Bell J, Bell S, Vahratian A, et al. Abdominal surgical incisions and perioperative morbidity among morbidly obese women undergoing cesarean delivery. Eur J Obstet Gynecol Reprod Biol 2011;154(1):16–9.
103. Brocato BE, Thorpe EM Jr, Gomez LM, et al. The effect of cesarean delivery skin incision approach in morbidly obese women on the rate of classical hysterotomy. J Pregnancy 2013;2013:890296.
104. McLean M, Hines R, Polinkovsky M, et al. Type of skin incision and wound complications in the obese parturient. Am J Perinatol 2012;29(4):301–6.
105. Marrs CC, Moussa HN, Sibai BM, et al. The relationship between primary cesarean delivery skin incision type and wound complications in women with morbid obesity. Am J Obstet Gynecol 2014;210(4):319.e1–4.
106. Durnwald CP, Ehrenberg HM, Mercer BM. The impact of maternal obesity and weight gain on vaginal birth after cesarean section success. Am J Obstet Gynecol 2004;191(3):954–7.
107. Chauhan SP, Magann EF, Carroll CS, et al. Mode of delivery for the morbidly obese with prior cesarean delivery: vaginal versus repeat cesarean section. Am J Obstet Gynecol 2001;185(2):349–54.
108. Carroll CS Sr, Magann EF, Chauhan SP, et al. Vaginal birth after cesarean section versus elective repeat cesarean delivery: Weight-based outcomes. Am J Obstet Gynecol 2003;188(6):1516–20 [discussion: 1520–2].
109. Hibbard JU, Gilbert S, Landon MB, et al. Trial of labor or repeat cesarean delivery in women with morbid obesity and previous cesarean delivery. Obstet Gynecol 2006;108(1):125–33.
110. Edwards RK, Harnsberger DS, Johnson IM, et al. Deciding on route of delivery for obese women with a prior cesarean delivery. Am J Obstet Gynecol 2003;189(2):385–9 [discussion: 389–90].

111. Fyfe EM, Thompson JM, Anderson NH, et al. Maternal obesity and postpartum haemorrhage after vaginal and caesarean delivery among nulliparous women at term: a retrospective cohort study. BMC Pregnancy Childbirth 2012;12:112.
112. Blomberg M. Maternal obesity and risk of postpartum hemorrhage. Obstet Gynecol 2011;118(3):561–8.
113. Hood DD, Dewan DM. Anesthetic and obstetric outcome in morbidly obese parturients. Anesthesiology 1993;79(6):1210–8.
114. Tan T, Sia AT. Anesthesia considerations in the obese gravida. Semin Perinatol 2011;35(6):350–5.
115. Butwick A, Carvalho B, Danial C, et al. Retrospective analysis of anesthetic interventions for obese patients undergoing elective cesarean delivery. J Clin Anesth 2010;22(7):519–26.
116. Kuczkowski KM, Benumof JL. Repeat cesarean section in a morbidly obese parturient: a new anesthetic option. Acta Anaesthesiol Scand 2002;46(6):753–4.
117. Saravanakumar K, Rao SG, Cooper GM. The challenges of obesity and obstetric anaesthesia. Curr Opin Obstet Gynecol 2006;18(6):631–5.
118. ACOG Committee on Gynecologic Practice. ACOG committee opinion. Number 319, October 2005. The role of obstetrician-gynecologist in the assessment and management of obesity. Obstet Gynecol 2005;106(4):895–9.
119. Getahun D, Ananth CV, Peltier MR, et al. Changes in prepregnancy body mass index between the first and second pregnancies and risk of large-for-gestational-age birth. Am J Obstet Gynecol 2007;196(6):530.e1–8.
120. Getahun D, Kaminsky LM, Elsasser DA, et al. Changes in prepregnancy body mass index between pregnancies and risk of primary cesarean delivery. Am J Obstet Gynecol 2007;197(4):376.e1–7.
121. Artal R, Lockwood CJ, Brown HL. Weight gain recommendations in pregnancy and the obesity epidemic. Obstet Gynecol 2010;115(1):152–5.
122. Flick AA, Brookfield KF, de la Torre L, et al. Excessive weight gain among obese women and pregnancy outcomes. Am J Perinatol 2010;27(4):333–8.
123. Ferraro Z, Barrowman N, Prud Homme D, et al. Excessive gestational weight gain predicts large for gestational age neonates independent of maternal body mass index. J Matern Fetal Neonatal Med 2012;25(5):538–42.
124. Cedergren MI. Optimal gestational weight gain for body mass index categories. Obstet Gynecol 2007;110(4):759–64.
125. Kiel DW, Dodson EA, Artal R, et al. Gestational weight gain and pregnancy outcomes in obese women: how much is enough? Obstet Gynecol 2007;110(4):752–8.
126. Wolff S, Legarth J, Vangsgaard K, et al. A randomized trial of the effects of dietary counseling on gestational weight gain and glucose metabolism in obese pregnant women. Int J Obes (Lond) 2008;32(3):495–501.
127. Guelinckx I, Devlieger R, Mullie P, et al. Effect of lifestyle intervention on dietary habits, physical activity, and gestational weight gain in obese pregnant women: a randomized controlled trial. Am J Clin Nutr 2010;91(2):373–80.
128. Thornton YS, Smarkola C, Kopacz SM, et al. Perinatal outcomes in nutritionally monitored obese pregnant women: a randomized clinical trial. J Natl Med Assoc 2009;101(6):569–77.
129. Quinlivan JA, Lam LT, Fisher J. A randomised trial of a four-step multidisciplinary approach to the antenatal care of obese pregnant women. Aust N Z J Obstet Gynaecol 2011;51(2):141–6.
130. Quinlivan JA, Julania S, Lam L. Antenatal dietary interventions in obese pregnant women to restrict gestational weight gain to institute of medicine recommendations: a meta-analysis. Obstet Gynecol 2011;118(6):1395–401.

131. American College of Obstetricians, Gynecologists. ACOG practice bulletin no. 105: bariatric surgery and pregnancy. Obstet Gynecol 2009;113(6):1405–13.

132. Schauer PR, Kashyap SR, Wolski K, et al. Bariatric surgery versus intensive medical therapy in obese patients with diabetes. N Engl J Med 2012;366(17): 1567–76.

133. Mingrone G, Panunzi S, De Gaetano A, et al. Bariatric surgery versus conventional medical therapy for type 2 diabetes. N Engl J Med 2012; 366(17):1577–85.

134. Maggard MA, Yermilov I, Li Z, et al. Pregnancy and fertility following bariatric surgery: a systematic review. JAMA 2008;300(19):2286–96.

135. Bennett WL, Gilson MM, Jamshidi R, et al. Impact of bariatric surgery on hypertensive disorders in pregnancy: retrospective analysis of insurance claims data. BMJ 2010;340:c1662.

136. Ducarme G, Revaux A, Rodrigues A, et al. Obstetric outcome following laparoscopic adjustable gastric banding. Int J Gynaecol Obstet 2007;98(3):244–7.

137. Lesko J, Peaceman A. Pregnancy outcomes in women after bariatric surgery compared with obese and morbidly obese controls. Obstet Gynecol 2012; 119(3):547–54.

138. Patel JA, Patel NA, Thomas RL, et al. Pregnancy outcomes after laparoscopic Roux-en-Y gastric bypass. Surg Obes Relat Dis 2008;4(1):39–45.

139. Burke AE, Bennett WL, Jamshidi RM, et al. Reduced incidence of gestational diabetes with bariatric surgery. J Am Coll Surg 2010;211(2):169–75.

140. Weintraub AY, Levy A, Levi I, et al. Effect of bariatric surgery on pregnancy outcome. Int J Gynaecol Obstet 2008;103(3):246–51.

141. Dixon JB, Dixon ME, O'Brien PE. Birth outcomes in obese women after laparoscopic adjustable gastric banding. Obstet Gynecol 2005;106(5 Pt 1):965–72.

142. Belogolovkin V, Salihu HM, Weldeselasse H, et al. Impact of prior bariatric surgery on maternal and fetal outcomes among obese and non-obese mothers. Arch Gynecol Obstet 2011;285(5):1211–8.

143. Sheiner E, Edri A, Balaban E, et al. Pregnancy outcome of patients who conceive during or after the first year following bariatric surgery. Am J Obstet Gynecol 2011;204(1):50.e1–6.

144. Kjaer MM, Lauenborg J, Breum BM, et al. The risk of adverse pregnancy outcome after bariatric surgery: a nationwide register-based matched cohort study. Am J Obstet Gynecol 2013;208(6):464.e1–5.

145. Berlac JF, Skovlund CW, Lidegaard O. Obstetrical and neonatal outcomes in women following gastric bypass: a Danish national cohort study. Acta Obstet Gynecol Scand 2014;93(5):447–53.

146. Wax JR, Cartin A, Wolff R, et al. Pregnancy following gastric bypass for morbid obesity: effect of surgery-to-conception interval on maternal and neonatal outcomes. Obes Surg 2008;18(12):1517–21.

147. Kjaer MM, Nilas L. Timing of pregnancy after gastric bypass—a national register-based cohort study. Obes Surg 2013;23(8):1281–5.

148. Miller AD, Smith KM. Medication and nutrient administration considerations after bariatric surgery. Am J Health Syst Pharm 2006;63(19):1852–7.

149. Skull AJ, Slater GH, Duncombe JE, et al. Laparoscopic adjustable banding in pregnancy: safety, patient tolerance and effect on obesity-related pregnancy outcomes. Obes Surg 2004;14(2):230–5.

150. Loar PV 3rd, Sanchez-Ramos L, Kaunitz AM, et al. Maternal death caused by midgut volvulus after bariatric surgery. Am J Obstet Gynecol 2005;193(5): 1748–9.

151. Brewer CJ, Balen AH. The adverse effects of obesity on conception and implantation. Reproduction 2010;140(3):347–64.
152. Reddy UM, Branum AM, Klebanoff MA. Relationship of maternal body mass index and height to twinning. Obstet Gynecol 2005;105(3):593–7.
153. Harper LM, Cahill AG, Smith K, et al. Effect of maternal obesity on the risk of fetal loss after amniocentesis and chorionic villus sampling. Obstet Gynecol 2012; 119(4):745–51.
154. Elsinga J, de Jong-Potjer LC, van der Pal-de Bruin KM, et al. The effect of preconception counselling on lifestyle and other behaviour before and during pregnancy. Womens Health Issues 2008;18(Suppl 6):S117–25.
155. Royal College of Obstetricians and Gynaecologists. Green-top guideline No. 37. Reducing the risk of thrombosis and embolism during pregnancy and the puerperium. London: Royal College of Obstetricians and Gynaecologists; 2009.
156. Liu B, Jorm L, Banks E. Parity, breastfeeding, and the subsequent risk of maternal type 2 diabetes. Diabetes Care 2010;33(6):1239–41.
157. Chuang CH, Chase GA, Bensyl DM, et al. Contraceptive use by diabetic and obese women. Womens Health Issues 2005;15(4):167–73.

Influenza
Threat to Maternal Health

 CrossMark

Elaine L. Duryea, MD*, Jeanne S. Sheffield, MD

KEYWORDS

- Influenza • Pregnancy • Respiratory illness • Maternal morbidity • Vaccination

KEY POINTS

- Increased morbidity and mortality have been associated with influenza infection in pregnancy, with infection in the third trimester the most common (approximately 50% of cases) and associated with a higher rate of complications.
- Prompt initiation of antiviral treatment decreases the likelihood of ICU admission and maternal mortality.
- Influenza vaccine is recommended in pregnancy regardless of trimester, with acceptance rates highest when the vaccine is offered at a physician's office.

INTRODUCTION

A maternal mortality rate of 1% was reported during the 2009–2010 influenza pandemic,[1] with influenza in pregnancy posing a serious risk to maternal health. A high level of suspicion coupled with prompt diagnosis and treatment is paramount to minimizing morbidity and mortality. Vaccination during pregnancy should be of high priority to improve both maternal and neonatal outcomes.

DISCUSSION

Influenza is an RNA virus of the Orthomyxoviridae family. There are 3 antigenic types of influenza: influenza A and influenza B both cause significant clinical disease and are associated with seasonal epidemics; influenza C causes only a mild respiratory illness without seasonality. Influenza A can be subtyped based on 2 surface glycoproteins— hemagglutinin (HA) and neuraminidase (NA). There are currently at least 16 antigenically distinct HAs and 9 distinct NAs and combinations of these 2 glycoproteins allow for the nomenclature of specific subtypes. Influenza B does not have these subtypes.

Financial Disclosure: The authors did not report any potential conflicts of interest.
Department of Obstetrics and Gynecology, University of Texas Southwestern Medical Center, 5323 Harry Hines Boulevard, Dallas, TX 75235-9032, USA
* Corresponding author.
E-mail address: Elaine.Duryea@UTSouthwestern.edu

Obstet Gynecol Clin N Am 42 (2015) 355–362
http://dx.doi.org/10.1016/j.ogc.2015.01.009
0889-8545/15/$ – see front matter © 2015 Elsevier Inc. All rights reserved.

obgyn.theclinics.com

Annual seasonal outbreaks occur with influenza cases first reported in approximately October with peak incidence in January–February and extension into May. Tropical climates may experience influenza activity throughout the year. Annual influenza vaccination is necessary to account for antigenic drift or subtle point mutations in surface antigens, which decrease host resistance to the pathogen. Occasionally with influenza A, an antigenic shift occurs. This is a significant change in the virus surface antigens (HA and NA), which leads to the emergence of a new subtype, often resulting in a global pandemic with increased morbidity and mortality. The last pandemic occurred with the emergence of the influenza A 2009 H1N1 strain.

INCREASED SEVERITY OF INFLUENZA IN PREGNANCY

Although pregnant women may not be more susceptible to influenza, higher morbidity and mortality have been associated with this infection in pregnancy. In a report of the influenza pandemic of 1918, pneumonia complicated approximately half of influenza infections in pregnancy and more than 20% of women died, with mortality highest in the third trimester.[2] Similar outcomes were reported during the pandemic of 1957.[3] Both immunologic and physiologic changes of pregnancy increase the potential severity of influenza in the gravid population. This was again highlighted during the 2009 H1N1 influenza A pandemic in which, despite aggressive hospitalization of pregnant women with influenza, 5% of deaths in the United States occurred among pregnant women whereas they composed only 1% of the population. Pregnant women are also more likely to experience severe disease requiring admission to an ICU. In comparison with years with only seasonal influenza, when only 40% of hospitalizations and 10% of deaths were among people age less than 65 years, in 2009 with the emergence of the H1N1 subtype, 90% of hospitalizations and 87% of deaths were among people less than 65 years,[4] highlighting the need for increased vigilance in the pregnant population, who more frequently experience adverse effects.

Gravid women experience a shift from helper T cell type 1 (T_H1) to helper T cell type 2 (T_H2) immunity with suppression of cell-mediated and increased humoral immunity, likely secondary to the increased levels of estradiol and progesterone during pregnancy. For example, there is an increase in T_H2-type cytokines, such as interleukin (IL)-4, IL-5, IL-10, and IL-13, with suppression of inflammatory cytokines (**Table 1**), which theoretically may decrease susceptibility to acquisition of an illness, such as influenza, but also can affect efficient clearance of the pathogen.[5] The normal physiologic changes of pregnancy, especially at advanced gestational ages, also may predispose women to worse disease and need for more intensive care. In pregnancy, there is a 20% to 30% decrease in pulmonary functional residual capacity due to diaphragm elevation. In addition, there is an increased oxygen requirement and possible increased critical closing volume (the volume at which dependent parts of the lung begin to close during expiration), which can worsen respiratory illness.[6] More than 60% of pregnant women admitted for influenza infection are in the third trimester, with a small minority (<10%) in the first trimester.[1]

Regardless of the various possible causes, there is no doubt that influenza in pregnancy may have devastating consequences, requiring rapid diagnosis and treatment by an informed clinician to best prevent complications.

CLINICAL PRESENTATION

The inoculation period for influenza is 1 to 4 days, with a majority of women reporting a known exposure, most of whom are immediate family members. Individuals are usually infectious the day before as well as for 5 days after symptom onset. In a prospective

Table 1
Pregnancy stage and immune function

Early Pregnancy	Mid- and Late Pregnancy

CD4+ T$_H$1 function response and cell-mediated immunity similar to nonpregnant state	Decrease in adaptive immune function
	  Decrease in number and function of CD4+, CD8+ T cells
	  Decrease in number and function of natural killer cells
	  Decrease in number and function of B cells
	Increase in innate immune function
	  Increase in monocytes, dendritic cells, and phagocytes
	  Increase in T-regulatory cells
	  Increase in α-defensin expression
	Decrease in interferon-γ, IL-2, monocyte chemotactic protein 1, eotaxin
	Increase in tumor necrosis factor α, IL-10, IL-4, IL-5, and granuloctye colony-stimulating factor

Adapted from Kourtis AP, Read JS, Jamieson DJ. Pregnancy and infection. N Engl J Med 2014;370:2215.

study of pregnant women diagnosed with seasonal (H3N2) influenza A in 2004, cough was the most commonly reported symptom, present in 93% of women. Fever was documented in most women (89%), although a temperature greater than 40°C was rare (<2%). Other common symptoms included myalgia, nausea/vomiting, rhinorrhea, pharyngitis, and headache (each present in at least 40% of cases). Tachycardia was prevalent and out of proportion to fever—a pulse greater than 100 beats per minute was documented in a majority of cases and a pulse greater than 130 beats per minute in 1 in 5 women.[7] Most symptoms, including fever, generally resolve within 1 week; however, cough and malaise may last for longer than 2 weeks. Symptoms and signs are similar with the 2009 H1N1 influenza subtype—either cough or fever was present in more than 90% of cases in one series.[8] Vaccination in the current season should not preclude consideration of influenza infection, especially if vaccine has been administered within the prior 2 weeks when antibody formation may not be complete.

DIAGNOSIS

The Centers for Disease Control and Prevention (CDC) definition of an influenza-like illness can be either clinical (fever of 100°F or higher and cough and/or sore throat) or laboratory (positive influenza test). Diagnostic testing should not delay initiation of treatment when clinical suspicion is high because the empirical treatment of pregnant women while awaiting results of testing is recommended. Many versions of rapid influenza diagnostic tests are available, all of which detect the qualitative presence of nucleoprotein antigens in specimens (ie, positive or negative), with some tests able to distinguish between influenza A and B. These rapid influenza tests yield results quickly, often within 15 minutes, with good specificity (85%–100%). The sensitivity is low, however, reported as 45% to 62% for both H3N2 and H1N1 subtypes, with a high rate of false-negative test results.[9] Certain factors may decrease the accuracy of these rapid tests, including poor specimen quality, location of specimen (lower respiratory tract samples may have a lower sensitivity than upper tract samples), and delayed collection (>72 hours from illness onset). A negative rapid test does not preclude influenza in a woman with a suspicious clinical presentation, especially during an influenza epidemic. Treatment should not be withheld from patients with suspected influenza when a rapid test is negative. Reverse transcription–polymerase chain reaction and viral cultures serve as reference standards for confirmation, with viral cultures recommended by the CDC for initial cases to identify strains within the population.

TREATMENT

Treatment of influenza in pregnancy includes antiviral therapy plus supportive care. Prompt treatment is associated with improved outcomes and shortened duration of symptoms. In a review of the 2009 H1N1 pandemic, antiviral treatment within 2 days of symptom onset decreased the likelihood of ICU admission and resulted in fewer maternal deaths.[10,11] Therefore, initiation of treatment as early as possible and preferably within 2 days of the onset of symptoms is recommended by the CDC. There is recent evidence, however, that initiation of antiviral therapy more than 2 days from the onset of symptoms may still improve the course of disease. Antiviral therapy should be given offered to acutely symptomatic pregnant women regardless of duration of symptoms.[12]

There are 4 antiviral medications with activity against influenza available in the United States (**Table 2**). Amantadine and rimantadine are M2 inhibitors that are active only against influenza A. More than 99% of currently circulating influenza A viruses, however, are resistant to the adamantanes and their use is not recommended. The current mainstays of treatment are the NA inhibitors. Oseltamivir is an oral NA inhibitor with activity against both influenza A and influenza B. Zanamivir is an inhaled NA inhibitor that can be used in pregnancy. Oseltamivir is preferred because there are more pharmacokinetic and outcome data available in pregnancy.[10] Zanamivir may also worsen pulmonary complications in certain pregnant women with respiratory issues. The CDC recommends the same dose of oseltamivir (75 mg twice daily for 5 days) for pregnant women as for nonpregnant patients, with pharmacokinetic studies demonstrating levels that remain constant across trimesters of pregnancy.[13] A higher

Table 2
Antiviral medications

Medication	Activity	Dose	Side Effects	Excretion
Neuraminadase inhibitors				
Oseltamivir	Influenza A and B	Treatment: 75 mg po bid Prophylaxis: 75 mg po qid × 10 d	Nausea/vomiting	Renal (hepatic metabolism)
Zanamivir	Influenza A and B	Treatment: 10 mg inhaled bid × 5 d	Bronchospasm	Renal
M2 inhibitors				
Amantadine[a]	Influenza A	Treatment: 100 mg po bid × 5 d Prophylaxis: 100 mg po bid × 5–7 d	Central nervous system: jitteriness, anxiety, concentration issues	Renal
Rimantadine[a]	Influenza A	Treatment: 100 mg po bid × 5 d Prophylaxis: 100 mg po bid × 5–7 d	Central nervous system, although less than amantadine	Renal (hepatic metabolism)

[a] Not currently recommended due to widespread resistance.

dose has been recommended by some (150 mg twice a day) in immunocompromised and severely ill patients, although limited data suggest that higher dosing may not provide additional benefit. Extended treatment may be warranted in severe cases and decision for treatment should be guided by virologic polymerase chain reaction testing. Intravenous peramivir and zanamivir are available in specific circumstances where administration of oseltamivir orally or via nasogastric tube is not possible or there is suspicion of oseltamivir resistance (rare).

Treatment in the peripartum period can be difficult. A recent study that evaluated hand hygiene, antiviral therapy for mothers, and encouragement of rooming-in and breastfeeding found no maternal-infant transmission in 42 cases of laboratory-confirmed influenza in the immediate postpartum period.[14] In addition, although oseltamivir is present in breast milk, levels are lower than maternal serum concentrations and well below the therapeutic range for infants. Breastfeeding is considered safe while taking oseltamivir.[15] Women should be considered at increased risk for influenza-related complications for up to 2 weeks postpartum and treated similarly to pregnant women during that time period.

Postexposure chemoprophylaxis with oseltamivir (75 mg once daily for 10 days) can be considered. Although there are few data on the efficacy of prophylaxis in pregnancy, oseltamivir in pregnancy is safe and the benefits often outweigh the risks. Prophylaxis is 70% to 90% effective in preventing influenza when administered within 2 days of the initial exposure. Women receiving prophylaxis should be instructed to contact their medical provider or seek immediate evaluation if they develop fever or other influenza symptoms.

COMPLICATIONS

Conventional risks factors for complications related to influenza infection, such as chronic lung disease, tobacco use, diabetes, chronic hypertension and cardiovascular disease, autoimmune disease, and immune suppression, place pregnant women at an increased risk of ICU admission and death in comparison with pregnant women without any underlying conditions (**Box 1**). A majority of pregnant women requiring ICU admission secondary to influenza infection, however, do not have preexisting medical conditions.[4] In a review of pregnant women infected with the 2009 H1N1 pandemic strain, these risk factors were found related to an increased risk of ICU admission and death; however, other underlying conditions complications, including thyroid disease, neurologic disease, and obesity, were also found more frequent in these women. In addition, timing of treatment was significantly associated with maternal mortality. Only 16% of women who required hospitalization and 4% who died received treatment within 2 days of the onset of symptoms.[11]

Complications of influenza include primary influenza pneumonia (discussed previously) and secondary bacterial pneumonia. Secondary bacterial pneumonias often present 2 to 3 days after a patient initially starts to improve. Fevers recur, sputum production increases, and lobar consolidations are often diagnosed on chest radiograph. *Staphylococcus aureus, Streptococcus pneumoniae*, and *Haemophilus influenzae* are the most common organisms identified. Appropriate antibiotic coverage for these organisms should be initiated. Other extrapulmonary complications, including rhabdomyolysis, myositis, myocarditis, and pericarditis, as well as evidence of CNS infections are far less common.

Influenza infection during pregnancy has also been associated with an increased risk of preterm delivery, small-for-gestational-age infants, and fetal death in addition to the maternal complications.[16-18]

Box 1
Risk factors associated with complications in pregnant women

Definite risk factors

- Existing pulmonary disease
- Smoking
- Diabetes
- Chronic hypertension
- Cardiovascular disease
- Autoimmune disease
- Use of immunosuppressive therapy
- Second or third trimester gestation
- Neurologic disease

Additional possible risk factors

- Thyroid disease
- Obesity

PREVENTION/VACCINATION

The CDC recommends influenza vaccination for all individuals over 6 months of age, regardless of risk factors. Universal vaccination in pregnancy has proved cost effective. Ideally vaccine should be received by October, because vaccination beyond November has been shown to result in overall decreased effectiveness and decreased cost-effectiveness.[19,20] Pregnant women are among the group of people at increased risk for complicated infections and should be given priority access to vaccine when supplies are limited.[21] The American Congress of Obstetricians and Gynecologists (ACOG) recommends influenza vaccine in pregnancy regardless of trimester as well as in the preconceptional and postpartum periods if not yet received for the current season.[22] The trivalent inactive influenza vaccine has been proved safe in the first trimester without increased risk of major fetal malformations or pregnancy loss.[23,24] Vaccination in any trimester is associated with a decreased risk of stillbirth, neonatal death, and preterm delivery. The quadrivalent vaccine, which provides increased immunity for an additional strain of influenza B, is also safe in pregnancy and is approved by the CDC and ACOG for use (no preference between the trivalent and quadrivalent vaccines is made by either organization). Contraindications to the influenza vaccine are rare and include a severe allergic reaction to any component of the vaccine (ie, eggs) or to a prior dose of vaccine. Consideration of vaccination deferment in individuals with moderate to severe illness with or without fever is reasonable; however, minor illness without fever is not a contraindication to receiving the vaccine. Live attenuated vaccine (FluMist, an intranasal suspension) is not recommended in pregnancy. There is no need, however, for pregnant women to avoid contact with those receiving live attenuated vaccine, and they may receive the live attenuated vaccine in the immediate postpartum period if the inactive vaccine was not given during the current season.[25]

Influenza vaccination in pregnancy results in the production of protective antibody titers in levels comparable to those in nonpregnant women. These antibodies can be transmitted via the placenta to the fetus and provide protection during the first few months of life when an infant is ineligible to receive vaccination.[26,27] Studies have recently demonstrated an increase in immunity and a decrease in influenza infections in infants born to mothers who received the vaccine during pregnancy even in populations thought at risk for poor vaccine response, such as those infected with HIV.[28,29]

In 2005, only 15% of pregnant women had been vaccinated for influenza in the previous 12 months.[25] Following the 2009 H1N1 pandemic, this percentage has risen, to 50% in 2012–2013; however, a great improvement can still be made in vaccination rates. Vaccine acceptance is affected by multiple factors. The most common reasons for declining vaccination are a lack of knowledge about the importance of vaccination and concern about risks to the fetus.[30] These issues may be easily addressed by a woman's physician, leading to increased acceptance of the vaccine. Acceptance rates are highest (65%) when the vaccine is offered on site at a physician's office. Recommendation for vaccination by a woman's physician does slightly increase vaccination rates but does not maximize compliance. In fact, 32% of women report never receiving a recommendation for vaccination from their medical provider.[31]

SUMMARY

Overall, influenza causes a disproportionate amount of morbidity and mortality among the pregnant population. Preventative measures are vital to decrease the disease incidence in this high-risk population. The CDC and the World Health Organization are currently monitoring several new avian influenza strains (eg, H5N1 and H7N9); although these strains normally do not infect humans, several cases recently have been reported with very high mortality rates. Human-to-human transmission is rare but these avian strains have the potential to change. Continued public health vigilance is needed on an international scale to help prevent the occurrence of the next pandemic.

REFERENCES

1. Varner MW, Rice MM, Anderson B, et al. Influenza-like illness in hospitalized pregnant and postpartum women durying the 2009–2010 H1N1 pandemic. Obstet Gynecol 2011;118(3):593–600.
2. Kilbourne ED. Influenza. New York: Plenum Publishing Corporation; 1987.
3. Greenberg M, Jacobziner H, Pakter J, et al. Maternal mortality in the epidemic of Asian influenza, New York city, 1957. Am J Obstet Gynecol 1958;76:897–902.
4. Creanga AA, Kamimoto L, Newsome K, et al. Seasonal and 2009 pandemic influenza A (H1N1) virus infection during pregnancy: a population-based study of hospitalized cases. Am J Obstet Gynecol 2010;204:S38–45.
5. Kourtis AP, Read JS, Jamieson DJ. Pregnancy and infection. N Engl J Med 2014; 370:2211–8.
6. Cunningham FG. Williams obstetrics. 24th edition. New York: McGraw Hill; 2014. Print.
7. Rogers VL, Sheffield JS, Roberts SW, et al. Presentation of seasonal influenza A in pregnancy. Obstet Gynecol 2010;115:924–9.
8. Louie JK, Acosta M, Jamieson DJ, et al. Severe 2009 H1N1 influenza in pregnancy and postpartum women in California. N Engl J Med 2010;362:27–35.
9. Guidance for Clinicians on the Use of Rapid Influenza Diagnostic Tests. Centers for Disease Control and Prevention. Available at: http://www.cdc.gov/flu/professionals/diagnosis/clinician_guidance_ridt.htm. Accessed August 22, 2014.
10. Greer LG, Sheffield JS, Rogers VL, et al. Maternal and neonatal outcomes after antepartum treatment of influenza with antiviral medications. Obstet Gynecol 2010;115:711–6.

11. Siston AM, Rasmussen SA, Honein MA, et al. Pandemic 2009 Influenza A (H1N1) virus illness among pregnant women in the United States. JAMA 2010;303: 1517–25.
12. Influenza Antiviral Medications: Summary for Clinicians. Centers for Disease Control and Prevention. Available at: http://www.cdc.gov/flu/professionals/antivirals/summary-clinicians.htm. Accessed August 22, 2014.
13. Greer LG, Leff RD, Rogers VL, et al. Pharmacokinetics of oseltamivir according the trimester of pregnancy. Am J Obstet Gynecol 2011;204:S89–93.
14. Cantey JB, Bascik SL, Heyne NG, et al. Prevention of mother-to-infant transmission of influenza during the postpartum period. Am J Perinatol 2013;30:233–40.
15. Greer LF, Leff RD, Rogers VL, et al. Pharmacokinetics of oseltamivir in breast milk and maternal plasma. Am J Obstet Gynecol 2011;204:524.e1–4.
16. Habery SE, Trogstad L, Funnes N, et al. Risk of fetal death after pandemic influenza virus infection or vaccination. N Engl J Med 2013;368:333–40.
17. McNeil SA, Dodds LA, Fell DB, et al. Effect of respiratory hospitalization during pregnancy on infant outcomes. Am J Obstet Gynecol 2011;204:S54–7.
18. Mendez-Figueroa H, Raker C, Anderson BL. Neonatal characteristics and outcomes of pregnancies complicated by influenza infection during the 2009 pandemic. Am J Obstet Gynecol 2011;204:S58–63.
19. Roberts S, Hollier LM, Sheffield JS, et al. Cost-effectiveness of universal influenza vaccination in a pregnant population. Obstet Gynecol 2006;107:1323–9.
20. Myers ER, Misurski DA, Swamy GK. Influence of timing of seasonal influenza vaccination on effectiveness and cost-effectiveness in pregnancy. Am J Obstet Gynecol 2011;204:S128–40.
21. Grohskopf LA, Shay DK, Shimabukuro TT, et al. Prevention and control of seasonal influenza with vaccines: recommendations of the advisory committee on immunization practices 2013–2014. MMWR Recomm Rep 2013;62:1–48.
22. American College of Obstetricians and Gynecologists. Committee opinion No. 608: influenza vaccination during pregnancy. Obstet Gynecol 2014;124:648–51.
23. Sheffield JS, Greer LG, Rogers V, et al. Effect of influenza vaccination in the first trimester of pregnancy. Obstet Gynecol 2012;120:532–7.
24. Moro PL, Museru OI, Broder K, et al. Safety of influenza A (H1N1) 2009 live attenuated monovalent vaccine in pregnant women. Obstet Gynecol 2013;122: 1271–8.
25. Centers for Disease Control and Prevention (CDC). Prevention and control of influenza. MMWR Morb Mortal Wkly Rep 2007;56:1–54.
26. Steinhoff MC, Omer SB, Roy E, et al. Influenza immunizations in pregnancy-antibody responses in mothers and infants. N Engl J Med 2010;362:1644–6.
27. Glezen WP. Effect of maternal antibodies on the infant immune response. Vaccine 2003;21:3389–92.
28. Poehling KA, Szilagyi PG, Staat MA, et al. Impact of maternal immunization on influenza hospitalizations in infants. Am J Obstet Gynecol 2011;204:S141–8.
29. Madhi SA, Cutland CL, Kuwanda L, et al. Influenza vaccination of pregnant women and protection of their infants. N Engl J Med 2014;371(10):918–31.
30. Fisher BM, Scott J, Hart J, et al. Behaviors and perceptions regarding seasonal and H1N1 influenza vaccination during pregnancy. Am J Obstet Gynecol 2011; 204:S107–11.
31. Centers for Disease Prevention and Control (CDC). Influenza vaccination coverage among pregnant women – United States, 2012–13 influenza season. MMWR Morb Mortal Wkly Rep 2013;62:787–92.

How to Approach Intrapartum Category II Tracings

Audra E. Timmins, MD, MBA*, Steven L. Clark, MD

KEYWORDS

- Fetal heart rate monitoring • Neonatal encephalopathy • Patient safety

KEY POINTS

- Standardized nomenclature for describing electronic fetal heart rate (eFHR) patterns has enabled better care.
- Category II FHR patterns are by far the most common and most diverse patterns, leading to broad variation in management.
- Standardization of management following an algorithm utilizing both FHR pattern and progress in labor should provide a starting point for both improved neonatal outcomes and new clinical trials.

INTRODUCTION

In 2008, a Eunice Kennedy Shriver National Institute of Child Health and Human Development (NICHD) consensus panel proposed a uniform system of terminology classifying fetal heart rate (FHR) patterns as category I, II, or III based on well-defined characteristics of the FHR.[1] This was done in an effort to standardize and thus improve the interpretation and management of FHR patterns. Since that time, the American Congress of Obstetricians and Gynecologists (ACOG) has issued specific guidelines for the management of category I (normal) and category III (pathologically abnormal) FHR patterns; the former are managed conservatively, and the latter are generally indications for prompt delivery.[2] However, ACOG guidelines for the management of category II FHR patterns are less specific and reflect the relatively low positive predictive value of many category II FHR patterns for the detection of fetal hypoxia/acidemia. The following is an attempt to provide a framework for the management of category II FHR tracings, which are seen in 80% of all fetuses in

The authors have nothing to disclose.
Texas Children's Hospital, Baylor College of Medicine, 6651 Main Street #1020, Houston, TX, 77030, USA
* Corresponding author.
E-mail address: atimmins@bcm.edu

Obstet Gynecol Clin N Am 42 (2015) 363–375
http://dx.doi.org/10.1016/j.ogc.2015.01.013
0889-8545/15/$ – see front matter © 2015 Elsevier Inc. All rights reserved.

labor. These recommendations are based on the best available evidence and are directed at optimizing fetal outcomes without significantly increasing rates of cesarean section.

DISCUSSION

Essential to any discussion of the management of FHR tracings is a standardized interpretation of those tracings. Based on the NICHD guidelines, a full description of external fetal monitoring requires evaluation of

- Uterine contractions
- Baseline FHR
- FHR variability
- Presence of accelerations
- Periodic or episodic decelerations
- Changes in FHR patterns over time

The uterine contraction pattern should be described in terms of frequency, duration, and intensity. For purposes of this discussion, the issue is contraction frequency:

- Normal: no more than 5 contractions in 10 minutes, averaged over 30 minutes
- Tachysystole: more than 5 contractions in 10 minutes, averaged over 30 minutes

Baseline FHR is based on the mean FHR in increments of 5 beats per minute during a 10 minute window, at least 2 minutes of which must be spent in identifiable baseline segments.

- Bradycardia: less than 100 beats per minute
- Normal: 110 to 160 beats per minute
- Tachycardia: greater than 160 beats per minute

Baseline FHR variability is defined as fluctuations in the baseline FHR (in that same 10-minute window) that are irregular in amplitude and frequency, exclusive of accelerations and decelerations:

- Absent: amplitude range undetectable
- Minimal: no more than 5 beats per minute
- Moderate: 6 to 25 beats per minute
- Marked: greater than 25 beats per minute

An acceleration is an abrupt increase in FHR lasting at least 15 seconds and rising at least 15 beats per minute above baseline. Abrupt is defined as reaching the peak/nadir in less than 30 seconds. Gradual is defined as reaching the peak/nadir in 30 seconds or more. Prolonged accelerations last at least 2 minutes but no more than 10 minutes. Beyond 10 minutes, such patterns are considered a change in baseline.

Decelerations are classified as variable, early, or late based on their timing and characteristics (**Box 1**).

Utilizing these definitions, the NICHD system classifies the FHR into 3 tiers. Category I tracings are normal:

- Baseline 110 to 160 beats per minute
- Variability: moderate
- No late or variable decelerations
- Early decelerations: present or absent
- Accelerations: present or absent

Box 1
Characteristics of decelerations

Late deceleration

- Visually apparent, usually symmetric gradual decrease and return of the FHR associated with a uterine contraction
- Delayed in timing, with the nadir occurring after the peak of the contraction
- Typically, the onset, nadir, and recovery of the deceleration occur after the beginning, peak, and ending of the contraction.

Early deceleration

- Visually apparent, usually symmetric gradual decrease and return of the FHR associated with a uterine contraction
- Nadir of the deceleration occurs at the same time as the peak of the contraction
- Typically, the onset, nadir, and recovery of the deceleration are coincident with beginning, peak, and ending of the contraction

Variable deceleration

- Visually apparent abrupt decrease in FHR
- Decrease is greater than 15 beats per minute, lasts greater than 15 seconds but less than 2 minutes
- If associated with contractions, appearance will vary with successive contractions

---

Category II tracings are indeterminate and account for about 80% of FHR tracings:

- Baseline rate tachycardia or bradycardia (not accompanied by absent variability)
- Baseline variability minimal, marked or absent (no accompanied by recurrent decelerations)
- Absent accelerations (even after stimulation)
- Periodic or episodic decelerations including recurrent variable decelerations, prolonged deceleration, recurrent late decelerations with moderate variability, variable decelerations with slow return to baseline, overshoots, or shoulders

Category III FHR tracings are abnormal:

- Absent variability and recurrent late decelerations, recurrent variable decelerations, or bradycardia
- Sinusoidal pattern

Although the management of category I and category III FHR patterns is clear, the breadth of category II FHR tracings makes strict delineation of management much more difficult. This is made even more problematic by the level of interobserver and intraobserver reliability, noted to be moderate for categories I and II and poor for category III FHR tracings (although the main variation was classifying minimal versus absent variability).[3] Additionally, although the amount of time spent with a category II tracing prior to delivery has been shown to increase short-term neonatal morbidity (higher rates of low Apgar scores and neonatal intensive care unit [NICU] admissions), there is no generally accepted stratification of risk within the category II tracings.[4] Also essential to the usefulness of any algorithm created will be its applicability across all clinical venues and all levels of practitioners The algorithm presented in the remainder of this article follows the one developed by Clark and colleagues[5] in 2013. Previously presented algorithms recognize many of the same issues but lack definitive recommendations for timing of intervention and are more subject to interobserver reliability.[6–8]

The goal of any algorithm should be to deliver a fetus prior to development of metabolic academia, thus reducing the risk of avoidable intrapartum neurologic injury. To achieve this goal, Miller and Miller presented several fundamental principles that have guided the development of all algorithms for intrapartum FHR interpretation:

1. Oxygen is carried from the environment to the fetus by maternal and fetal blood along a pathway that includes the maternal heart, lungs, vasculature, uterus, placenta, and umbilical cord.
2. Interruption of fetal oxygenation has the potential to result in hypoxic neurologic injury.
3. Acute intrapartum interruption of fetal oxygenation does not result in neurologic injury in the absence of significant fetal metabolic academia.

Prior to any discussion of a specific algorithm, a review of the pathophysiology of decelerations is warranted to explain why the algorithm is structured the way it is. Since 1967, decelerations have been referred to as early, late, or variable based on their timing and shape.[9] These were thought to be caused by head compression, placental insufficiency, and cord compression, respectively. Early decelerations are likely of no clinical importance. Late decelerations, especially with minimal-to-absent variability, represent a protective fetal response to contraction-induced hypoxia, and often represent an already compromised fetus (**Fig. 1**). In reality, most decelerations that occur in labor are variables. Although most of these are benign, there is good evidence that deep, frequent variable decelerations may lead to significant fetal compromise.[10,11]

Although there is no direct relationship between uterine artery blood flow and umbilical venous blood flow, a reduction in maternal blood flow to the placenta may negatively affect oxygenation of fetal blood flowing from the placenta. Janbu and Nesheim demonstrated a nearly linear fall in uterine artery blood flow during contractions.[12] In fetal lambs, there is good evidence that fetal hypoxia results from decreased umbilical venous blood flow.[13] Although such repetitive contraction-induced hypoxia is a feature of normal labor, and is tolerated well in most cases, the marginally oxygenated or developmentally compromised fetus may exhibit a protective hypoxia-induced reduction in FHR (late deceleration) in response to such stress.

Variable decelerations resulting from umbilical cord compression are at the heart of any discussion of category II FHR tracing management. Fletcher and colleagues[14] showed that the initial fall in FHR is an adaptation that decreases myocardial work and oxygen requirements. Fetal lamb studies have shown that the depth of the deceleration is related to the severity of the hypoxia.[15,16] The frequency of decelerations is also important, as umbilical cord occlusion studies in fetal sheep show that fetuses exposed to more frequent cord occlusion (1 every 2.5 minutes vs 1 every 5 minutes) experience a larger fall in pH and increase in base deficit.[17,18] Additionally, Hamilton and colleagues[19] showed that only 3 subtypes of variables were associated with increased risk of fetal acidosis: those with prolonged duration, those with loss of internal variability, and those with "sixties" criteria. "Sixties" criteria are met if 2 or more of the following conditions are present in a variable deceleration: depth of 60 beats per minute or more, nadir of 60 beats per minute or less, and duration of 60 seconds or longer. Thus, any useful algorithm would need take into account the frequency, length, and depth of variable decelerations.

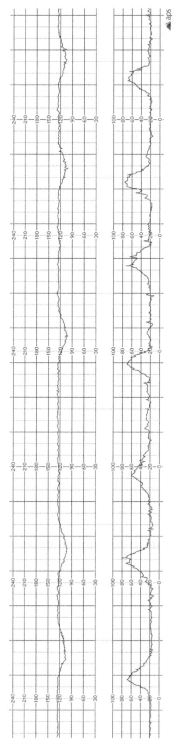

Fig. 1. FHR tracing exhibiting minimal variability with recurrent late decelerations. Expedited delivery is indicated. (*Courtesy of* Advanced Practice Strategies Inc, Boston, MA; with permission.)

What happens between decelerations is likely an even better predictor of fetal well being. Parer and colleagues[20] recently demonstrated that a fetus with moderate variability is coping well with the demands of labor and is unlikely to have significant acidosis. That same review noted that the most consistent predictor of newborn academia was absent or minimal variability with late or variable decelerations. In a similar manner, spontaneous or induced accelerations reliably exclude significant fetal metabolic acidemia.[5] With this background, the authors present an algorithm for the management of category II FHR patterns that requires only standard cardiotocography equipment available in all labor and delivery units (**Fig. 2**). It utilizes standard NICHD definitions and is consistent with, but more specific than, that document with respect to management recommendations. The algorithm begins with an assessment of baseline variability, as the presence of moderate variability allows one to effectively rule out clinically significant metabolic acidemia. Because variability within decelerations cannot reliably exclude fetal acidemia, this type of variability is not considered when evaluating the FHR. Then, with the goal of predicting/preventing the development of significant acidemia prior to delivery, the focus shifts to decelerations. The algorithm cannot change the outcome for a previously injured fetus or one that experiences a catastrophic event during labor (abruption, uterine rupture, cord prolapse) (**Box 2**, see **Fig. 2**).

While following the algorithm, it is often appropriate to first make conservative attempts to relieve potential causes of the category II tracing. Amnioinfusion for oligohydramnios-associated variable decelerations is well supported.[21] Maternal positioning out of the supine position may also increase fetal oxygenation. On the other hand, the commonly utilized administration of oxygen to the mother, in concentrations

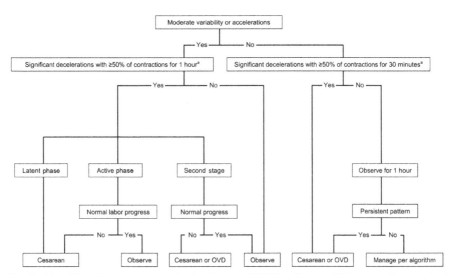

Fig. 2. Algorithm for management of category II FHR patterns. OVD, operative vaginal delivery. [a] That have not resolved with appropriate conservative corrective measures, which may include supplemental oxygen, maternal position changes, intravenous fluid administration, correction of hypotension, reduction or discontinuation of uterine stimulation, administration of uterine relaxant, amnioinfusion, and/or changes in second-stage breathing and pushing techniques. (*From* Clark SL, Nageotte MP, Garite TJ, et al. Intrapartum management of category II fetal heart rate tracings: towards standardization of care. Am J Obstet Gynecol 2013;209(2):90; with permission.)

Box 2
Management of category II fetal heart rate patterns: clarifications for use in algorithm

1. Variability refers to predominant baseline FHR pattern (marked, moderate, minimal, absent) during a 30-minute evaluation period, as defined by NICHD

2. Marked variability is considered same as moderate variability for purposes of this algorithm

3. Significant decelerations are defined as any of the following:
   - Variable decelerations lasting longer than 60 seconds and reaching a nadir more than 60 beats per minute below baseline
   - Variable decelerations lasting longer than 60 seconds and reaching a nadir less than 60 beats per minute regardless of the baseline.
   - Any late decelerations of any depth
   - Any prolonged deceleration, as defined by the NICHD; because of the broad heterogeneity inherent in this definition, identification of a prolonged deceleration should prompt discontinuation of the algorithm until the deceleration is resolved

4. Application of algorithm may be initially delayed for up to 30 minutes while attempts are made to alleviate category II pattern with conservative therapeutic interventions (eg, correction of hypotension, position change, amnioinfusion, tocolysis, reduction, or discontinuation of oxytocin)

5. Once a category II FHR pattern is identified, FHR is evaluated and algorithm applied every 30 minutes

6. Any significant change in FHR parameters should result in reapplication of algorithm

7. For category II FHR patterns in which algorithm suggests delivery is indicated, such delivery should ideally be initiated within 30 minutes of decision for cesarean section

8. If at any time tracing reverts to category I status, or deteriorates for even a short time to category III status, the algorithm no longer applies; however, algorithm should be reinstituted if category I pattern again reverts to category II

9. In fetus with extreme prematurity, neither significance of certain FHR patterns of concern in more mature fetus (eg, minimal variability) nor ability of such fetuses to tolerate intrapartum events leading to certain types of category II patterns is well defined; this algorithm is not intended as guide to management of fetus with extreme prematurity

10. Algorithm may be overridden at any time if, after evaluation of patient, physician believes it is in best interest of the fetus to intervene sooner

From Clark SL, Nageotte MP, Garite TJ, et al. Intrapartum management of category II fetal heart rate tracings: towards standardization of care. Am J Obstet Gynecol 2013;209(2):91; with permission.

---

normally available on labor and delivery units, does not improve fetal oxygen saturation; no evidence exists that such therapy improves neonatal outcomes.[22,23] Finally, attempts to reduce uterine tachysystole or tetanic contractions should also be made, especially if the labor is being augmented.

Phase of labor and expected time to delivery also play important roles in the algorithm. A fetus exhibiting deep variables in a rapidly progressing second stage may be able to tolerate them until spontaneous delivery, while a fetus with the same FHR pattern in latent labor is less likely to be able to tolerate them for the expected amount of time to delivery (**Fig. 3**). This is important to consider when evaluating a patient with a potential arrest disorder, as recent data suggest that a more conservative approach with longer periods of observation is warranted before that diagnosis is made in the fetus with a reassuring heart rate pattern. For purposes of this algorithm, which

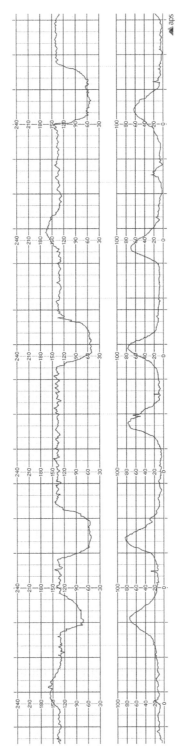

Fig. 3. When close to delivery, with normal progress in the second stage, this fetus may be watched or considered for operative vaginal delivery if the pattern persists. When remote from delivery, cesarean section should be done per the algorithm. (*Courtesy of* Advanced Practice Strategies Inc, Boston, MA; with permission.)

applied only to fetuses with a category II FHR pattern, normal progress in labor refers to the older Friedman time limits.[5]

Although no management algorithm for FHR tracings will ever predict unexpected sentinel events, 2 clinical situations should be specifically addressed. Patients with vaginal bleeding and a category II FHR tracing should be considered for expedited delivery, as abruption may be the underlying cause and may progress precipitously to frank fetal asphyxia.[24] Patients undergoing a trial of labor after cesarean section should also be carefully watched for any sudden FHR tracing changes, as the further decline may be much more rapid in the case of uterine rupture than in a patient with an otherwise similar FHR tracing.[25]

Decelerations may fall outside the strict parameter of the algorithm, yet still be clinically important (**Fig. 4**). Prolonged decelerations as defined by the NICHD are not addressed by the algorithm, as the variability in causation, timing, and management is too great to be addressed by any single algorithm. Additionally, in a mixed pattern including variable and late decelerations, precedence should always be given to the late decelerations.

Minimal variability and absent variability in the FHR are considered as one for the purposes of this algorithm for 3 reasons. First, discussed earlier, is the lack of interobserver and intraobserver reliability in distinguishing between the two. The other is the presumption that a fetus with a moderate variability will pass through a stage of minimal variability as its condition worsens. Finally, while variability must be absent to correlate with severe fetal acidemia with a high degree of statistical reliability, the goal of electronic FHR monitoring during labor is to deliver infants prior to the development of such acidemia. Any concerns about the quality of the tracing and the ability to determine variability should be addressed by the placement of a fetal scalp electrode unless contraindicated.

Some fetuses may present with persistent minimal-to-absent variability but have no significant decelerations (**Fig. 5**). This most likely represents pre-existing insults, and a brief period of observation is reasonable and appropriate. Although the fetus may have been damaged, no further damage is occurring in the absence of significant decelerations.

As noted previously, this algorithm is designed for use in any obstetric unit. Other technologies such as fetal scalp sampling and fetal pulse oximetry have been evaluated and found not to offer a significant advantage over eFHR.[26] Newer technologies may arise that will alter the use of the algorithm.

In 1990, Roger Freeman observed that the saga of electronic FHR monitoring had been "a disappointing story" in that such monitoring had failed to result in any significant reduction in rates of neonatal encephalopathy and subsequent neurologic impairment but had contributed to the rise in cesarean section delivery rate. A quarter of a century later, the situation remains unchanged, yet the approach to FHR interpretation and management has remained static. Recent data suggest that variation in interpretation and response to abnormal FHR patterns is largely to blame and that, as in many other areas of medicine, standardization will yield improved outcomes. In a series of over 14,000 patients undergoing oxytocin induction of labor, those women who were managed with a standardized protocol that included unambiguous definition of normal and abnormal FHR patterns and prescribed specific actions in response to specific patterns experienced fewer low 1- and 5-minute Apgar scores, fewer infant NICU admissions and a lower cesarean section delivery rate.[27] Along with the authors of the original algorithm discussed here, the authors believe that such an approach to the management of category II FHR patterns is likely to yield similar results. In addition, such an algorithm represents 1 approach to FHR

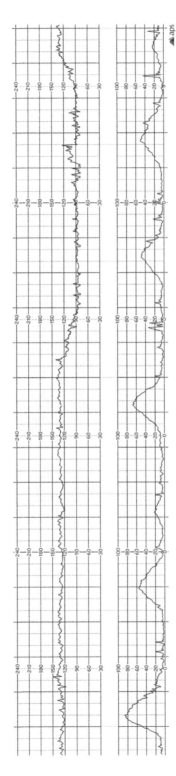

Fig. 4. The etiology of this prolonged deceleration is unknown. The management of this type of FHR pattern is not covered by the algorithm and needs to be tailored to the clinical picture. (*Courtesy of* Advanced Practice Strategies Inc, Boston, MA; with permission.)

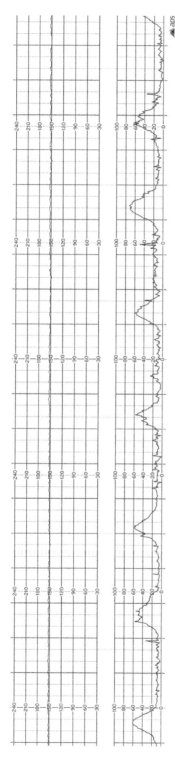

Fig. 5. The absence of decelerations exc udes ongoing hypoxia in a neurologically intact fetus, but this fetus may not tolerate labor; delivery should be considered if the pattern persists for 1 hour. (Courtesy of Advanced Practice Strategies Inc, Boston, MA; with permission.)

interpretation that is, in the opinion of the 18 clinician–investigators responsible for the bulk of authoritative work on this subject in the past 30 years, reasonable given the current understanding and available data, and it should be viewed as such during any scientifically valid, objective review of such tracings. Although other approaches may be equally reasonable, the authors feel this approach will be particularly useful to clinicians and provide a starting point for well-designed clinical trials to further refine a uniform approach to this issue.

REFERENCES

1. Macones GA, Hankins GD, Spong CY, et al. The 2008 National Institutes of Child Health and Human Development workshop report on electronic fetal monitoring; update on definitions, interpretation and research guidelines. Obstet Gynecol 2008;112:661–6.
2. American College of Obstetricians and Gynecologists. Practice Bulletin No. 116: Management of intrapartum fetal heart rate tracings. Obstet Gynecol 2010;116: 1232–40.
3. Blackwell SC, Grobman WA, Antoniewicz L, et al. Interobserver and intraobserver reliability of the NICHD 3-Tier Fetal Heart Rate Interpretation System. Am J Obstet Gynecol 2011;205:378.e1–5.
4. Jackson M, Holmgren C, Esplin MS, et al. Frequency of fetal heart rate categories and short-term neonatal outcome. Obstet Gynecol 2011;118:803–8.
5. Clark SL, Nageotte MP, Garite TJ, et al. Intrapartum management of category II fetal heart rate tracings: towards standardization of care. Am J Obstet Gynecol 2013;209(2):89–97.
6. Chandrahan E, Arulkumaran S. Prevention of birth asphyxia: responding appropriately to cardiotocograph (CTG) traces. Best Pract Res Clin Obstet Gynaecol 2007;21:609–24.
7. Parer JT, Ikeda T. A framework for standardized management of intrapartum fetal heart rate patterns. Am J Obstet Gynecol 2007;197:26.e1–6.
8. Miller DA, Miller LA. Electronic fetal heart rate monitoring: applying principles of patient safety. Am J Obstet Gynecol 2012;206:278–83.
9. Hon E, Quilligan EJ. The classification of fetal heart rate: II, a revised working classification. Conn Med 1967;31:779–84.
10. Westgate JA, Harris M, Curnow JS, et al. Randomised trial of cardiotocography alone or with ST waveform analysis for intrapartum monitoring. Lancet 1992; 340:194–8.
11. de Hann HH, Gunn AJ, Williams CE, et al. Brief repeated umbilical cord occlusions cause sustained cytotoxic cerebral edema and focal infarcts in near term fetal lambs. Pediatr Res 1997;41:96–104.
12. Janbu T, Nesheim BI. Uterine artery blood velocities during contractions in pregnancy and labour related to intrauterine pressure. BJOG 1987;94:1150–5.
13. Tchirikov M, Eisermann K, Rybakowski C, et al. Doppler ultrasound evaluation of ductus venosus blood flow during acute hypoxemia in fetal lambs. Ultrasound Obstet Gynecol 1998;11:426–31.
14. Fletcher AJ, Gardner DS, Edwards M, et al. Development of the ovine fetal cardiovascular defense to hypoxemia towards term. Am J Physiol Heart Circ Physiol 2006;291:H3023–34.
15. Itskovitz J, LaGamma EF, Rudolph AM. Heart rate and blood pressure responses to umbilical cord compression in fetal lambs with special reference to the mechanism of variable deceleration. Am J Obstet Gynecol 1983;147:451–7.

16. Baan J Jr, Boekkooi PF, Teitel DF, et al. Heart rate fall during acute hypoxemia: a measure of chemoreceptor response in fetal sheep. J Dev Physiol 1993;19: 105–11.
17. de Haan HH, Gunn AJ, Gluckman PD. Fetal heart rate changes do not reflect cardiovascular deterioration during brief repeated umbilical cord occlusions in near term fetal lambs. Am J Obstet Gynecol 1997;176:8–17.
18. Westgate JA, Bennet L, Gunn AJ. Fetal heart rate variability changes during brief repeated umbilical cord occlusion in near term fetal sheep. BJOG 1999;106: 664–71.
19. Hamilton EF, Daly MV, Townsend K. New perspectives in electronic fetal surveillance. J Perinat Med 2012;0(0):1–10.
20. Parer JT, King T, Flanders S, et al. Fetal academia and electronic fetal heart rate patterns: is there evidence of an association? J Matern Fetal Neonatal Med 2006; 19:289–94.
21. Simpson KR, James DC. Efficacy of intrauterine resuscitation techniques in improving fetal oxygen status during labor. Obstet Gynecol 2005;105:1362–8.
22. Hayden M, Gorenberg D, Nageotte M, et al. The effect of maternal oxygen administration on fetal pulse oximetry during labor in fetuses with non-reassuring fetal heart rate tracings. Am J Obstet Gynecol 2006;195:735–8.
23. Dildy GA, Clark SL. Effects of maternal oxygen administration on fetal pulse oximetry. Am J Obstet Gynecol 2007;196:13–6.
24. Oyelse Y, Ananth CV. Placental abruption. Obstet Gynecol 2006;108:1005–16.
25. Leung AS, Leung EK, Paul RH. Uterine rupture after previous cesarean delivery: maternal and fetal consequences. Am J Obstet Gynecol 1993;169:945–50.
26. East CE, Begg L, Colditz PB, et al. Fetal pulse oximetry for fetal assessment in labour. Cochrane Database Syst Rev 2014;(10):CD004075.
27. Clark SL, Meyers JA, Garthwaite T, et al. Recognition and response to electronic fetal heart rate patterns – impact on newborn outcomes and primary cesarean delivery rate in women undergoing induction of labor. Am J Obstet Gynecol 2014. http://dx.doi.org/10.1016/j,ajog.2014.11.019.

Prevention of the First Cesarean Delivery

Catherine Y. Spong, MD

KEYWORDS

- Prevention • Cesarean • Vaginal delivery • Maternal and fetal health

KEY POINTS

- Prevention of the first cesarean is a major driver to reducing overall cesarean rates.
- There are numerous obstetric, fetal, and maternal factors that are modifiable and impact cesarean delivery rates.
- Patience is necessary to allow normal labor; recent data demonstrate that the labor course is longer than previously taught.

INTRODUCTION

Cesarean childbirth began as a practice to remove the infant from a dead or dying mother, it was a measure of last resort and was not intended to preserve the mother's life.[1] From these origins, cesarean delivery has moved in the twenty-first century to become one of the most common major abdominal surgeries performed, and has a variety of obstetric and medical indications.

Of the almost 4 million births in the United States in 2012, 32.8% were delivered by cesarean, a rate unchanged since 2010. From 1996 to 2010 the rate had steadily increased from 20.7% in 1996 to the current 32%.[2] In parallel with the rise in total cesarean births from 1996 to 2010 is a rise in primary cesarean deliveries. Before 1996, the rate was flat or declining from the mid-1980s, in part because of the increasing use of vaginal birth after cesarean; however, the vaginal birth after cesarean rate peaked in the mid-1990s and now accounts for less than 10% of deliveries despite evidence supporting the method.[3]

Internationally, rates of cesarean vary dramatically ranging from less than 20% in northwestern European countries to 50% in southeastern Europe and more than 60% in some Latin-American countries.[4]

The author has nothing to disclose.
National Institute of Child Health and Human Development, National Institutes of Health, 31 Center Drive, Room 2A03, Bethesda, MD 20892, USA
E-mail address: spongc@mail.nih.gov

Obstet Gynecol Clin N Am 42 (2015) 377–380
http://dx.doi.org/10.1016/j.ogc.2015.01.010
0889-8545/15/$ – see front matter Published by Elsevier Inc.

obgyn.theclinics.com

Although overall cesarean is considered safe, it is generally accepted that there are increases in morbidity and mortality with cesarean[5–9]:

- Two-fold increase in maternal mortality
- Greater blood loss
- Impaired neonatal respiratory function
- Increased incidence of maternal postpartum infections
- Fetal lacerations
- Affects maternal-infant interaction
- Longer recovery
- Rehospitalization

Fetal risks include 1% to 2% risk of laceration, 1% to 4% risk of respiratory morbidity in those delivered by cesarean, and 1% to 2% risk of shoulder dystocia in those delivered vaginally. Although the initial cesarean is associated with increases in maternal morbidity and mortality, such as a rate of severe morbidity of 9.2% versus 8.6% in vaginal deliveries and mortality of 2.7% versus 0.9%, respectively, the downstream effects are even greater because of the risks of repeat cesareans in subsequent pregnancies, and associated placentation complications.[10] Multiple repeat cesareans are associated with a dose-dependent increase in placenta accreta, placenta previa, hysterectomy, transfusion of greater than or equal to four units, and maternal intensive care unit admission.[11]

Solheim and colleagues[12] performed a decision analysis model of the downstream consequences of rising cesarean rates and if they continue at current rates, by 2020 there will be a cesarean section rate of 56.2%, an additional 6236 previas per year, an additional 4504 accretas per year, and an additional 130 maternal deaths per year.

Given the fall in vaginal birth after cesarean, the risks associated with multiple cesareans, and the current trends, the most effective approach to reducing the overall cesarean delivery rate is to prevent the first cesarean. Major indications for primary cesarean include those occurring before labor and those during labor. Before labor the major cause is malpresentation and during labor first-stage and second-stage arrest.[13]

To identify points for intervention, obstetric, fetal, and maternal factors can be considered to identify those that are modifiable and may impact the overall cesarean rate. An expert panel convened to evaluate these factors and bin them into their diagnostic accuracy, the size of the effect if it were to be successful, and preventative strategies for each factor.[14] Of these many had limited diagnostic accuracy and small overall effects.

Failed induction and arrest of labor had the greatest potential effect, although the diagnostic accuracy was considered limited. Other obstetric factors with smaller impact include the use of external cephalic version for malpresentation; efforts to limit maternal weight gain to impact suspected macrosomia; and education for preeclampsia, cardiovascular disease, maternal request, and inadequate pelvis.

The definitions of failed induction and arrest of labor were reviewed and rethought based on current information to provide practitioners guidance. Failed induction should be diagnosed only after an adequate attempt, which is defined as least 24 hours of oxytocin with artificial membrane rupture (if feasible) with the failure to generate regular contractions and cervical change. Limiting the use of induction of labor to avoid elective inductions, recognizing the association of cesarean with cervical status (less favorable cervix = higher risk of cesarean), and the importance of allowing the induction sufficient time to progress all may result in lower cesarean rates.[14] The obstetric care consensus went even further than the expert panel recommendations stating that induction of labor should only be used for maternal or fetal indications before 41 weeks of gestation.[10]

The recent data demonstrating contemporary labor curves reinforce the need for patience during the labor process. It is critical to allow adequate time for normal latent and active phases of the first and second stages of labor, unless expeditious delivery is indicated. Zhang and colleagues[15] studied more than 60,000 women with singleton pregnancies at term, all with spontaneous onset of labor, vaginal deliveries, and normal neonatal outcomes. They found that the inflection point was at 6 cm dilation, not the traditionally taught 4 cm, defining the active phase of labor, and that this only occurred in multiparous women. In addition, the dilation at admission to labor and delivery affected the pattern of labor progression. First- and second-stage arrest were also redefined to allow longer time and these were confirmed by the recent obstetric care consensus document.[10,14]

Thus contemporary labor is not what was previously taught; spontaneous labor progresses more slowly. A measured, nuanced approach is needed along with consideration of the new definitions of the active phase of labor and definitions of labor arrest. Other considerations, such as the dilation at admission, need to be considered in evaluating labor progress. In addition, other strategies to reduce cesarean in the second stage of labor need to be encouraged and taught including operative vaginal delivery and manual rotation of the fetal occiput. Despite the well-known benefits of these approaches, many are not routinely taught or embraced by providers given the acceptance of cesarean. It is critical that not only are these taught but also that providers and patients are comfortable with their use.

In addition to the opportunities afforded by the obstetric, fetal, and maternal factors, there are many other influences on delivery method. Practice models including different models of care, such as collaborative practice,[16] hospitalists, and integration of midwifery, should be considered as opportunities to impact the cesarean rate. Several studies have demonstrated that the use of models that enhance flexibility and reduce financial incentives influence delivery route. In addition, studies have shown that malpractice is associated with cesarean rates. States with higher malpractice rates correlated to lower vaginal delivery and higher cesarean deliveries.[17]

Another important component is accountability for the provider and clear hospital policies on indications for inductions, definitions, and protocols. For providers, the use of audits, feedback and tracking of vertex, singleton term gestation delivery method including nonmedically indicated cesarean, nonmedically indicated induction of labor, labor arrest, failed induction and cesarean delivery for nonreassuring fetal heart rate.

Education of providers and patients on the importance of vaginal delivery, for the current and future pregnancies, is essential to reverse the current trend of primary cesareans. When discussing cesarean with patients, counseling should include the effect on subsequent pregnancy risks including possibility of uterine rupture and placentation abnormalities. In addition, counseling must include the concept that normal labor takes time. In the current era of information available instantaneously and instant gratification, the concept of allowing labor to occur naturally without interventions to initiate or augment unless medically necessary is not prevalent. Societal expectations are for rapid and positive outcomes. Re-education on the natural process of labor, the importance of allowing the time needed, and patience with the duration of pregnancy and process of labor is essential.

REFERENCES

1. Sewell JE. Cesarean section: a brief history. A brochure to accompany an exhibition on the history of cesarean section at the National Library of Medicine, 30

April 1993–31 August 1993. Available at: http://www.nlm.nih.gov/exhibition/cesarean/. Accessed February 18, 2015.

2. Martin JA, Bamilton BE, Osterman MJ, et al. Births: final data for 2012. Natl Vital Stat Rep 2013;62(9):1–68.

3. National Institutes of Health Consensus Development Conference Panel. National Institutes of Health Consensus Development Conference statement: vaginal birth after cesarean: new insights March 8-10, 2010. Obstet Gynecol 2010;115(6): 1279–95.

4. Visser GH. Women are designed to deliver vaginally and not by cesarean section: an obstetrician's view. Neonatology 2015;107:8–13.

5. Hall MH, Bewley S. Maternal mortality and mode of delivery. Lancet 1999; 354(9180):776.

6. Levine EM, Ghai V, Barton JJ, et al. Mode of delivery and risk of respiratory diseases in newborns. Obstet Gynecol 2001;97(3):439–42.

7. Dessole S, Cosmi E, Balata A, et al. Accidental fetal lacerations during cesarean delivery: experience in an Italian level III university hospital. Am J Obstet Gynecol 2004;191(5):1673–7.

8. Buhimschi CS, Buhimschi I. Advantages of vaginal delivery. Clin Obstet Gynecol 2006;49(1):167–83.

9. Lydon-Rochelle M, Holt VL, Martin DP, et al. Association between method of delivery and maternal rehospitalization. JAMA 2000;283(18):2411–6.

10. American College of Obstetricians and Gynecologists (College), Society for Maternal-Fetal Medicine, Caughey AB, et al. Safe prevention of the primary cesarean delivery. Am J Obstet Gynecol 2014;201(3):179–93.

11. Silver RM, Landon MB, Rouse DJ, et al, National Institute of Child Health and Human Development Maternal-Fetal Medicine Units Network. Maternal morbidity associated with multiple repeat cesarean deliveries. Obstet Gynecol 2006; 107(6):1226–32.

12. Solheim KN, Esakoff TF, Little SE, et al. The effect of cesarean delivery rates on the future incidence of placenta previa, placenta accreta, and maternal mortality. J Matern Fetal Neonatal Med 2011;24(11):1341–6.

13. Barber EL, Lundsberg LS, Belanger K, et al. Indications contributing to the increasing cesarean delivery rate. Obstet Gynecol 2011;118:29–38.

14. Spong CY, Berghella V, Wenstrom K, et al. Preventing the first cesarean delivery: summary of a joint Eunice Kennedy Shriver National Institute of Child Health and Human Development, Society for Maternal-Fetal Medicine, and American College of Obstetricians and Gynecologists workshop. Obstet Gynecol 2012;120: 1181–93.

15. Zhang J, Landy H, Branch W, et al. Contemporary patterns of spontaneous labor with normal neonatal outcomes. Obstet Gynecol 2010;116:1281–7.

16. Larsen JW, Pinger WA. Primary cesarean delivery prevention. Obstet Gynecol 2014;123(5):152S–3S.

17. Johnson CT, Werner EF. The nationwide relationship between malpractice rates of vaginal and cesarean delivery. Obstet Gynecol 2014;123(5):119S–20S.

Placenta Accreta Spectrum
Accreta, Increta, and Percreta

Robert M. Silver, MD, Kelli D. Barbour, MD, MSc*

KEYWORDS

- Abnormal placentation • Accreta • Increta • Percreta • Placenta • Hemorrhage
- Cesarean hysterectomy • Indicated preterm delivery

KEY POINTS

- The incidence of placenta accreta is increasing. Major risk factors include history of cesarean delivery, placenta previa, and prior uterine surgery.
- Antenatal diagnosis can decrease morbidity and mortality; ultrasound is the best imaging modality and has good accuracy.
- A multidisciplinary team in a center of excellence can optimize maternal and neonatal outcomes with accreta.
- Timing of delivery should be individualized, but is typically done between 34 and 36 weeks. Planned cesarean-hysterectomy is the standard management for placenta accreta.
- Conservative management may allow for fertility preservation. However, risks are substantial and optimal candidates and management strategies have not been identified.

INTRODUCTION

Normal placentation results from adherence of the blastocyst to the decidualized endometrium. Abnormal placentation includes placental abruption, placenta previa, cesarean scar ectopic pregnancy, cervical pregnancy, and the accreta spectrum. Placenta accreta occurs secondary to abnormal adherence of the placenta to the myometrium, instead of the decidua. This abnormal adherence has important clinical implications that can result in severe maternal and neonatal morbidity and mortality. This typically occurs when the placenta does not separate from the uterus after delivery, leading to massive hemorrhage and associated complications such as disseminated intravascular coagulation (DIC), multiorgan dysfunction and/or failure, and death.[1] Correction and treatment of hemorrhage often requires massive transfusion, intensive care unit (ICU) admission, interventional radiologic procedures, and hysterectomy, which also increase morbidity.[1] Fetal morbidity and mortality, as with placenta previa, is related to complications of premature birth.[2]

The authors have nothing to disclose.
Division of Maternal-Fetal Medicine, Department of Obstetrics & Gynecology, University of Utah Health Sciences Center, 30 North 1900 East 2B200 SOM, Salt Lake City, UT 84132, USA
* Corresponding author.
E-mail address: kelli.barbour@hsc.utah.edu

With increased recognition of risk factors and obstetric ultrasonography, many cases of placenta accreta spectrum disorders are diagnosed prenatally.[3] However, not all populations have access to ultrasound, qualified ultrasonographers, or experienced radiologists or obstetricians who can make these diagnoses antenatally. Because of these limitations, placenta accreta, increta, and percreta, may be encountered at the time of delivery. It is, therefore, important for all obstetricians and other providers of obstetric care to be familiar with the epidemiology, risk factors, diagnosis, and management of these potentially highly morbid and fatal disorders of abnormal placentation. Ideally, cases with suspected accreta should be referred to centers of excellence in the care of accreta.

DEFINITIONS

The term 'placenta accreta' has been used to describe a single pathologic entity, as well as a generic term for the disease spectrum. Used singly, a placenta accreta (vera) occurs if the placenta attaches to, but does not invade into, myometrium (**Fig. 1**). If the placenta invades into the myometrium, but not beyond, the placenta is described as a placenta increta. When the placenta invades through the serosal layer and potentially beyond, the term placenta percreta is employed.[4] On this spectrum, placenta accreta is the most common and placenta percreta the least common. For this article, we use the term 'placenta accreta' to refer to the single entity as well as to placenta accreta spectrum. The term should be considered to refer to the spectrum, unless specifically noted in the text.

EPIDEMIOLOGY

The rate of cesarean delivery has increased substantially over the past few decades, both within and outside of the United States.[5,6] As the cesarean rate increased, so has the incidence of pregnancies complicated by placenta accreta spectrum disorders.[7–9] Between the 1960s and 2002, the incidence increased from 1 in 30,000 pregnancies to 1 in 533; this constitutes a nearly 60-fold increase in a matter of 5 decades.[6] As placenta accretas have increased, the indications for peripartum hysterectomy have changed, with accreta accounting for up to 47% of indications.[10]

RISK FACTORS

The pathophysiology of placenta accreta disorders is uncertain. Nonetheless, the result is abnormal adherence of the trophoblasts surrounding the blastocyst to

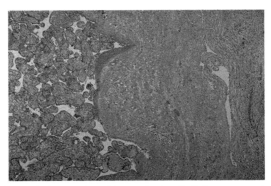

Fig. 1. Histopathology of placenta invading to the level of the myometrium (H&E stain, 40× [forty magnification]).

and/or through the myometrium. In pregnancies not complicated by accreta, tropho-blast invades the endometrium until they reach Nitabuch's layer (spongiosus layer of the decidua).[11] Upon reaching this layer, cytotrophoblasts cease invasion and begin to differentiate into the placental tissue needed for a successful pregnancy. Although advances are being made in understanding these processes, many details of normal and abnormal placentation remain uncertain.

As mentioned, there is an association between the increasing numbers of cesarean deliveries and the risk of subsequent placenta accreta. This association is thought to be owing to malrepair of the endometrium and/or decidua basalis. With the subse-quent pregnancy, cytotrophoblasts invade decidualized endometrium, but fail to encounter the spongiosus layer and do not encounter the normal signal to stop inva-sion. Instead, trophoblasts continue their invasion to an abnormal degree. Histopath-ologic evaluation of placenta accreta specimens support this theory; they show trophoblast invasion of the myometrium without evidence of a decidual layer in bet-ween.[11] Trophoblast inclusions (inner layer of syncytiotrophoblasts, outer layer of cytotrophoblasts contained solely within chorionic villi) also are more common in placenta accreta specimens compared with normal placentas.[12] Decidual natural killer cells also are fewer in patient with placenta accreta.[13]

Relative hypoxia of cesarean scar tissue (resulting from fibroblast-based repair and decreased vessel concentration) may also be involved in the pathophysiology of accreta.[14] Cytotrophoblast invasion is stimulated by invasion—not until they reach spiral arterioles do the trophoblasts differentiate and change behavior, allowing for spiral arteriole reorganization and increased oxygen tension and delivery.[15] The rela-tive hypoxia of the cesarean scar tissue may recruit preferentially the blastocyst to implant in areas that result in an increased risk of placenta accreta. The increased inci-dence of previas and accretas in women with multiple cesareans (and therefore increased relatively hypoxic tissue) supports this theory.

Whatever the true pathophysiology of abnormal placentation, multiple studies sup-port the substantially increased risk of placenta accreta in women with a history of multiple cesarean deliveries. The majority of placenta accretas occur in multiparous women, especially in those with at least 1 prior cesarean delivery. As the number of prior cesarean's increase, so does the risk of encountering a placenta accreta, increta, or percreta. For example, women with a history of 3 or 4 cesareans have at least a 2% chance of accreta; women underdoing their sixth or greater cesarean delivery (having had at least 5 previous cesarean sections) have a more than 3-fold higher risk of accreta ($\sim$7%; **Table 1**).[7]

Although placenta accreta can occur without a placenta previa, the presence of a placenta previa and a history of multiple cesareans increase drastically the risk of abnormal placentation involving a previous cesarean scar. A 2006 cohort study estimated the risk of placenta accreta in women with a known placenta previa to be 3%, 11%, 40%, 61%, and 67% for first, second, third, fourth, and fifth or more cesarean deliveries, respectively (**Table 2**).[7] Even with just 1 previous cesarean delivery, the presence of a placenta previa should increase the clinician's suspicion for a possible placenta accreta.

Cesarean deliveries are not the only manner in which uterine histology can be dis-rupted. Other forms of uterine surgery are a risk factor for placenta accreta. Placenta accretas have been seen after uterine curettage, myomectomy, and hysteroscopic surgery, although it is difficult to ascertain an absolute risk.[16] If Asherman's syndrome develops (most commonly after, but not limited to, uterine curettage), the risk of accreta seems to be particularly high. Prior endometrial ablation, uterine embolization (arterial or fibroid specific), and pelvic irradiation also are risk factors for developing a placenta accreta.[17,18]

Table 1
Odds ratios with 95% CIs for placenta accreta and hysterectomy by number of cesarean deliveries compared with first cesarean delivery

No. of Cesarean Deliveries	Accreta, n (%)	OR (95% CI)	Hysterectomy, n (%)	OR (95% CI)
First[a]	15 (0.2)	—	40 (0.7)	—
Second	49 (0.3)	1.3 (0.7–2.13)	67 (0.4)	0.7 (0.4–0.97)
Third	36 (0.6)	2.4 (1.3–4.3)	57 (0.9)	1.4 (0.9–2.1)
Fourth	31 (2.1)	9.0 (4.8–16.7)	35 (2.4)	3.8 (2.4–6.0)
Fifth	6 (2.3)	9.8 (3.8–25.5)	9 (3.5)	5.6 (2.7–11.6)
≥6	6 (6.7)	29.8 (11.3–78.7)	8 (9.0)	15.2 (6.9–33.5)

Abbreviation: OR, odds ratio.
[a] Primary cesarean delivery.
From Silver RM, Landon MB, Rouse DJ, et al. Maternal morbidity associated with multiple repeat cesarean deliveries. Obstet Gynecol 2006;107(6);1229; with permission.

A history of abnormal placentation in a previous pregnancy (specifically placenta accreta spectrum disorders) or a current placenta previa without history of cesarean delivery also increases the risk of accreta. In addition to these disorders that result in or indicate abnormal endometrial histologic architecture, advanced maternal age and increasing parity have been identified in some, but not all, studies as risk factors.[19,20]

PREVENTION

Prevention of placenta accreta requires "upstream" or primary prevention: avoiding multiple cesarean deliveries or other uterine surgeries. Strategies are beyond the scope of this article, but societal and economic as well as medical issues need to be considered. Goals include both prevention of the first cesarean (primary prevention) and in identifying and encouraging appropriate trial of labor after cesarean (secondary prevention). A recent non-Markov decision and cost-effectiveness analysis shows that maternal and neonatal benefits accrue with each subsequent successful

Table 2
Placenta previa and placenta accreta by number of cesarean deliveries

No. of Cesarean Deliveries	Previa	Previa[a]:Accreta,[b] n (%)	No Previa[c]:Accreta,[c] n (%)
First[d]	398	13 (3.3)	2 (0.03)
Second	211	23 (11)	26 (0.2)
Third	72	29 (40)	7 (0.1)
Fourth	33	20 (61)	11 (0.8)
Fifth	6	4 (67)	2 (0.8)
≥6	3	2 (67)	4 (4.7)

[a] Percentage of accreta in women with placenta previa.
[b] Increased risk with increasing number of cesarean deliveries (P<.001).
[c] Percentage of accreta in women without placenta previa.
[d] Primary cesarean.
From Silver RM, Landon MB, Rouse, DJ, et al. Maternal morbidity associated with multiple repeat cesarean deliveries. Obstet Gynecol 2006;107(6);1230; with permission.

vaginal birth after cesarean and that a trial of labor after cesarean was the preferred method in at least 75% of simulations.[21]

Potential secondary prevention methods include alterations in surgical technique and use of revascularization-promoting topical agents. For example, does double-layer versus single-layer or incorporation of the endometrium versus nonincorporation result in better reconstitution of the decidua basalis with subsequent decreased risk of accreta? Intraoperative secondary prevention strategies are an active area of investigation. For noncesarean uterine surgeries, providers and patients should understand and be educated regarding the risks of subsequent accrete; this knowledge should be incorporated into counseling and decision making before the index procedure.

DIAGNOSIS

The gold standard continues to be histologic examination of the placenta and uterus with documentation of abnormal trophoblast invasion of the myometrium. However, this is only possible when a hysterectomy is performed. Although this is often done, it does not occur in every case. A clinical diagnoses of focal or complete accreta can be made in the setting of abnormally adherent placenta managed conservatively. Accreta is considered to be present when the placenta is "abnormally adherent."[22] Of course, this is extremely subjective and can be controversial. Most authorities only consider cases that require additional surgical interventions to control bleeding, such as hysterectomy, uterine curettage, and embolization of pelvic vessels, to have clinical evidence of accreta.

PRENATAL DIAGNOSIS

Obstetric ultrasonography has improved dramatically the antenatal diagnosis of placenta accreta spectrum. This is highly desirable, given the high morbidity and mortality associated with placenta accreta. Several studies suggest that outcomes can be optimized with prenatal diagnosis to levels similar of less complicated accretas.[23]

Imaging

Imaging modalities for antenatal diagnosis include ultrasonography and MRI.

Ultrasonography

Ultrasonography is reported to have a sensitivity of 80% to 90% and a specificity of nearly 98% for diagnosis and exclusion of diagnosis of placenta accreta, respectively.[24] More recent studies noted worse performance characteristics.[25] A 2011 study reported a positive predictive value of only 68%, although the negative predictive value was 98%. A 2014 series conducted in an accreta referral center showed sensitivity to be closer to 55% and specificity to be 88%. The overall accuracy was only 65%.[26] It is noteworthy that the individuals interpreting the sonograms in this study were "blinded" to the clinical status of the cases. Knowledge of the clinical scenario and risk factors clearly improves the accuracy of ultrasound. Also, pretest probability affects predictive values and the majority of studies assessing diagnostic accuracy of ultrasonography have been conducted in women at high risk for accreta. First trimester ultrasonography is also noted to be less sensitive.[27] In populations with a smaller pretest probability, the accuracy of ultrasonography for evaluation of accreta is likely lesser. Location of the accreta likely also affects sonographic accuracy.[28] Ultrasonographic quality, ultrasonographer skill, and clinician experience are further contributors to sensitivity and specificity. The majority of studies of ultrasonography are from tertiary care centers with particular expertise in the diagnosis of placenta accreta. Performance is assuredly worse in low-volume centers.

Ultrasound findings suggestive of accreta can vary and depend on gestational age and placental development. In the first trimester, a finding of a gestational sac implanted low and anterior in the uterus is concerning for accreta.[29] Loss of the retroplacental–myometrial zone can also potentially be seen in the first trimester.[30,31] The most helpful finding on ultrasonography is to identify the presence of a placenta previa; as previously discussed, the presence of a placenta previa drastically changes the likelihood of placenta accreta. Ultrasonographic findings of normal placentation include a uniform, homogenous placenta and bladder. There should be a distinct intervening echolucent zone (myometrial zone) between the placenta and bladder. In contrast, in many cases of placenta accreta there is a complete loss or disruption of the myometrial zone continuity.[32] With the more invasive forms of placenta accreta, disruption of the bladder wall can be seen and occasionally the placenta is noted to protrude into the bladder. The abnormal placenta of an accreta often seems to be irregular (nonhomogenous) secondary to lacunae (irregularly shaped vascular spaces); the lack of a homogenous appearance and the varying sizes of lacunae give the placenta a "Swiss cheese" appearance (**Fig. 2**).[33] Doppler velocimetry often detects lacunar turbulence (**Fig. 3**).[34] Additional ultrasonographic findings include increased vascularity of the bladder–placenta interface and vessel crossing of placenta–uterine wall interface.[35,36] Of all ultrasonographic findings, turbulent flow and the presence of lacunae are most consistently associated with accreta.[26]

In the 2014 study discussed, a true positive (the ultrasonographer diagnosing an accreta when it was actually present) was increased in the presence of lacunae, loss of retroplacental myometrial zone space, or when color Doppler abnormalities were present.[26] Nonanterior location of a placenta accreta may make diagnosis by ultrasound more difficult.[37] Some investigators also use 3-dimensional Doppler as an adjunct for imaging, especially when placenta percreta is suspected.[38]

MRI

MRI is a newer modality for diagnosis of accreta and is not performed routinely in all centers. In studies from centers with expertise in accreta, the sensitivity and specificity of MRI is reported to be more than 90% and 98%, respectively.[39] In contrast, others

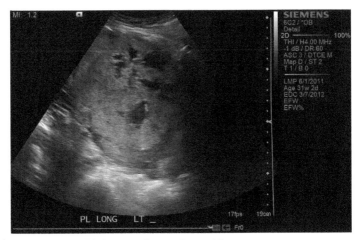

Fig. 2. Placenta accreta with lacunae (hypoechogenic).

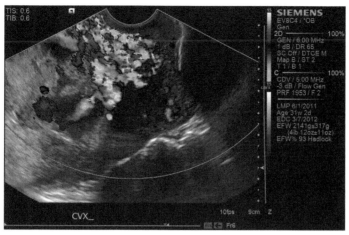

Fig. 3. Placenta accreta with increased vascularity between placenta and bladder; turbulent flow within placental lacunae.

have shown the sensitivity to be as low as 67%.[40] A 2014 systematic review and meta-analysis of MRI in identifying invasive placentation showed a sensitivity of 94.4%, specificity of 84.0%, a positive likelihood ratio of 5.91, and a negative likelihood ratio of 0.07. According to this study, MRI also had highly predictive accuracy in assessing depth of invasion and topography of invasion using uterine bulging, heterogeneous signal intensity, focal interruption of the myometrium, bladder tenting, and dark intraplacental bands on T2-weighted images (**Fig. 4**). The review compared MRI to ultrasonography and found no difference in sensitivity or specificity.[41] Where invasion of other structures is often difficult to determine on ultrasound, MRI may provide clearer delineation of the extent of placental invasion.[42] It also may be useful in cases of posterior previa/accreta. Importantly, it is not clear that MRI improves diagnosis above and beyond that achieved with ultrasonography; in addition, it is expensive and not available widely. Like ultrasonography, experience with using this modality to diagnose placenta accreta affects accuracy. Because of the varied accuracy and unproven benefit of MRI, MRI is not recommended as a routine screening test for placenta accreta (National Institutes of Health ultrasound workshop). It is advised when findings are inconclusive on ultrasonography, posterior previas, and in suspected percreta.

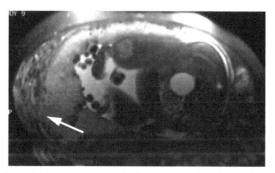

Fig. 4. MRI with placental invasion through the myometrium (*arrow*).

MATERNAL BLOOD

Biomarkers in maternal blood may aid in the diagnosis of placenta accreta. Current putative markers include alpha-fetoprotein, cell-free fetal/placental DNA, placental mRNA, cell-free human placental lactogen mRNA, β-human chorionic gonadotropin, pregnancy-associated plasma protein A, and creatinine kinase. These analytes are generally markers of placental damage and/or abnormal placental development. Although these markers show promise in accreta diagnoses, they are not accurate enough to use clinically at this time.

MANAGEMENT OF PLACENTA ACCRETA

Prenatal diagnosis provides multiple advantages for the management of a pregnancy complicated by placenta accreta. First, delivery without attempting to remove the placenta decreases blood loss significantly, and is accomplished by making a hysterotomy away from the placenta (typically fundal), delivering the infant, closing the hysterotomy and proceeding with planned hysterectomy.[43,44] Rarely, hysterectomy is deferred in hopes of conserving the uterus and hence fertility (see below). Second, prenatal diagnosis allows for care in an accreta center of excellence. Several cohort studies have demonstrated improved outcomes and less blood loss in accretas managed by multidisciplinary teams with experience and expertise in accreta.[45,46] A high index of suspicion, based on an individual woman's risk factors, is essential to enable early diagnosis.

Optimal antepartum and intrapartum management of placenta accreta is not standardized. There are no published, randomized, controlled trials showing that 1 strategy is superior to others. Thus, management is based on retrospective case series (often small), expert opinion, and numerous biases. Fortunately, efforts are under way to organize multicenter, collaborative efforts and higher quality data should be forthcoming.

Current guidelines suggest delivery in a hospital with the needed resources and expertise needed to decrease morbidity and mortality, which includes a fully stocked blood bank capable of massive transfusion of multiple forms of blood products, anesthesiologists experienced in the care of critically ill obstetric patients, and surgeons with training in accreta and with the skills to work with the retroperitoneal space, bladder, ureter, and bowel. Multiple studies indicate that the multidisciplinary team approach in a tertiary care center with experience in managing placenta accreta results in improved morbidity and mortality outcomes (blood loss, transfusion volume, ICU admission).[47] Detailed criteria for an accreta center of excellence are available.[48] It is noteworthy that, even with adequate planning and optimal management, it is still possible for significant morbidity and mortality to occur.

TIMING OF DELIVERY

No randomized, controlled trials have been conducted to identify the optimal gestational age of delivery. As mentioned, outcomes are optimized when the delivery is conducted under "ideal" circumstances, usually requiring a scheduled delivery. Extending the accreta-complicated pregnancy toward term increases the likelihood of vaginal bleeding, labor, or both. Delivery earlier in gestation increases neonatal morbidity and mortality owing to prematurity. The ideal time of delivery balances maternal and neonatal risks and benefits, including the risks of delivery in an unscheduled and suboptimal setting. Generally, a late preterm birth before the onset of labor or bleeding is indicated. A decision analysis of women with placenta previa and placenta accreta estimated the optimal timing of delivery to be at 34 weeks of gestation when neonatal morbidity and mortality decrease, but before the risk of labor or bleeding increases substantially.[49] Because of the increased risk for bleeding, especially after 36 weeks, indicated preterm delivery is often suggested before 36 completed weeks of gestation; optimal timing of delivery must also take individual patient risk factors (such as bleeding) into account.[50]

Risk factors for unscheduled delivery of women with a placenta accreta include bleeding, contractions and premature preterm rupture of membranes. In a recent retrospective cohort study, women more likely to deliver unscheduled if they have had any vaginal bleeding, had multiple episodes of vaginal bleeding (increasing risk with increasing number of episodes), experienced uterine activity, or were diagnosed with preterm premature rupture of membranes.[51] Importantly, many women with no bleeding or contractions had uncomplicated scheduled deliveries at 36 weeks gestation.[51] Thus, it is our practice to individualize timing of delivery based on several factors including, premature preterm rupture of membranes, labor, bleeding, and suspicion of percreta. We scheduled delivery between 34 and 36 weeks' gestation, based on the stability of the clinical course. Conversely, we may schedule delivery between 32 and 34 weeks gestation in women with chronic bleeding or uterine activity. Delivery before 32 weeks gestation is reserved for emergent cases. Corticosteroids should always be administered in cases of suspected accreta.

INTRAOPERATIVE DIAGNOSIS

Unfortunately, placenta accreta is not always suspected or diagnosed before the intrapartum period. This is more likely in less complicated forms of accreta, in cases without classic risk factors, or pregnancies complicated by limited prenatal care.[52] Placenta accreta may be diagnosed at the time of vaginal or cesarean delivery. Findings in the third stage that should raise suspicion for an undiagnosed accreta include continued vaginal bleeding, inability to remove the placenta, or endometritis.[53] Diagnosis at the time of cesarean section may be easier in that invasion is visualized more easily. As might be suspected, blood loss is often greater when the diagnosis of accreta is not made before delivery.[44,54,55]

Regardless, quick action in required once an accreta is recognized. An attempt at multidisciplinary approach should be made with activation of the blood bank, additional anesthesia and critical care support, and surgical backup as needed based on the provider's experience. We recommend the included algorithm for management at the time of surgical diagnosis (see **Box 4**).

COMPLICATIONS OF SURGICAL MANAGEMENT

Despite scheduled delivery in a well-resourced setting with a highly experienced and adequately prepared multidisciplinary team, significant complications can occur. The most common are massive and/or persistent hemorrhage, cystotomy, ureteral damage, and bowel injury. These complications often result in ICU admission (25%–50% of cases), which carries additional risks of infection from pneumonia and invasive catheters.[56] Postpartum status and major complicated surgery put the patient at risk of venous thromboembolism. Manipulation of the urinary tract with a Foley catheter and/or stents may increase the risk of pyelonephritis. Additional complications include injury to large vessels or pelvic nerves; wound, abdominal, and vaginal cuff infections; and the possible need for reoperation.

The most common complication of placenta accreta is hemorrhage, which can lead to DIC, hypovolemic shock, and multiorgan dysfunction or failure. A 2009 series of 76 cases of placenta accreta treated surgical noted that blood transfusion was required in more than 80% of cases; at least one- half required 4 or more units of packed red blood cells. Twenty-eight percent experienced DIC.[43] Another cohort reported a mean blood loss of 3 L; 44% of women required up to 5 U of blood with another 23% requiring between 5 and 9 units.[57] Women receiving multiple types of blood products are at greater risk of respiratory, renal, and hematologic complications.

Whether from placental invasion into the bladder, unintentional injury owing to impaired visualization and poor dissection planes, or intentional injury (to facilitate visualization), cystotomy is the most common surgical complication in the management of accreta. One review identified the risk as high as 17%.[58] Even when a planned delivery and hysterectomy are conducted in a nonemergent setting, cystotomy and hemorrhage are common.[59] Iatrogenic ureteral injury can also occur for the same reasons as iatrogenic cystotomy; the estimated prevalence of ureteral injury during cesarean hysterectomy in the setting of accreta is 10% to 15%. A 2012 systematic review showed that antenatal diagnosis of accreta, revised surgical technique, methotrexate therapy, as well as placement of ureteral stents are associated with decreased ureteral injuries.[60] However, clear proof of efficacy for stents is lacking. An important late complication of cesarean hysterectomy is a vesicovaginal fistula. The obstetric provider should keep this complication in mind when a postpartum patient complains of urinary incontinence or watery vaginal discharge.

Maternal mortality has been reported to be as high as 7%, but seems to be less in larger series.[61] In less well-resourced settings, mortality has been found to be even higher.[62] The rates of morbidity, complications, and mortality are influenced by the type of accreta spectrum disorder present.[63] Because of their more extensive invasion through the uterus and into surrounding tissues, percretas are associated with an higher incidence of morbidity and mortality. Expertise of the delivery center also affects patient outcome.[63] Publication bias and underreporting of outcomes for low-volume facilities likely further increase the discrepancy in outcomes between low- and high-volume centers.

Although the majority of fetal/neonatal morbidity and mortality results from indicated preterm birth, maternal hemorrhage can result in fetal compromise from compromised uteroplacental oxygenation with resultant fetal hypoxemia and acidosis.[2] Perinatal mortality has been quoted as high as 25%.[11]

CONTROVERSIES IN SURGICAL MANAGEMENT

Owing to a lack of data from appropriate trials, there are several controversies regarding optimal surgical management of accreta. One area of debate is the type of incision. Classically, a vertical skin incision is used in suspected cases of accreta. There is no question that adequate visualization can be extremely helpful when performing a difficult hysterectomy on a large, pregnant uterus. Nonetheless, case series note good results with Pfannenstiel-, Maylard-, and Cherney-type incisions. We have had excellent results using a Cherney incision. There also is considerable variation in the types of uterine incisions, which may include transverse fundal incisions, classical vertical incisions, and posterior incisions, among others. The key issue with regard to uterine incision is the avoidance of the placenta. Accordingly, we find it helpful to use ultrasonography to visualize the placenta and to individualize the incision in each case.

Some obstetricians and anesthesiologists routinely use general anesthesia, whereas others advocate for regional anesthesia in well-chosen patients. Regional anesthesia is desirable owing to fewer adverse effects, easier recovery, better postoperative pain relief, and the ability for the mother to be awake and "experience" the birth. However, the large incision, complex surgery, and often critically ill patients favor general anesthesia with a controlled airway. Other options include a regional anesthetic that is "converted" to general if needed and a planned "combined" epidural and general anesthetic. The former makes good sense in cases of possible accreta wherein the diagnosis is uncertain and hysterectomy may not be required. It is ideal to discuss each case preoperatively with the anesthesiologist and the patient to decide upon the best approach.

Prophylactic ureteral stent placement is a hot area of debate. Evidence from studies conducted in benign and malignant gynecologic surgeries indicate that stent placement helps to identify a ureteral injury, but does not aid in prevention of ureteral injury. Studies in patients with placenta accreta yield mixed results; moreover, they are observational and include small numbers of women. One retrospective cohort study showed no difference in ureteral injury with the use of stents, but all 3 cases of injury occurred in women who did not have stents placed.[43]

Intraoperative cell salvage has also been supported by some and is routine care in some countries.[64] Autologous blood transfusion is another option, but given the likelihood of needing multiple units of blood products, it may not be a reliable or cost-effective strategy to decrease transfusion morbidities.[65]

Delayed hysterectomy also is controversial. The theory behind delayed hysterectomy is that keeping the placenta in situ may allow for involution of the gravid vascularity, possibly decreasing blood loss, facilitating hysterectomy, and avoiding bladder resection. This approach also allows for the postcesarean use of pelvic artery embolization. Ideally, this would allow for 2 surgeries with less combined morbidity than a planned cesarean hysterectomy. However, efficacy is uncertain. Although several groups have used this approach successfully with percretas (unpublished communication), our experience has been poor. We are aware of 2 cases of planned delayed hysterectomy that had life-threatening hemorrhage and intrauterine infection weeks after the initial cesarean. Also, delayed surgeries were no less morbid than those performed at the time of cesarean. As such, the approach should be considered experimental.

Another option is the use of supracervical hysterectomy. Removal of the cervix is often the most difficult part of a hysterectomy associated with accreta and may prolong needlessly the surgery in critically ill or unstable patients. This option should always be considered in such cases. Conversely, the majority of accretas involve the lower uterine segment and/or the cervix. Thus, it may not be possible to control hemorrhage adequately without removing the cervix.

The use of interventional radiology to embolize pelvic vessels on a prophylactic basis also is a major area of debate. Typically, catheters are placed in the internal iliac or uterine arteries before a planned cesarean hysterotomy. This is done in a suite capable of fluoroscopy, typically in a radiology department, but occasionally in an equipped operating room. Deflated balloons are placed through the catheters. They are then inflated after delivery of the infant so as to not compromise uterine blood flow. Advocates of this technique claim decreased blood loss with the hysterectomy. However, considerable morbidity, such as occlusion of major arteries owing to thrombosis or endothelial damage, may occur.[66] Moreover, it is not clear that prophylactic embolization decreases blood loss because routine hypogastric artery ligation does not impact clearly blood loss.[43] Hence, the use of prophylactic hypogastric artery embolization remains controversial.

Management of Intrapartum/Postpartum Hemorrhage

As mentioned, placenta accreta can result in a life-threatening hemorrhage. Median blood loss for placenta accreta has been reported as anywhere from 2000 to

7800 mL.[57] Median units of blood transfused is 5.[57] In 1 older study, more than 90% of patients lost more than 3 L of blood.[67] The blood bank at the delivering facility should be prepared for a large-volume blood product transfusion. Ideally, all products should be appropriately typed and crossed to decrease morbidity. The need for packed red blood cells, fresh frozen plasma, or platelets transfused does not change based on the extent of the accreta (accreta vs percreta).[68] In the setting of acute hemorrhage, it is ideal to use a "massive transfusion" protocol. This protocol typically involves transfusing packed red blood cells and fresh frozen plasma in a 1:1 ratio and keeping several units ahead with regard to cross-matching and blood product availability. The specifics of the protocol are less important than the establishment of a protocol with well-functioning logistics.

In addition to packed red blood cells, platelets, fresh frozen plasma, and cryoprecipitate, consideration should be given to the utilization of recombinant activated factor VII. Recombinant activated factor VII is a relatively newer therapy utilized in the setting of massive hemorrhage. It has been studied in massive hemorrhage resulting from obstetric complications, trauma, dilutional coagulopathy, and DIC. In the obstetric setting, its administration can decrease the need for additional blood products as well as the need for a peripartum hysterectomy.[69,70] It is quite expensive and, in current practice, is one of the last treatments used in an attempt to stem hemorrhage.

ALTERNATIVE SURGICAL AND CONSERVATIVE THERAPIES

Although hysterectomy and removal of invading placental tissue with or without adjunctive therapies is considered "generally accepted" management, several cases have been managed conservatively (no hysterectomy) in hopes of preserving fertility.[71] In a US survey, up to 32% of maternal–fetal medicine specialists have attempted conservative management of accreta.[72] This strategy includes delayed surgical removal of the uterus and/or placenta or medical management without surgical management beyond the cesarean portion. Proponents of conservative management cite benefits such as decreased blood loss, fertility preservation, and decreased morbidity.[73] Strategies include leaving the placenta in situ, oversewing of the placental vascular bed, uterine compression sutures, utilizing surgical uterine devascularization, intrauterine tamponade balloon, uterine vessel embolization, hysteroscopic resection of retained placental tissue, use of mifepristone and misoprostol, and administering methotrexate.

Placenta in Situ

Leaving the placenta in situ after delivery of the fetus has been utilized in multiple studies, but generally in conjunction with other conservative modalities.

Uterine Compression Sutures

Uterine compression sutures include the B lynch stitch, multiple squares techniques, and superposition suturing.

Vessel Embolization

The aorta, common iliac, internal iliac, and uterine vessels can be occluded. In the case of the aorta, common iliac artery and internal iliac artery, occlusion is temporary.[74] Vessel embolization utilizes balloon catheter placement and/or other embolization techniques. Balloon placement preoperatively followed by hysterectomy in an unstable patient or subsequent embolization (via coils, gel, or particles) with delayed hysterectomy has shown some promise.[75] A 2010 study showed staged surgery was possible in 8 of 26 cases—1 case required subsequent unplanned hysterectomy and overall blood loss was less in the staged group.[76] A 2011 study that evaluated temporary catheterization also showed a possible decrease in blood loss.[77] In a 2006 study, however, balloon-assisted occlusion did not result in less blood loss and 2 patients incurred a cystotomy.[78] Similarly, a 1999 study showed no difference in outcomes, including blood loss.[79] Studies of isolated uterine vessel embolization show some success in either delay of or complete avoidance of hysterectomy.[80]

Methotrexate

Methotrexate has also been used by some clinician investigators as a conservative therapy.[71] It can be used with or without plans for surgical intervention in mind. Its utility derives from the antimetabolic effect on trophoblast cells and therefore on trophoblast growth, resulting in more rapid placental involution. On the other hand, there are few actively dividing trophoblast cells in the third trimester and treatment may be inconsequential.

A 2011 systematic review of 60 articles (only 10 cohort studies) addressing conservative management of placenta accreta assessed secondary hysterectomy rates, mortality, return of menses, and subsequent pregnancy. In patients managed expectantly, 19% underwent subsequent hysterectomy, 0.3% died, 90% had return of menses, and 67% had a subsequent pregnancy. For embolization-managed patients, those numbers were similar for hysterectomy and mortality (18% and 0%, respectively), but less encouraging for return of menses (62%) and subsequent pregnancy (15%). Methotrexate event incidence was similar to expectant management, although fewer women required subsequent hysterectomy (6%). Uterus-preserving surgery (not defined) had the highest incidence of subsequent hysterectomy at 31%, the highest mortality (4%), a higher return to menses (82%), and a high success in subsequent pregnancies (73%).[81]

Success and complications vary by protocol, institution, and study. As with hysterectomy, complications include the need for reoperation, ICU admission, infection/sepsis, shock, and necrosis of the uterus or surrounding tissues.[82,83] Other risks of conservative therapy include delayed hemorrhage, multiple transfusions, thrombus formation, limb ischemia, vessel injury, and subsequent abnormal uterine bleeding.[66,84] Combinations of conservative management approaches have had various success rates as well as morbidities.[85] The ideal surveillance in conservatively managed patients remains to be determined, but may include serial β-human chorionic gonadotropin, ultrasonographic, or MRI studies.[86,87]

DEBATE SURROUNDING CONSERVATIVE MANAGEMENT

Although several successful cases have been reported, success is not guaranteed and risks (such as sepsis or delayed hemorrhage) may be significant. There is likely a publication bias in favor of successful cases of conservative management. Because efforts at conservative management are relatively new, the risk of recurrent accreta in general and stratified by type of management is unknown.[88] A 2014 study from Israel found a relative risk of recurrence at 15.41.[89] A few studies suggest that conservative management may result in better outcomes in women with more tissue involvement.[90]

The largest problem with assessing the pros and cons of conservative management is the fact that it is impossible to be certain that conservatively managed cases truly have placenta accreta. In such cases, placental histology and/or clinical evidence of morbidly adherent placenta cannot be used to vet the diagnosis. Accordingly, it is possible (and even likely) that many cases of successful conservatively managed accretas are not truly accretas (or at least are "different" than the cases included in most series of documented accretes). There is a need for consensus regarding criteria for antenatal diagnosis of accreta.

Given these issues, conservative management is best undertaken after appropriate and honest counseling, and in centers with the ability to deal with potential complications.[91] Patients opting for and allowed a trial of conservative management need to be monitored closely in the postpartum period. The "best" candidates for conservative management include women with posterior placenta previa and accreta, a fundal accreta, a partial accrete, or when the diagnosis of accreta is uncertain.[92]

LOCATION OF DIAGNOSIS, ANTEPARTUM MANAGEMENT, AND DELIVERY: ACCRETA CENTER OF EXCELLENCE

As discussed, a facility and provider's expertise with placenta accreta disorders directly impact maternal outcomes. Given this correlation, it makes good sense for care of patients with suspected accreta to be conducted at accreta centers of excellence.[48] The availability of appropriate facilities, experience, multidisciplinary expertise, and resources will optimize maternal and fetal outcomes. Criteria for accreta centers of excellence are outlined in **Box 1**.

Box 1
Criteria for accreta referral center

1. Multidisciplinary team
   a. Experienced maternal–fetal medicine physician or obstetrician
   b. Imaging experts (ultrasound and MRI)
   c. Pelvic surgeon (ie, gynecologic oncology or urogynecology)
   d. Anesthesiologist (ie, obstetric anesthesia or cardiac anesthesia)
   e. Urologist
   f. Trauma surgeon or general surgeon
   g. Interventional radiologist
   h. Neonatologist
2. ICU and facilities
   a. Interventional radiology
      i. Capability within the operating suite—hybrid operating room
   b. Surgical or medical ICU
      i. 24-hour availability of intensive care specialists
   c. Neonatal ICU
      i. Gestational age appropriate for neonate
3. Blood services
   a. Massive transfusion capabilities
   b. Cell-saver and perfusionists
   c. Experience and access to alternative blood products
   d. Guidance of transfusion medicine specialists or blood bank pathologists

From Silver RM, Fox KA, Barton JR, et-al. Center of excellence for placenta accreta. Am J Obstet Gynecol. 2014. http://dx.doi.org/10.1016/j.ajog.2014.11.018; with permission.

FOLLOW-UP

The multiple morbidities of placenta accreta, including psychosocial effects, should prompt close postpartum follow-up. It is reasonable to consider additional postpartum visits starting at 1 week after delivery. Close follow-up enables monitoring of delayed and late complications, assessment of emotional well-being, and the ability to offer needed support. Difficulties with recovery from major surgery, neonatal morbidities and possible mortality, adjustment to lost fertility should all be assessed; appropriate counseling can be helpful and should be offered and made easily available. Counseling should also consider subsequent gynecologic care (ie, need for cervical cancer screening in the setting of retained cervix and possible need for hormone replacement therapy in case of oophorectomy). For women managed without hysterectomy, counseling should include a discussion of the uncertain risk of recurrent accreta and recommended interpregnancy intervals. Subsequent pregnancy in a patient with a previous accreta should prompt early and close monitoring with careful, advanced preparation for antepartum and intrapartum management.

SUMMARY

As the incidence of cesarean deliveries have increased, placenta accreta also has increased and is an important cause of maternal and fetal/neonatal morbidity and mortality. Although multiple cesarean deliveries are the largest risk factor for placenta accreta, previa, increasing maternal age and parity, as well as other uterine surgeries are also important. In patients at risk for accreta, obstetric ultrasonography performed by an experienced provider should be obtained. A multidisciplinary team in a center with expertise in managing placenta accreta should care for cases of suspected

---

Box 2
Proposed algorithm for antepartum management of suspected accreta

1. Obstetric sonogram to assess the probability of accreta.

2. Consideration of MRI to assess the probability of accreta if unclear based on sonogram, in cases of posterior previa or if suspected percreta.

3. Pelvic rest.

4. Consideration of bed rest and/or hospitalization if stable.

5. Administration of corticosteroids to enhance fetal pulmonary maturity in cases of antepartum bleeding at the time of hospital admission.

6. If there is no antepartum bleeding, empiric administration of corticosteroids to enhance fetal pulmonary maturity at 34 weeks of gestation.

7. Consultation with the patient and her family to discuss delivery options, risks of the disease, potential complications, and impact of treatment on fertility.

8. Consultation with a multidisciplinary team to plan the delivery (see **Box 3**).

9. The optimal timing of delivery is uncertain. Ideally, it should be accomplished in a scheduled and controlled fashion. The risk of maternal hemorrhage must be weighed against the fetal risk of prematurity. In cases without antepartum bleeding, delivery at 34–35 weeks of gestation is advised. It is not necessary to assess fetal pulmonary maturity with amniocentesis.

10. In cases with episodic bleeding, delivery between 32 and 34 weeks of gestation is advised, depending on the severity of bleeding.

11. Heavy bleeding may require earlier delivery.

Box 3
Proposed algorithm for surgical management of suspected accreta

1. Care should be provided with a multidisciplinary team. This team should include surgeons with experience in accreta, critical care specialists, anesthesiologists, and blood bank specialists. Gynecologic oncologists are ideal because of their experience with bladder and ureteral surgery in addition to difficult pelvic surgery. Interventional radiologists and vascular surgeons should be available.

2. If all of the requirements under (1) are not available, consider transfer to a center with appropriate expertise.

3. If possible, the case should be performed in the 'main' operating room rather than in the labor and delivery unit. In most centers, the staff in the 'main' operating room is considerably more experienced with the care of critically ill patients than labor and delivery personnel.

4. Adequate blood products should be available. Ideally, this should include 20 U of packed red blood cells and fresh frozen plasma and 12 U of platelets. Additional blood products should be available in reserve. Recombinant activated factor VII also should be available.

5. A vertical skin incision should be made, regardless of prior abdominal or pelvic scars. A Cherney incision is a reasonable alternative.

6. General anesthesia should be used. It is reasonable to use a regional anesthetic for the delivery of the infant, followed by general anesthetic for the hysterectomy in stable patients.

7. The patient should be kept warm and a (relatively) normal pH maintained.

8. Strong consideration should be given to preoperative placement of ureteral stents. Our group has found this to be extremely helpful with minimal risk.

9. Consideration should be given to using an autologous blood salvage device. Although there are theoretic risks of contamination with amniotic fluid, blood obtained with a cell saver at time of cesarean delivery seems to be safe for maternal transfusion.

10. Consideration should be given to preoperative placement of either regular or balloon catheters in the uterine arteries. These can be infused with material for embolization or the balloons inflated after the delivery of the fetus. In turn, this may decrease blood loss at the time of hysterectomy or allow for the avoidance of hysterectomy (see **Box 4**). Alternatively, catheters can be placed and only used if needed. This practice is controversial and serious adverse events with balloon placement have been reported.

11. Ideally, in cases of strongly suspected accreta, planned cesarean hysterectomy should be accomplished. A classical hysterotomy that does not compromise the placenta should be used to deliver the infant. *No attempt should be made to remove the placenta*. Placental removal has the potential to increase dramatically the risk of life-threatening hemorrhage. The hysterotomy should be quickly sutured to achieve some measure of hemostasis, followed by hysterectomy. If the case is difficult to accomplish or if the patient is unstable, consideration should be given to supracervical hysterectomy.

12. Umbrella packs or other tamponade devices such as a Bakri balloon should be available.

13. Consideration may be given to hypogastric artery ligation. Our group has not found this to be helpful.

14. Consideration may be given to leaving the placenta in situ, closing the hysterotomy, and planning a "delayed" hysterectomy in 6 weeks. In theory, this may allow some of the enhanced vascularity associated with pregnancy to regress, facilitating the hysterectomy. This approach has been advocated in women with percretas to avoid bladder resection. Our group has not found this to be helpful.

Box 4

Proposed algorithm for surgical management of previously unsuspected accreta

1. Once an accreta is recognized, help should be summoned. This help should include surgeons with experience in accreta, critical care specialists, anesthesiologists, and blood bank specialists. Gynecologic oncologists are ideal because of their experience with bladder and ureteral surgery in addition to difficult pelvic surgery. Interventional radiologists and vascular surgeons should be considered.

2. If the surgeon or medical center is not capable of caring for the patient, consideration should be given to performing a stabilizing procedure and transferring the patient to an appropriate center for definitive therapy. This may require packing the abdomen to control bleeding, transfusion, and medical stabilization of the patient. Stabilization and transfer is not always possible.

3. If labor and delivery personnel are uncomfortable with the case, personnel from the main operating room should be recruited. Instruments and equipment may need to be obtained from the main operating room as well.

4. The blood bank should be alerted to the need for adequate blood products. Many hospitals have a massive transfusion protocol. If so, this should be activated. Recombinant activated factor VII also should be available.

5. If a Pfannenstiel incision is used; a Mallard or Cherney incision can be used to allow better pelvic access.

6. The patient should be kept warm and a (relatively) normal pH maintained.

7. Consideration should be given to converting to general anesthesia.

8. Consideration should be given to using an autologous blood salvage device. Although there are theoretic risks of contamination with amniotic fluid, blood obtained with a cell saver at time of cesarean delivery seems to be safe for maternal transfusion.

9. The hysterotomy should be sutured quickly to achieve some measure of hemostasis, followed by hysterectomy. If the case is difficult to accomplish or if the patient is unstable, consideration should be given to supracervical hysterectomy.

10. Umbrella packs or other tamponade devices such as a Bakri balloon should be available.

11. Consideration may be given to hypogastric artery ligation. Our group has not found this to be helpful.

12. Consideration may be given to leaving the placenta in situ, closing the hysterotomy, and planning a "delayed" hysterectomy in 6 weeks. In theory, this course of action may allow some of the enhanced vascularity associated with pregnancy to regress, facilitating the hysterectomy. This approach has been advocated in women with percretas to avoid bladder resection. Our group has not found this to be helpful.

---

accreta. Suggested algorithms for the management of suspected accreta are shown in **Boxes 2–4**.[48] Most cases should be managed by planned cesarean hysterectomy before the onset of labor or bleeding. Additional research is needed to identify optimal methods of secondary prevention, alternative modalities for diagnosis, surgical techniques, and appropriate conservative management strategies.

REFERENCES

1. Upson K, Silver RM, Greene R, et al. Placenta accreta and maternal morbidity in the Republic of Ireland, 2005–2010. J Matern Fetal Neonatal Med 2014;27(1):24–9.
2. Vinograd A, Wainstock T, Mazor M, et al. Placenta accreta is an independent risk factor for late pre-term birth and perinatal mortality. J Matern Fetal Neonatal Med 2014;1–7.

3. Palacios-Jaraquemada JM. Diagnosis and management of placenta accreta. Best Pract Res Clin Obstet Gynaecol 2008;22(6):1133–48.
4. Garmi G, Salim R. Epidemiology, etiology, diagnosis, and management of placenta accreta. Obstet Gynecol Int 2012;2012(8):873929.
5. MacDorman MF, Menacker F, Declercq E. Cesarean birth in the United States: epidemiology, trends, and outcomes. Clin Perinatol 2008;35(2):293–307, v.
6. Khong TY. The pathology of placenta accreta, a worldwide epidemic. J Clin Pathol 2008;61(12):1243–6.
7. Silver RM, Landon MB, Rouse DJ, et al. Maternal morbidity associated with multiple repeat cesarean deliveries. Obstet Gynecol 2006;107(6):1226–32.
8. Klar M, Michels KB. Cesarean section and placental disorders in subsequent pregnancies–a meta-analysis. J Perinat Med 2014;42(5):571–83.
9. Silver RM. Implications of the first cesarean: perinatal and future reproductive health and subsequent cesareans, placentation issues, uterine rupture risk, morbidity, and mortality. Semin Perinatol 2012;36(5):315–23.
10. Rossi AC, Lee RH, Chmait RH. Emergency postpartum hysterectomy for uncontrolled postpartum bleeding: a systematic review. Obstet Gynecol 2010;115(3): 637–44.
11. Breen JL, Neubecker R, Gregori CA, et al. Placenta accreta, increta, and percreta. A survey of 40 cases. Obstet Gynecol 1977;49(1):43–7.
12. Adler E, Madankumar R, Rosner M, et al. Increased placental trophoblast inclusions in placenta accreta. Placenta 2014;35(12):1075–8.
13. Laban M, Ibrahim EA, Elsafty MS, et al. Placenta accreta is associated with decreased decidual natural killer (dNK) cells population: a comparative pilot study. Eur J Obstet Gynecol Reprod Biol 2014;181:284–8.
14. Jauniaux E, Jurkovic D. Placenta accreta: pathogenesis of a 20th century iatrogenic uterine disease. Placenta 2012;33(4):244–51.
15. Hannon T, Innes BA, Lash GE, et al. Effects of local decidua on trophoblast invasion and spiral artery remodeling in focal placenta creta - an immunohistochemical study. Placenta 2012;33(12):998–1004.
16. Gyamfi-Bannerman C, Gilbert S, Landon MB, et al. Risk of uterine rupture and placenta accreta with prior uterine surgery outside of the lower segment. Obstet Gynecol 2012;120(6):1332–7.
17. Bowman ZS, Simons M, Sok C, et al. Cervical insufficiency and placenta accreta after prior pelvic radiation. J Obstet Gynaecol 2014;34(8):735.
18. Pron G, Mocarski E, Bennett J, et al. Pregnancy after uterine artery embolization for leiomyomata: the Ontario multicenter trial. Obstet Gynecol 2005;105(1):67–76.
19. Bowman ZS, Eller AG, Bardsley TR, et al. Risk factors for placenta accreta: a large prospective cohort. Am J Perinatol 2014;31(9):799–804.
20. Miller DA, Chollet JA, Goodwin TM. Clinical risk factors for placenta previa-placenta accreta. Am J Obstet Gynecol 1997;177(1):210–4.
21. Wymer KM, Shih YC, Plunkett BA. The cost-effectiveness of a trial of labor accrues with multiple subsequent vaginal deliveries. Am J Obstet Gynecol 2014;211(1):56.e1–12.
22. Belfort MA. Placenta accreta. Am J Obstet Gynecol 2010;203(5):430–9.
23. Koai E, Hadpawat A, Gebb J, et al. Clinical outcomes and efficacy of antenatal diagnosis of placenta accreta using ultrasonography and magnetic resonance imaging. Obstet Gynecol 2014;123(Suppl 1):61S.
24. Japaraj RP, Mimin TS, Mukudan K. Antenatal diagnosis of placenta previa accreta in patients with previous cesarean scar. J Obstet Gynaecol Res 2007; 33(4):431–7.

25. Riteau AS, Tassin M, Chambon G, et al. Accuracy of ultrasonography and magnetic resonance imaging in the diagnosis of placenta accreta. PLoS One 2014;9(4):e94866.
26. Bowman ZS, Eller AG, Kennedy AM, et al. Accuracy of ultrasound for the prediction of placenta accreta. Am J Obstet Gynecol 2014;211(2):177.e1–7.
27. Rahimi-Sharbaf F, Jamal A, Mesdaghinia E, et al. Ultrasound detection of placenta accreta in the first trimester of pregnancy. Iran J Reprod Med 2014; 12(6):421–6.
28. Laifer Narin SL. OP03.09: MRI evaluation of pregnancies with an indeterminate location on ultrasound. Ultrasound Obstet Gynecol 2007;30(4):466.
29. Comstock CH, Bronsteen RA. The antenatal diagnosis of placenta accreta. BJOG 2014;121(2):171–81 [discussion: 181–2].
30. Chen YJ, Wang PH, Liu WM, et al. Placenta accreta diagnosed at 9 weeks' gestation. Ultrasound Obstet Gynecol 2002;19(6):620–2.
31. Moretti F, Merziotis M, Ferraro ZM, et al. The importance of a late first trimester placental sonogram in patients at risk of abnormal placentation. Case Rep Obstet Gynecol 2014;2014(9):345348.
32. Comstock CH, Love JJ, Bronsteen RA, et al. Sonographic detection of placenta accreta in the second and third trimesters of pregnancy. Am J Obstet Gynecol 2004;190(4):1135–40.
33. Chou MM, Ho ES, Lee YH. Prenatal diagnosis of placenta previa accreta by transabdominal color Doppler ultrasound. Ultrasound Obstet Gynecol 2000;15(1): 28–35.
34. Chou MM, Tseng JJ, Hwang JI, et al. Sonographic appearance of tornado blood flow in placenta previa accreta/increta. Ultrasound Obstet Gynecol 2001;17(4): 362–3.
35. Chou MM, Tseng JJ, Ho ES, et al. Three-dimensional color power Doppler imaging in the assessment of uteroplacental neovascularization in placenta previa increta/percreta. Am J Obstet Gynecol 2001;185(5):1257–60.
36. Wong HS, Cheung YK, Zuccollo J, et al. Evaluation of sonographic diagnostic criteria for placenta accreta. J Clin Ultrasound 2008;36(9):551–9.
37. Koai E, Hadpawat A, Gebb J, et al. Clinical outcomes of anterior compared with posterior placenta accreta. Obstet Gynecol 2014;123(Suppl 1):60S.
38. Warshak CR, Eskander R, Hull AD, et al. Accuracy of ultrasonography and magnetic resonance imaging in the diagnosis of placenta accreta. Obstet Gynecol 2006;108(3 Pt 1):573–81.
39. Esakoff TF, Sparks TN, Kaimal AJ, et al. Diagnosis and morbidity of placenta accreta. Ultrasound Obstet Gynecol 2011;37(3):324–7.
40. Bauwens J, Coulon C, Azaïs H, et al. Placenta accreta: can prenatal diagnosis be performed? Ultrasound and MRI interests. About 27 cases. Gynecol Obstet Fertil 2014;42(5):306–11 [in French].
41. D'Antonio F, Iacovella C, Palacios-Jaraquemada J, et al. Prenatal identification of invasive placentation using magnetic resonance imaging: systematic review and meta-analysis. Ultrasound Obstet Gynecol 2014;44(1):8–16.
42. Palacios-Jaraquemada JM, Bruno CH. Magnetic resonance imaging in 300 cases of placenta accreta: surgical correlation of new findings. Acta Obstet Gynecol Scand 2005;84(8):716–24.
43. Eller AG, Porter TF, Soisson P, et al. Optimal management strategies for placenta accreta. BJOG 2009;116(5):648–54.
44. Warshak CR, Ramos GA, Eskander R, et al. Effect of predelivery diagnosis in 99 consecutive cases of placenta accreta. Obstet Gynecol 2010;115(1):65–9.

45. Eller AG, Bennett MA, Sharshiner M, et al. Maternal morbidity in cases of placenta accreta managed by a multidisciplinary care team compared with standard obstetric care. Obstet Gynecol 2011;117(2 Pt 1):331–7.

46. Wright JD, Herzog TJ, Shah M, et al. Regionalization of care for obstetric hemorrhage and its effect on maternal mortality. Obstet Gynecol 2010;115(6):1194–200.

47. Al-Khan A, Gupta V, Illsley NP, et al. Maternal and fetal outcomes in placenta accreta after institution of team-managed care. Reprod Sci 2014;21(6):761–71.

48. Silver RM, Fox KA, Barton JR, et al. Center of excellence for placenta accreta. Am J Obstet Gynecol 2014. http://dx.doi.org/10.1016/j.ajog.2014.11.018.

49. Robinson BK, Grobman WA. Effectiveness of timing strategies for delivery of individuals with placenta previa and accreta. Obstet Gynecol 2010;116(4): 835–42.

50. Belfort MA. Indicated preterm birth for placenta accreta. Semin Perinatol 2011; 35(5):252–6.

51. Bowman ZS, Manuck TA, Eller AG, et al. Risk factors for unscheduled delivery in patients with placenta accreta. Am J Obstet Gynecol 2014;210(3):241.e1–6.

52. Hall T, Wax JR, Lucas FL, et al. Prenatal sonographic diagnosis of placenta accreta–impact on maternal and neonatal outcomes. J Clin Ultrasound 2014; 42(8):449–55.

53. Ryan GL, Quinn TJ, Syrop CH, et al. Placenta accreta postpartum. Obstet Gynecol 2002;100(5 Pt 2):1069.

54. Asıcıoglu O, Şahbaz A, Güngördük K, et al. Maternal and perinatal outcomes in women with placenta praevia and accreta in teaching hospitals in Western Turkey. J Obstet Gynaecol 2014;34(6):462–6.

55. Fitzpatrick KE, Sellers S, Spark P, et al. The management and outcomes of placenta accreta, increta, and percreta in the UK: a population-based descriptive study. BJOG 2014;121(1):62–70 [discussion: 70–1].

56. Bretelle F, Courbiere B, Mazouni C, et al. Management of placenta accreta: morbidity and outcome. Eur J Obstet Gynecol Reprod Biol 2007;133(1):34–9.

57. Wright JD, Pri-Paz S, Herzog TJ, et al. Predictors of massive blood loss in women with placenta accreta. Am J Obstet Gynecol 2011;205(1):38.e1–6.

58. Clausen C, Lönn L, Langhoff-Roos J. Management of placenta percreta: a review of published cases. Acta Obstet Gynecol Scand 2014;93(2):138–43.

59. Hoffman MS, Karlnoski RA, Mangar D, et al. Morbidity associated with nonemergent hysterectomy for placenta accreta. Am J Obstet Gynecol 2010;202(6):628.e1–5.

60. Tam Tam KB, Dozier J, Martin JN. Approaches to reduce urinary tract injury during management of placenta accreta, increta, and percreta: a systematic review. J Matern Fetal Neonatal Med 2012;25(4):329–34.

61. Clark SL, Belfort MA, Dildy GA, et al. Maternal death in the 21st century: causes, prevention, and relationship to cesarean delivery. Am J Obstet Gynecol 2008; 199(1):36.e1–5 [discussion: 91–2.e7–11].

62. Guleria K, Gupta B, Agarwal S, et al. Abnormally invasive placenta: changing trends in diagnosis and management. Acta Obstet Gynecol Scand 2013;92(4): 461–4.

63. Tan SG, Jobling TW, Wallace EM, et al. Surgical management of placenta accreta: a 10-year experience. Acta Obstet Gynecol Scand 2013;92(4):445–50.

64. Catling S. Blood conservation techniques in obstetrics: a UK perspective. Int J Obstet Anesth 2007;16(3):241–9.

65. Pregazzi R, Levi D'Ancona R, Ricci G, et al. The donation of autologous blood in pregnancy. Observations on its safety and the cost-benefit relationship. Minerva Ginecol 1994;46(3):95–8 [in Italian].

66. Bishop S, Butler K, Monaghan S, et al. Multiple complications following the use of prophylactic internal iliac artery balloon catheterisation in a patient with placenta percreta. Int J Obstet Anesth 2011;20(1):70–3.
67. Hudon L, Belfort MA, Broome DR. Diagnosis and management of placenta percreta: a review. Obstet Gynecol Surv 1998;53(8):509–17.
68. Brookfield KF, Goodnough LT, Lyell DJ, et al. Perioperative and transfusion outcomes in women undergoing cesarean hysterectomy for abnormal placentation. Transfusion 2014;54(6):1530–6.
69. Bouma LS, Bolte AC, van Geijn HP. Use of recombinant activated factor VII in massive postpartum haemorrhage. Eur J Obstet Gynecol Reprod Biol 2008; 137(2):172–7.
70. Alfirevic Z, Elbourne D, Pavord S, et al. Use of recombinant activated factor VII in primary postpartum hemorrhage: the Northern European Registry 2000–2004. Obstet Gynecol 2007;110(6):1270–8.
71. Khan M, Sachdeva P, Arora R, et al. Conservative management of morbidly adherent placenta - a case report and review of literature. Placenta 2013; 34(10):963–6.
72. Esakoff TF, Handler SJ, Granados JM, et al. PAMUS: placenta accreta management across the United States. J Matern Fetal Neonatal Med 2012;25(6):761–5.
73. Sentilhes L, Ambroselli C, Kayem G, et al. Maternal outcome after conservative treatment of placenta accreta. Obstet Gynecol 2010;115(3):526–34.
74. Panici PB, Anceschi M, Borgia ML, et al. Intraoperative aorta balloon occlusion: fertility preservation in patients with placenta previa accreta/increta. J Matern Fetal Neonatal Med 2012;25(12):2512–6.
75. Dinkel HP, Dürig P, Schnatterbeck P, et al. Percutaneous treatment of placenta percreta using coil embolization. J Endovasc Ther 2003;10(1):158–62.
76. Angstmann T, Gard G, Harrington T, et al. Surgical management of placenta accreta: a cohort series and suggested approach. Am J Obstet Gynecol 2010; 202(1):38.e1–9.
77. Carnevale FC, Kondo MM, de Oliveira Sousa W Jr, et al. Perioperative temporary occlusion of the internal iliac arteries as prophylaxis in cesarean section at risk of hemorrhage in placenta accreta. Cardiovasc Intervent Radiol 2011;34(4): 758–64.
78. Bodner LJ, Nosher JL, Gribbin C, et al. Balloon-assisted occlusion of the internal iliac arteries in patients with placenta accreta/percreta. Cardiovasc Intervent Radiol 2006;29(3):354–61.
79. Levine AB, Kuhlman K, Bonn J. Placenta accreta: comparison of cases managed with and without pelvic artery balloon catheters. J Matern Fetal Neonatal Med 1999;8(4):173–6.
80. Descargues G, Douvrin F, Degré S, et al. Abnormal placentation and selective embolization of the uterine arteries. Eur J Obstet Gynecol Reprod Biol 2001; 99(1):47–52.
81. Bisschop CN, Schaap TP, Vogelvang TE, et al. Invasive placentation and uterus preserving treatment modalities: a systematic review. Arch Gynecol Obstet 2011; 284(2):491–502.
82. Alanis M, Hurst B, Marshburn P, et al. Conservative management of placenta increta with selective arterial embolization preserves future fertility and results in a favorable outcome in subsequent pregnancies. Fertil Steril 2006;86(5): 1514.e3–7.
83. Chiang YC, Shih JC, Lee CN. Septic shock after conservative management for placenta accreta. Taiwan J Obstet Gynecol 2006;45(1):64–6.

84. Pather S, Strockyj S, Richards A, et al. Maternal outcome after conservative management of placenta percreta at caesarean section: a report of three cases and a review of the literature. Aust N Z J Obstet Gynaecol 2014;54(1):84–7.

85. Butt K, Gagnon A, Delisle MF. Failure of methotrexate and internal iliac balloon catheterization to manage placenta percreta. Obstet Gynecol 2002;99(6):981.

86. Kim TH, Lee HH. Conservative management of abnormally invasive placenta after vaginal delivery. Acta Obstet Gynecol Scand 2014;93(1):123–4.

87. Roulot A, Barranger E, Morel O, et al. Two- and three-dimensional power Doppler ultrasound in the follow-up of placenta accreta treated conservatively. J Gynecol Obstet Biol Reprod (Paris) 2015;44(2):176–83.

88. Provansal M, Courbiere B, Agostini A, et al. Fertility and obstetric outcome after conservative management of placenta accreta. Int J Gynaecol Obstet 2010; 109(2):147–50.

89. Kabiri D, Hants Y, Shanwetter N, et al. Outcomes of subsequent pregnancies after conservative treatment for placenta accreta. Int J Gynaecol Obstet 2014; 127(2):206–10.

90. Cali G, Forlani F, Giambanco L, et al. Prophylactic use of intravascular balloon catheters in women with placenta accreta, increta and percreta. Eur J Obstet Gynecol Reprod Biol 2014;179:36–41.

91. Lo TK, Yung WK, Lau WL, et al. Planned conservative management of placenta accreta - experience of a regional general hospital. J Matern Fetal Neonatal Med 2014;27(3):291–6.

92. Pinho S, Sarzedas S, Pedroso S, et al. Partial placenta increta and methotrexate therapy: three case reports. Clin Exp Obstet Gynecol 2008;35(3):221–4.

Index

Note: Page numbers of article titles are in **boldface** type.

Obstet Gynecol Clin N Am 42 (2015) 403–413
http://dx.doi.org/10.1016/S0889-8545(15)00038-8
0889-8545/15/$ – see front matter © 2015 Elsevier Inc. All rights reserved.

obgyn.theclinics.com

Moving?

Make sure your subscription moves with you!

To notify us of your new address, find your **Clinics Account Number** (located on your mailing label above your name), and contact customer service at:

Email: journalscustomerservice-usa@elsevier.com

800-654-2452 (subscribers in the U.S. & Canada)
314-447-8871 (subscribers outside of the U.S. & Canada)

Fax number: 314-447-8029

Elsevier Health Sciences Division
Subscription Customer Service
3251 Riverport Lane
Maryland Heights, MO 63043

*To ensure uninterrupted delivery of your subscription, please notify us at least 4 weeks in advance of move.

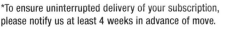

Printed and bound by CPI Group (UK) Ltd, Croydon, CR0 4YY

03/10/2024

01040488-0005